Study Guide for

Maternal Child Nursing Care

Fifth Edition

Karen A. Piotrowski, RNC, MSN
Associate Professor of Nursing
D'Youville College
Buffalo, New York

David Wilson, MS, RNC, NIC
Staff & PALS Coordinator
Children's Hospital at Saint Francis
Tulsa, Oklahoma

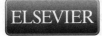

ELSEVIER
MOSBY

Study Guide for
Maternal Child Nursing Care, Fifth Edition

ISBN: 978-0-323-09607-2

Notices

Knowledge and best practice in this field are constantly changing. As new research and experience broaden our understanding, changes in research methods, professional practices, or medical treatment may become necessary.

Practitioners and researchers must always rely on their own experience and knowledge in evaluating and using any information, methods, compounds, or experiments described herein. In using such information or methods they should be mindful of their own safety and the safety of others, including parties for whom they have a professional responsibility.

With respect to any drug or pharmaceutical products identified, readers are advised to check the most current information provided (i) on procedures featured or (ii) by the manufacturer of each product to be administered, to verify the recommended dose or formula, the method and duration of administration, and contraindications. It is the responsibility of practitioners, relying on their own experience and knowledge of their patients, to make diagnoses, to determine dosages and the best treatment for each individual patient, and to take all appropriate safety precautions.

To the fullest extent of the law, neither the Publisher nor the authors, contributors, or editors, assume any liability for any injury and/or damage to persons or property as a matter of products liability, negligence or otherwise, or from any use or operation of any methods, products, instructions, or ideas contained in the material herein.

Content Manager: Laurie K. Gower
Senior Content Development Specialist: Heather Bays
Content Coordinator: Hannah Corrier
Publishing Services Manager: Hemamalini Rajendrababu
Project Manager: Nisha Selvaraj

Printed in the United States of America

Last digit is the print number: 9 8 7 6 5 4 3 2 1

Working together
to grow libraries in
developing countries

www.elsevier.com • www.bookaid.org

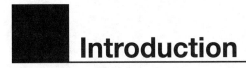# Introduction

Maternal Child Nursing Care, fifth edition, is a comprehensive textbook of maternity and pediatric nursing. This *Study Guide* is designed to help students use the textbook more effectively. In addition to reviewing content of the text, this *Study Guide* encourages students to think critically in applying their knowledge.

ORGANIZATION

Each chapter in this *Study Guide* is designed to incorporate learning activities that will help students meet the objectives of the corresponding textbook chapter. The content is organized as follows:

- **Learning Key Terms**—Matching or fill-in-the-blank questions give students the opportunity to test their ability to define all key terms in the corresponding textbook chapter.

- **Reviewing Key Concepts**—A variety of questions (matching, fill-in-the-blank, true/false, short answer, and multiple choice) are used to provide students with ample opportunity to assess their knowledge and comprehension of the information covered in the text. These activities are specifically designed to help students identify the important content of the chapter and test their level of knowledge and understanding after reading the chapter.

- **Thinking Critically**—Students are required to apply concepts found in the chapter to solve problems, make decisions concerning care management, and provide responses to patients' questions and concerns.

- **Answer Key**—Answers to all questions are provided at the end of this *Study Guide*.

Contents

PART 1: MATERNITY NURSING

Unit 1 Introduction to Maternity Nursing

1. 21st Century Maternity Nursing **1**
2. Community Care: The Family and Culture **5**

Unit 2 Reproductive Years

3. Assessment and Health Promotion **13**
4. Reproductive System Concerns **24**
5. Infertility, Contraception, and Abortion **35**

Unit 3 Pregnancy

6. Genetics, Conception, and Fetal Development **42**
7. Anatomy and Physiology of Pregnancy **48**
8. Nursing Care of the Family During Pregnancy **53**
9. Maternal and Fetal Nutrition **62**
10. Assessment of High Risk Pregnancy **67**
11. High Risk Perinatal Care: Preexisting Conditions **72**
12. High Risk Perinatal Care: Gestational Conditions **80**

Unit 4 Childbirth

13. Labor and Birth Processes **90**
14. Pain Management **93**
15. Fetal Assessment During Labor **99**
16. Nursing Care of the Family During Labor and Birth **104**
17. Labor and Birth Complications **112**

Unit 5 Postpartum Period

18. Maternal Physiologic Changes **121**
19. Nursing Care of the Family During the Postpartum Period **124**
20. Transition to Parenthood **130**
21. Postpartum Complications **135**

Unit 6 Newborn

22. Physiologic and Behavioral Adaptations of the Newborn **143**
23. Nursing Care of the Newborn and Family **149**
24. Newborn Nutrition and Feeding **155**
25. The High Risk Newborn **160**

PART 2: PEDIATRIC NURSING

Unit 7 Children, Their Families, and the Nurse

26. 21st Century Pediatric Nursing **167**
27. Family, Social, Cultural, and Religious Influences on Child Health Promotion **171**
28. Developmental and Genetic Influences on Child Health Promotion **176**

Unit 8 Assessment of the Child and Family

29. Communication, History, and Physical Assessment **181**
30. Pain Assessment and Management **187**

Unit 9 Health Promotion and Special Health Problems

31. The Infant and Family **190**
32. The Toddler and Family **194**
33. The Preschooler and Family **197**
34. The School-Age Child and Family **200**
35. The Adolescent and Family **203**

Unit 10 Special Needs, Illness, and Hospitalization

36. Chronic Illness, Disability, and End-of-Life Care **207**
37. Cognitive and Sensory Impairment **210**
38. Family-Centered Care of the Child During Illness and Hospitalization **214**
39. Pediatric Variations of Nursing Interventions **217**

Unit 11 Health Problems of Children

40. Respiratory Dysfunction **221**
41. Gastrointestinal Dysfunction **226**
42. Cardiovascular Dysfunction **231**
43. Hematologic and Immunologic Dysfunction **237**
44. Genitourinary Dysfunction **240**
45. Cerebral Dysfunction **244**
46. Endocrine Dysfunction **248**
47. Integumentary Dysfunction **252**
48. Musculoskeletal or Articular Dysfunction **258**
49. Neuromuscular or Muscular Dysfunction **263**

Answer Key 266

21st Century Maternity Nursing

I. LEARNING KEY TERMS

MATCHING: Match each term with its corresponding description.

1. _____ Number of live births in 1 year per 1000 population.

2. _____ All deaths during pregnancy and within 1 year following the end of pregnancy.

3. _____ Number of maternal deaths from births and complications of pregnancy, childbirth, and puerperium (the first 42 days after termination of the pregnancy) per 100,000 live births.

4. _____ An infant who, at birth, demonstrates no signs of life, such as breathing, heartbeat, or voluntary muscle movements.

5. _____ Number of stillbirths and number of neonatal deaths per 1000 live births.

6. _____ Number of births per 1000 women between the ages of 15 and 44 years (inclusive), calculated on an annual basis.

7. _____ An embryo or fetus that is removed or expelled from the uterus at 20 weeks of gestation or less, weighs 500 g or less, or measures 25 cm or less.

8. _____ Number of deaths of infants younger than 1 year of age per 1000 live births.

9. _____ Number of deaths of infants younger than 28 days of age per 1000 live births.

10. _____ Deaths that are a complication of pregnancy, an aggravation of an unrelated condition by the physiology of pregnancy, or a chain of events initiated by the pregnancy.

a. Fertility rate

b. Infant mortality rate

c. Birth rate

d. Maternal mortality rate

e. Neonatal mortality rate

f. Perinatal mortality rate

g. Pregnancy-associated deaths

h. Pregnancy-related deaths

i. Stillbirth

j. Abortus

FILL IN THE BLANKS: Insert the term that corresponds to each of the following definitions or descriptions.

11. _____ Specialty area of nursing practice that focuses on the care of childbearing women and their families through all stages of pregnancy and childbirth, as well as the first 4 weeks after birth.

12. _____ A set of goals based on assessments of major risks to health and wellness, changes in public health priorities, and issues related to the health preparedness and prevention of our nation.

13. _____ A set of eight goals to be achieved by 2015 that respond to the world's main development challenges and are adopted by 189 nations under the auspices of the United Nations.

1

14. _____ Approach to health care that encompasses complementary and alternative therapies in combination with conventional Western modalities of treatment.

15. _____ An umbrella term for the use of communication technologies and electronic information to provide or support health care when the participants are separated by distance.

16. _____ Trained and experienced female labor attendants who provide a continuous one-on-one caring presence throughout the labor and birth process.

17. _____ Term that refers to a spectrum of abilities, ranging from reading an appointment slip to interpreting medication instructions.

18. _____ Health care that is based on information gained through research and clinical trials.

19. _____ Guidelines for nursing practice that reflect current knowledge, represent levels of practice agreed on by leaders in the specialty, and can be used for clinical benchmarking.

20. _____ An evolving process that is used to identify risks, establish preventive practices, develop reporting mechanisms, and delineate procedures for managing lawsuits.

21. _____ Term used by The Joint Commission to describe an unexpected occurrence involving death or serious physical or psychological injury, or risk thereof.

22. _____ Failure to recognize or act on early signs of distress. Key components include careful surveillance and identification of complications and quick action to initiate appropriate interventions and activate a team response.

23. _____ Level of practice that a reasonably prudent nurse would provide in the same or similar circumstances.

24. _____ An effort to provide nurses with the competencies to improve the quality and safety of the systems of health care in which they practice. They were delineated by the IOM.

25. _____ A teamwork system for health professionals to provide higher quality, safer patient care. It provides an evidence base to improve communication and teamwork skills.

II. REVIEWING KEY CONCEPTS

1. When assessing pregnant women, what factors would you recognize as having the potential to contribute to the rate of infant mortality in the United States?

2. The number of high risk pregnancies occurring in the United States is increasing. Briefly discuss several factors that have been identified as contributing to this increase in incidence of high risk pregnancies.

3. An integrative health care approach implies which of the following? (Circle all that apply.)
   a. The focus is on the whole person.
   b. Conventional Western modalities of treatment are not included.
   c. The beliefs, values, and desires of the patient in terms of health and health care are respected.
   d. Patient autonomy is limited in terms of choosing alternative therapies.
   e. The patient's disease complex is the primary consideration when choosing treatment approaches.

4. A nurse manager of a prenatal clinic should recognize that the most significant barrier encountered by pregnant women in accessing health care would be which of the following?
   a. Lack of transportation to the clinic
   b. Child care responsibilities
   c. Inability to pay
   d. Deficient knowledge related to the benefits of prenatal care

5. In the United States, the leading cause of maternal mortality is which one of the following?
   a. Unsafe abortion
   b. Infection
   c. Gestational hypertension
   d. Diabetes

6. Pregnant women who are obese are more likely to develop one or both of the two most frequently reported maternal risk factors. These factors include which of the following combinations?
   a. Premature labor and infection
   b. Hemorrhage and hypertension associated with pregnancy
   c. Infection and diabetes
   d. Diabetes and hypertension associated with pregnancy

III. THINKING CRITICALLY

1. Imagine that you are the nursing director of an inner-city prenatal clinic that serves a large number of minority women, many of whom are younger than 20 years of age. Describe five nursing services you would provide for these women that would help reduce the potential for maternal and infant morbidity and mortality and low birth weight. Use the statistical data and risk behaviors presented in Chapter 1 to support the types of services you propose.

2. Support the accuracy of the following statement: An emphasis on high-technology medical care and lifesaving techniques will not reduce the rate of preterm and low-birth-weight infants in the United States.

3. Explain how a nurse could use social media to improve the health care provided to pregnant women and their families. Identify the precautions the nurse must take to ensure that patient confidentiality and privacy are respected.

4. Many barriers interfere with a woman's participation in early and ongoing prenatal care. Describe incentives and services that you would offer to pregnant women to encourage their participation in prenatal care. State the rationale for your proposals. Your answer should reflect an understanding of the barriers.

5. As a nurse manager of an in-hospital perinatal unit, what care approaches would you implement to ensure quality family-centered care?

6. Discuss measures that can be taken to ensure that the health literacy needs of patients are met.

7. Medical errors are the leading cause of death in the United States. Explain the process that you will use as a student to prevent medical errors.

8. Discuss two international concerns that have serious detrimental effects on the health and safety of women. Explain how nurses can address these concerns.

2 Community Care: The Family and Culture

I. LEARNING KEY TERMS

MATCHING: Match the family described with the appropriate family category.

1. _____ Miss M. lives with her 4-year-old adopted Korean daughter, Kim.

2. _____ Anne and Duane are married and live with their daughter, Susan, and Duane's aunt and uncle.

3. _____ Gloria and Andy are a married couple living with their new baby girl, Annie.

4. _____ Carl and Allan are a gay couple living with Carl's daughter, Sally, whom they are raising together.

5. _____ The S. family consists of Jim; his second wife, Jane; and Jim's two daughters by a previous marriage.

6. _____ Tammy and Joseph live with their grandmother Irene who has been caring for them since their mother died.

7. _____ Ruth lives with her son, Peter, his wife Anne, and their twin sons.

a. Multigenerational family

b. Single-parent family

c. Homosexual family

d. Nuclear family

e. Extended family

f. Married-blended family

g. No-parent family

MATCHING: Match the description with the appropriate cultural concept.

8. _____ Mrs. M., a Mexican-American who just gave birth, tells the nurse not to include certain foods on her meal tray because her mother told her to avoid those foods while breastfeeding. The nurse tells her that she doesn't have to avoid any foods and should eat whatever she desires.

9. _____ Ms. P., an immigrant from Vietnam, has lived in the United States for 1 year. She tells you that while she enjoys the comfort of wearing blue jeans and sneakers for casual occasions, like shopping, she still wears traditional or "conservative" clothing for family gatherings.

10. _____ A Cambodian family immigrated to the United States and has been living in Denver for over 5 years. The parents express concern about their children, ages 10, 13, and 16, stating, "The children act so differently now. They are less respectful to us, want to eat only American food, and go to rock concerts. It's hard to believe they are our children."

11. _____ The Amish represent an important ethnic community in Lancaster, Pennsylvania.

12. _____ The nurse is preparing a healthy diet plan for Mrs. O. In doing so, she takes the time to include the Polish foods that Mrs. O. enjoys.

a. Cultural relativism

b. Ethnocentrism

c. Assimilation

d. Subculture

e. Acculturation

5

FILL IN THE BLANKS: Insert the cultural concept that corresponds to each of the following definitions.

13. _____ An ongoing process that influences a person throughout his or her life. It provides an individual with beliefs and values about each facet of life that are passed from one generation to the next.

14. _____ A group existing within a larger cultural system that retains its own characteristics.

15. _____ Recognizing that people from different cultural backgrounds comprehend the same objects and situations differently; that a culture determines a person's viewpoint.

16. _____ Changes that occur within one group or among several groups when people from different cultures come in contact with one another and exchange and adopt each other's mannerisms, styles, and practices.

17. _____ Process in which one cultural group loses its identity and becomes a part of the dominant culture.

18. _____ A belief that one's cultural way of doing things is the right way, supporting the notion that "My group is the best."

19. _____ Approach that involves the ability to think, feel, and act in ways that acknowledge, respect, and build upon ethnic, cultural, and linguistic diversity; to act in ways that meet the needs of the patient and are respectful of ways and traditions that may be different from one's own.

20. _____ Type of time orientation that maintains a focus on achieving long-term goals; families or people who practice this time orientation are more likely to return for follow-up visits related to health care and to participate in primary prevention activities.

21. _____ Type of time orientation of families or people who are more likely to strive to maintain tradition or the status quo and have little motivation for formulating future goals.

22. _____ Type of time orientation of families or people who may have difficulty adhering to strict schedules and are often described as living for the moment.

23. _____ Cultural concept that reflects dimensions of personal comfort zones. Actions such as touching, placing the woman in proximity to others, taking away personal possessions, and making decisions for the woman can decrease personal security and heighten anxiety.

24. _____ A unit of socialization and nurturing within a community that preserves and transmits culture. It is a social network that acts as a potent support system for its members.

25. _____ Family category in which male and female partners and their children live as an independent unit, sharing roles, responsibilities, and economic resources.

26. _____ Family category that includes the nuclear family and other people related by blood (kin) such as grandparents, aunts, uncles, and cousins.

27. _____ Family category in which an unmarried biologic or adoptive parent heads the household; it is becoming an increasingly recognized structure in our society. These families tend to be vulnerable both socially and economically.

28. _____ Family category that forms as a result of divorce and remarriage. It includes stepparents, stepchildren, and stepsiblings who join to create a new household.

29. _____ Family category comprised of gay or lesbian couples who live together with or without children.

30. _____ Family category consisting of grandparents, children, and grandchildren. This family form is becoming increasingly common.

31. _____ Family category in which children live independently in foster or kinship care such as living with a grandparent.

32. _____ Family category in which children live with two unmarried biologic parents or two adoptive parents.

33. _____ Term for the family tree format that depicts relationships of family members over at least three generations; it provides valuable information about a family and its health.

34. _____ Term for a graphic portrayal of social relationships of the patient and family including school, work, religious affiliations, and club memberships.

35. _____ Groups within the community who are more likely to experience health status problems and negative health outcomes as a result of a variety of sociocultural, economic, and environmental risk factors that contribute to disparities in health.

36. _____ Level of preventive care that involves health promotion and disease prevention activities to decrease the occurrence of illness and enhance general health and quality of life.

37. _____ Level of preventive care that targets populations at risk and involves early detection of a disease and prompt treatment, with the goal of curing the disease or slowing its progression and preventing subsequent disability.

38. _____ Level of preventive care that focuses on rehabilitation; it follows the occurrence of a defect or disability and is aimed at preventing disability through restoration of optimal functioning.

II. REVIEWING KEY CONCEPTS

1. Discuss why the nurse should take each of the following "products of culture" into consideration when providing care within a cultural context:

   a. Communication

   b. Personal space

   c. Time orientation

   d. Family roles

2. State the rationale for the increasing emphasis on home- and community-based health care. How has this trend changed the demands placed on the community-based nurse?

3. Community health promotion requires the collaborative efforts of many individuals and groups within a community. Cite several programs that could be established to promote the health of a community's childbearing families.

4. Explain why each of the groups listed below have been identified as vulnerable populations:

   • Women in general

   • Adolescent girls and older women

   • Racial and ethnic minorities

   • Incarcerated women

   • Refugee, immigrant, and migrant women

5. Describe the ways that nurses can provide care to perinatal patients using the telephone.

6. Which one of the following nursing actions is most likely to reduce a patient's anxiety and enhance the patient's personal security as it relates to the concept of personal space needs?
   a. Touching the patient before and during procedures
   b. Providing explanations when performing tasks
   c. Making eye contact as much as possible
   d. Reducing the need for the patient to make decisions

7. A Native-American woman gave birth to a baby girl 12 hours ago. The nurse notes that the woman keeps her baby in the bassinet except for feeding and states that she will wait until she gets home to begin breastfeeding. The nurse recognizes that this behavior is most likely a reflection of:
   a. embarrassment.
   b. delayed attachment.
   c. disappointment that the baby is a girl.
   d. cultural beliefs regarding the care of newborns.

8. When caring for a pregnant woman who is Hispanic, the nurse should recognize that the woman may be guided by which of the following cultural beliefs and practices during her pregnancy? (Circle all that apply.)
   a. Warm breezes can be dangerous during pregnancy.
   b. Prenatal care should begin very early in pregnancy.
   c. Milk should be avoided because it results in big babies and difficult births.
   d. Drinking chamomile tea should be avoided because it can cause preterm labor.
   e. The advice of both mother and mother-in-law should be followed during pregnancy.
   f. Pelvic examinations should not be performed by a male health care provider.

9. European-American women are likely to believe which of the following regarding pregnancy and childbirth? (Circle all that apply.)
   a. The father of the baby should be actively involved in the labor and birth.
   b. Pregnancy requires medical attention so prenatal care should begin early in pregnancy.
   c. Birthing at home should be valued.
   d. Pregnant women should participate in childbirth education.
   e. The doctor is the head of the obstetrical care team.
   f. Mothers should not begin to breastfeed until milk comes in.

10. A student nurse is planning to communicate with her postpartum patient using an interpreter. Her instructor should provide further guidance if the student does which of the following?
    a. Chooses a female interpreter from the woman's country of origin.
    b. Stops periodically during the interaction to ask the interpreter how things are going.
    c. Asks questions while looking at the interpreter.
    d. Gathers culturally appropriate learning aids and reading materials to use during the interaction.

11. Which of the following health services represents the primary level of preventive care? (Circle all that apply.)
    a. Breast self-examination and testicular self-examination education programs
    b. Providing flu immunizations in pharmacies
    c. A safer-sex informational pamphlet provided to adolescents during a health education class
    d. Blood pressure and cholesterol screening at a health fair
    e. Instituting a wheelchair, cane, and walker exchange program for persons whose health insurance does not cover these items
    f. A car-seat fitting fair at local auto dealerships

12. A student nurse's association is planning a health fair that will emphasize secondary level prevention activities. Which of the following activities would their faculty advisor tell them to eliminate because it does not fit into their stated focus?
    a. Teaching participants how to check their radial pulse for rate and regularity
    b. Blood glucose monitoring
    c. Demonstration of relaxation measures to manage stress
    d. Breast models that participants can use to learn breast palpation techniques

13. When making a home visit, it is essential that the nurse use appropriate infection control measures. Of the measures listed below, which one is the most important?
    a. Including personal protective equipment in the home care bag
    b. Designating a dirty area with a trash bag to collect soiled equipment and supplies
    c. Wearing clean vinyl gloves for procedures that involve touching the patient
    d. Performing hand hygiene using either soap and running water or a self-drying antiseptic solution.

III. THINKING CRITICALLY

1. Imagine that you are a nurse working in a clinic that provides prenatal services to a multicultural community predominated by Hispanic, African-American, and Asian-American families. Describe how you would adapt care measures to reflect the cultural beliefs and practices of pregnant women and their families from each of the following cultural groups.

   a. Hispanic

   b. African-American

   c. Asian-American

2. Pamela is a 20-year-old Native-American woman. She is 3 months pregnant and has come to the prenatal clinic on the reservation where she lives for her first visit to obtain some prenatal vitamins, which her friends at work told her are important.

   a. State the questions the nurse should ask to determine Pamela's cultural expectations about childbearing.

   b. Describe the communication approach you would consider when interviewing Pamela.

   c. Identify the Native-American beliefs and practices regarding childbearing that may influence Pamela's approach to her pregnancy and the birth of her child.

3. A nurse has been providing care to a Hispanic family. This family recently experienced the birth of twin girls at 38 weeks of gestation. It is the first birth experience for both parents and the first grandchildren for the extended family. Both newborns are healthy and living at home. Describe the cultural beliefs and practices that the family, being Hispanic, might use as guidelines to provide care to their newborn twin girls.

4. The nurse-midwife at a prenatal clinic has been assigned to care for a Sunni refugee couple from Iraq who recently immigrated to the United States. The woman has just been diagnosed as being 2 months pregnant. Neither she nor her husband speaks English. Outline the process that this nurse should use when working with a translator to facilitate communication with this couple to enhance care management.

5. Imagine that you are a nurse who has just been hired to provide in-home health care. Before you begin seeing your patients, you realize that it would be helpful for you to become familiar with the neighborhood and resources in the community where your patients live. You decide to conduct a walking survey of this community.

   a. Describe how you would go about conducting this survey and gathering data.

   b. List the data you believe it would be essential to gather.

   c. Discuss how you would use the findings from your walking survey when providing health care to the patients you will be visiting.

6. Marie is a single parent of two young children ages 4 years and 1 year. She and her children have been homeless for 3 months because her husband abandoned her and she lost her job because she had no one to help her care for her children.

   a. Discuss the basis for the types of health problems to which Marie and her children are most vulnerable.

   b. What factors related to being homeless could increase Marie's risk for becoming pregnant? If she did become pregnant, explain why it would be considered a high risk pregnancy.

   c. How would you, as a nurse, provide health care services to Marie and her children?

7. Consuelo is the wife of a migrant laborer. She and her husband, along with their two children, have been working on a California farm for 2 weeks. She has arrived at a health center established for migrant laborers. Consuelo states that she is 4 months pregnant. As the women's health nurse practitioner assigned to care for Consuelo, what approaches would you use to ensure that she obtains quality health care that addresses her unique health risks as a migrant worker?

8. Write a series of questions that you would ask when making a postpartum follow-up call to a woman who gave birth 3 days ago.

9. Eileen gave birth to a son 36 hours ago. A home care nurse has been assigned to visit Eileen and her husband in their home to assess the progress of her recovery after birth, the health status of her newborn son, and the adaptation of family processes to the responsibilities of newborn care.

   a. Outline the approach the nurse should take in preparing for this visit.

   b. Describe the nurse's actions during the visit using the care management process as a format.

   c. Discuss how the nurse should end the visit.

   d. Identify interventions the nurse should implement at the conclusion of the visit with Eileen and her husband.

   e. Specify how the nurse should protect her personal safety both outside and inside Eileen's home.

f. Cite the infection control measures the nurse should use when conducting the visit and providing care in Eileen's home.

10. Angela has recently been diagnosed with hyperemesis gravidarum and has been hospitalized to stabilize her fluid and electrolyte balance. The hospital-based nurse must evaluate Angela for referral to home care.

a. State the criteria that this nurse should follow to determine Angela's readiness for discharge from hospital to home care.

b. Angela has been discharged and will be receiving parenteral nutrition in her home. Discuss the additional information required related to high technology home care.

c. Identify specific home environment criteria that must be met to ensure the safety and effectiveness of Angela's treatment.

11. A nurse is seeking funding to start a home care agency designed to provide home visits to postpartum women and their families within 1 week of birth and follow-up visits as indicated. State the points the nurse should emphasize as a rationale for the importance of this health care service and the cost-effectiveness of funding such a service.

3 Assessment and Health Promotion

I. LEARNING KEY TERMS

FILL IN THE BLANKS: Insert the term that corresponds to each of the following definitions related to the female reproductive system and breasts. Use the anatomic drawings (Figs. 3-1, 3-2, 3-4, 3-5, and 3-6 in your textbook) to visualize each of the structures as you are inserting the terms.

1. _____ Fatty pad that lies over the anterior surface of the symphysis pubis.

2. _____ Two rounded folds of fatty tissue covered with skin that extend downward and backward from the mons pubis; their purpose is to protect the inner vulvar structures.

3. _____ Two flat, reddish folds composed of connective tissue and smooth muscle, which are supplied with nerve endings that are extremely sensitive.

4. _____ Hood-like covering of the clitoris.

5. _____ Fold of tissue under the clitoris.

6. _____ Thin flat tissue formed by the joining of the labia minora; it lies underneath the vaginal opening at the midline.

7. _____ Small structure underneath the prepuce composed of erectile tissue with numerous sensory nerve endings; it increases in size during sexual arousal.

8. _____ Almond-shaped area enclosed by the labia minora that contains openings to the urethra, Skene's glands, vagina, and Bartholin's glands.

9. _____ Bladder opening found between the clitoris and the vagina.

10. _____ Skin-covered muscular area between the fourchette and the anus that covers the pelvic structures.

11. _____ Fibromuscular, collapsible tubular structure that extends from the vulva to the uterus and lies between the bladder and rectum. Its mucosal lining is arranged in transverse folds called _____. _____ glands (located on each side of the urethra), and _____ glands (located on each side of the vagina) secrete mucus that lubricates the vagina. The _____ is a connective tissue membrane that surrounds the vaginal opening and can be perforated during strenuous exercise, insertion of tampons, masturbation, and vaginal intercourse.

12. _____ Anterior, posterior, and lateral pockets that surround the cervix.

13. _____ Muscular pelvic organ located between the bladder and the rectum and just above the vagina. The _____ is a deep pouch, or recess, posterior to the cervix formed by the posterior ligament.

14. _____ Upper triangular portion of the uterus.

15. _____ Also known as the lower uterine segment, it is the short constricted portion that separates the corpus of the uterus from the cervix.

16. _____ Dome-shaped top of the uterus.

17. _____ Highly vascular lining of the uterus.

18. _____ Layer of the uterus composed of smooth muscles that extend in three different directions.

19. _____ Lower cylindric portion of the uterus composed of fibrous connective tissue and elastic tissue.

20. _____ Canal connecting the uterine cavity to the vagina. The opening between the uterus and this canal is the _____. The opening between the canal and the vagina is the _____.

21. _____ Location in the cervix where the squamous and columnar epithelium meet; it is also known as the _____ zone; it is the most common site for neoplastic changes; cells from this site are scraped for the Pap smear.

22. _____ Passageways between the ovaries and the uterus; they are attached at each side of the dome-shaped uterine fundus.

23. _____ Almond-shaped organs located on each side of the uterus; their two functions are _____ and the production of the hormones _____, _____, and _____.

24. _____ Structure that protects the bladder, uterus, and rectum; accommodates the growing fetus during pregnancy; and anchors support structures.

25. _____ The paired mammary glands.

26. _____ Segment of mammary tissue that extends into the axilla.

27. _____ Mammary papilla.

28. _____ Pigmented section of the breast that surrounds the nipple.

29. _____ Sebaceous glands that secrete a fatty substance to lubricate the nipple and cause the areola to appear rough.

FILL IN THE BLANKS: Insert the term that corresponds to each of the following definitions related to the menstrual cycle. Use the illustration of the Menstrual Cycle (Fig. 3-7 in your textbook) to visualize the cycle as you are inserting the terms.

30. _____ The first menstruation.

31. _____ Transitional stage between childhood and sexual maturity.

32. _____ Transitional phase during which ovarian function and hormone production decline.

33. _____ The last menstrual period dated with certainty once one year has passed after menstruation ceases.

34. _____ Period preceding the last menstrual period that lasts about 4 years; during this time ovarian function declines, ova diminish, more menstrual cycles become anovulatory, and irregular bleeding occurs.

35. _____ Periodic uterine bleeding that begins approximately 14 days after ovulation. It is controlled by the feedback system of three cycles, namely _____, _____, and _____. The average length of each menstrual cycle is _____ but variations are normal. Day one of the cycle is considered to be _____. The average duration of menstrual flow is _____ with a range of _____.

36. _____ Cycle that involves cyclic changes in the lining of the uterus. It consists of four phases, namely _____, _____, _____, and _____.

37. _____ Cycle that involves secretion of hormones required to stimulate ovulation.

38. _____ Cycle that involves the changes in the ovary leading to ovulation. It consists of two phases, namely _____ and _____.

39. _____ Hormone secreted by the hypothalamus when ovarian hormones are reduced to a low level. It stimulates the pituitary gland to secrete two critical hormones for the menstrual cycle, namely _____ and _____.

40. _____ Pituitary hormone that stimulates the development of graafian follicles in the ovary.

41. _____ Pituitary hormone that stimulates the expulsion of the ovum from the graafian follicle and formation of the corpus luteum.

42. _____ Ovarian hormone that stimulates the thickening of the endometrium that occurs after menstruation and prior to ovulation; it is also responsible for changes in the cervix and the stretchable quality of the cervical mucus called _____.

43. _____ Ovarian hormone that is responsible for the changes in the endometrium that occur after ovulation to facilitate implantation should fertilization occur; it is also responsible for the rise in _____ temperature that occurs after ovulation.

44. _____ Localized, lower abdominal pain that coincides with ovulation. Some vaginal spotting may occur.

45. _____ Oxygenated fatty acids classified as hormones. They are thought to play an essential role in ovulation, transport of sperm, regression of the corpus luteum, and menstruation. By increasing the myometrial response to oxytocin, they also play a role in labor and dysmenorrhea.

FILL IN THE BLANKS: Insert the term that corresponds to each of the following definitions or descriptions related to women's health care.

46. _____ Type of health care that provides women and their partners with information that is needed to make decisions about their reproductive future.

47. _____ Term that describes a body mass index (BMI) of 30 or greater.

48. _____ Term that describes a chronic eating disorder in which women undertake strict and severe diets and rigorous, extreme exercise as a result of a distorted view of their bodies as being much too heavy.

49. _____ Term that describes an eating disorder characterized by secret, uncontrolled binge eating alternating with practices that prevent weight gain, which can include self-induced vomiting, laxatives or diuretics, strict diets, fasting, and rigorous exercise.

50. _____ or _____ The intentional removal of all or part of the external female genitalia.

51. _____, _____, _____, and _____ or _____ violence are terms applied to a pattern of assaultive and coercive behaviors inflicted by a male partner in a marriage or other heterosexual, significant, intimate relationship.

52. According to the cycle of violence theory, battering occurs in cycles. The three-phase cyclic pattern that occurs begins with a period of _____ leading to the _____, which is then followed by a period of _____ known as the _____ phase.

II. REVIEWING KEY CONCEPTS

1. It is essential that guidelines for laboratory and diagnostic procedures be followed exactly in order to ensure the accuracy of the results obtained. Outline the guidelines that should be followed when performing a Papanicolaou smear in terms of each of the following:

   a. Patient preparation

   b. Timing during examination when the specimen is obtained

   c. Sites for specimen collection

   d. Handling of specimens

   e. Frequency of performance

2. Although women may recognize the need for reproductive health care, they may encounter barriers to accessing this type of care. Identify one barrier represented by each of the following issues and describe a solution you would propose for helping women overcome the barrier identified.

   • Financial issues

   • Cultural issues

   • Gender issues

3. A nurse is preparing a pamphlet designed to alert adolescents to the dangers of sexually transmitted infections and what they can do to prevent their transmission.

    a. Describe what information the pamphlet should provide about STI transmission prevention.

    b. As an impetus to motivate adolescents to use prevention measures, the nurse decides to include a section on the consequences of sexually transmitted infections. Discuss the points that should be emphasized in this section of the pamphlet.

4. What are the essential questions that should be asked when providing health care to women to assess them for abuse?

5. Eating disorder screening tools can be used to determine whether a woman is experiencing an eating disorder and to what degree. Explain the SCOFF tool and how you would use it when providing well woman care.

6. Using and abusing some substances while pregnant can increase the risk for adverse outcomes for the woman and her fetus-newborn. Identify the maternal-fetal-newborn effects for each of the substances listed below.

    • Alcohol

    • Tobacco

    • Caffeine

    • Cocaine

    • Marijuana

    • Opiates

    • Methamphetamines

    • Phencyclidine

7. A 20-year-old woman tells the nurse that she performs breast self-examination (BSE) on a regular basis. The nurse evaluates the woman's understanding of BSE and ability to perform the technique correctly. Which of the following actions by the woman indicate that she needs further instructions regarding BSE? (Circle all that apply.)
    a. Performs BSE every month on the first day of her menstrual cycle
    b. Observes the size of her breasts, the direction of her nipples, and appearance of her skin including the presence of dimpling when looking at her breasts in the mirror
    c. Lies down on her bed and puts a pillow under the shoulder of the breast she is going to palpate; then she places the arm on that side under her head
    d. Uses the tips of her four fingers to palpate her breast
    e. Palpates her breast, using an overlapping circular pattern around her entire breast
    f. Palpates her breasts and up into her axilla while taking a shower

8. A nurse instructed a female patient regarding vulvar self-examination (VSE). Which of the statements made by the patient will require further instruction?
    a. "I will perform this examination at least once a month, especially if I change sexual partners or am sexually active."
    b. "I will become familiar with how my genitalia look and feel so that I will be able to detect changes."
    c. "I will use the examination to determine when I should get medications at the pharmacy for infections."
    d. "I will wash my hands thoroughly before and after I examine myself."

9. A women's health nurse practitioner is going to perform a pelvic examination on a female patient. Which of the following nursing actions would be least effective in enhancing the patient's comfort and relaxation during the examination?
    a. Encourage the patient to ask questions and express feelings and concerns before and after the examination.
    b. Ask the patient questions as the examination is performed.
    c. Allow the patient to keep her shoes and socks on when placing her feet in the stirrups.
    d. Instruct the patient to place her hands over her diaphragm and take deep, slow breaths.

10. To enhance the accuracy of the Papanicolaou (Pap) test, the nurse should instruct the patient to do which of the following?
    a. Schedule the test just prior to the onset of menses.
    b. Stop taking birth control pills for 2 days before the test.
    c. Avoid intercourse for 24 to 48 hours before the test.
    d. Douche with a specially prepared antiseptic solution the night before the test.

11. When assessing women, it is important for the nurse to keep in mind the possibility that they are victims of violence. The nurse should:
    a. use an abuse assessment screen during the assessment of every woman.
    b. recognize that abuse rarely occurs during pregnancy.
    c. assess a woman's legs and back as the most commonly injured areas.
    d. notify the police immediately if abuse is suspected.

12. A 52-year-old woman asks the nurse practitioner about how often she should be assessed for the common health problems women of her age could experience. The nurse would recommend which of the following screening measures? (Circle all that apply.)
    a. An endometrial biopsy every 2 to 3 years
    b. A fecal occult blood test every year
    c. A mammogram every other year
    d. Clinical breast examination every year
    e. Bone mineral density testing every year beginning when she is 55
    f. Vision examination every 2 to 4 years

13. Which of the following group descriptions is most accurate regarding those persons who should participate in preconception counseling?
    a. All women and their partners as they make decisions about their reproductive future, including becoming parents
    b. All women during their childbearing years
    c. Sexually active women who do not use birth control
    d. Women with chronic illnesses such as diabetes who are planning to get pregnant

14. A newly married 25-year-old woman has been smoking since she was a teenager. She has come to the women's health clinic for a checkup before she begins trying to get pregnant. The woman demonstrates a need for further instruction about the effects of smoking on reproduction and health when she makes which of the following statements? (Circle all that apply.)
    a. "Smoking can interfere with my ability to get pregnant."
    b. "My husband also needs to stop smoking because secondhand smoke can have an adverse effect on my pregnancy and the development of the baby."
    c. "Smoking can make my pregnancy last longer than it should."
    d. "Smoking can reduce the amount of calcium in my bones."
    e. "Smoking will mean I will experience menopause at an older age than my friends who do not smoke."

15. A pregnant woman in her first trimester tells her nurse midwife that although she does drink during pregnancy, she does so only on the weekend and only a little bit. What should the nurse's initial response be to this woman's comment?
    a. "You need to realize that use of alcohol, in any amount, will result in your child being mentally retarded."
    b. "I am going to refer you to a counseling center for women with alcohol problems."
    c. "Tell me what you mean by drinking a little on the weekend."
    d. "Antioxidants can reduce the effect of alcohol exposure for your baby. I will tell you what you can take."

16. A nurse is teaching a class of young women in a drug rehabilitation program about the risks associated with using illicit drugs during pregnancy. Which of the following statements if made by the students indicate that they understood the nurse's instructions? (Circle all that apply.)
    a. "My baby won't get enough oxygen if I smoke marijuana."
    b. "Cocaine can make my baby grow too big and make my pregnancy last too long."
    c. "Cocaine can make the placenta separate from my baby too early."
    d. "If I use heroin during pregnancy my baby will go through withdrawal after birth."
    e. "Methamphetamine exposure can make my baby's head too big."
    f. "My baby might get birth defects, especially in the heart and lungs, if I use PCP."

17. When communicating with an abused woman, which of the following statements should be avoided? (Circle all that apply.)
    a. "Why do you think your husband hits you even though you are pregnant?"
    b. "I cannot believe how terrible your husband is being to you."
    c. "The violence you are experiencing now is likely to continue and to get even worse as your pregnancy progresses."
    d. "Tell me why you did not go to the shelter I recommended to you; they are very helpful and you would have avoided this beating if you had gone."
    e. "Next time you come in for care, I want you to be sure to bring your husband so I can talk to him myself."
    f. "I am afraid for your safety and the safety of your other children."

18. A women's health nurse practitioner is preparing an education presentation on the topic of intimate partner violence (IPV) to a group of women who come to the clinic where she practices. As part of the presentation, she plans to dispel commonly held myths regarding IPV. Which of the following statements represent the facts related to IPV? (Circle all that apply.)
    a. Battering almost always affects women who are poor.
    b. Of women who experience battering, 25% are battered by an intimate partner.
    c. Women usually are safe from battering while they are pregnant, although the battering will resume after they have the baby.
    d. Women tend to leave the relationship if the battering is bad.
    e. Counseling may be successful in helping the batterer stop his behavior.
    f. Women do not like to be beaten and will often do anything to avoid a confrontation.

III. THINKING CRITICALLY

1. An inner-city women's health clinic serves a diverse population in terms of age, ethnic background, and health problems. Describe how each of the following factors should influence a women's health nurse practitioner's approach when assessing the health of the women who come to the clinic for care.

    a. Culture

    b. Age

    c. Disabilities

    d. Abuse

2. Imagine that you are a nurse working at a clinic that provides health care to women. Describe how you would respond to each of the following concerns or questions of women who have come to the clinic for care.

    a. Jane, a newly married woman, is concerned that she did not bleed during her first coital experience with her husband. She states, "I was a virgin and always thought you had to bleed when you had sex for the first time. Do you think my husband will still believe I was a virgin on our wedding night?"

    b. Serena, a 17-year-old woman, has just been scheduled for her first women's health checkup, which will include a pelvic examination and Pap smear. She nervously asks if there is anything she needs to do to get ready for the examination.

c. Andrea is trying to get pregnant. She wonders if there are signs she could observe in her body that would indicate that she is ovulating and therefore able to conceive a baby with her partner.

d. Anne, a 24-year-old woman, asks the nurse about a recommended douche to use a couple of times a week to stay "nice and clean down there."

3. Julie, a 21-year-old woman, has come to the women's health clinic for a women's health checkup. During the health history interview she becomes very anxious and states, "I have to tell you this is my first examination. I am very scared; my friends told me that it hurts a lot to have this examination." Describe how the nurse should respond in an effort to reduce Julie's anxiety.

4. As a nurse working in a women's health clinic, you have been assigned to interview Angie, a 25-year-old new patient, to obtain her health history.

a. List the components that should be emphasized in gathering Angie's history.

b. Write a series of questions that you would ask to obtain data related to Angie's reproductive and sexual health and practices.

c. Give an example of how you would use each of the following therapeutic communication techniques to develop trust, to facilitate the collection of data, and to provide support during the assessment process.

Facilitation

Reflection

Clarification

Empathy

Confrontation

Interpretation

Open-ended questions and statements

5. Self-examination of the breasts and vulva (genitalia) are important assessment techniques to teach a woman. Outline the procedure that you would use to teach each technique to one of your patients. Include the teaching methodologies that you would use to enhance learning.

   a. Breast self-examination

   b. Vulvar (genital) self-examination

6. Lu is a 25-year-old exchange student from China who has been living in the United States for 3 months. This is the first time that she is away from home. She comes to the university women's health clinic for a checkup and to obtain birth control. Describe how the nurse assigned to Lu would approach and communicate with her in a culturally sensitive manner.

7. Nurses working in women's health care must be aware of the growing problem of violence against women. All women should be screened when being assessed during health care for the possibility of abuse.

   a. Describe how you as a nurse would adjust the environment and your communication style when conducting the health history interview and physical examination in order to elicit a woman's confidence and trust.

   b. Identify indicators of possible abuse that you would look for before the appointment and then during the health history interview and physical examination.

   c. State the questions you would ask to screen for abuse.

   d. Discuss the approach you would take if abuse is confirmed during the assessment.

8. As a student you may be assigned to assist a health care provider during the performance of a pelvic examination for one of your patients.

   a. Describe how you would do each of the following:

   Prepare your patient for the examination

   Support your patient during the examination

   Assist your patient after the examination

   b. Describe how you would assist the health care provider who is performing the examination.

9. A nurse is teaching a group of young adult women about health promotion activities. As part of the discussion, the nurse identifies preconception care and counseling as an important health promotion activity. One woman in the class asks, "I know you need to go for checkups once you are pregnant, but why would you need to see a doctor before you get pregnant? Isn't that a big waste of time and money?" Explain how the nurse should respond to this woman's question.

10. During a routine checkup for her annual Pap smear, Julie, a 26-year-old woman, asks the nurse for advice regarding nutrition and exercise. She is considered to be overweight with a body mass index (BMI) of 27.4 and wants to lose weight sensibly. Discuss the advice the nurse should give to Julie.

11. You are a nurse midwife working in a prenatal clinic. As part of your role, you need to teach newly diagnosed pregnant women about the importance of coming for their prenatal care visits. What would you tell them?

12. Alice, a 30-year-old woman, comes to the women's health clinic complaining of fatigue, insomnia, and feeling anxious. She works as a stockbroker for a major Wall Street brokerage firm. Alice states that, although she enjoys the challenge of her job, she never can seem to find time for herself or to socialize with her friends. Alice tells the nurse practitioner that she has been drinking more and started to smoke again to help her relax. She is glad that she has lost some weight, attributing this occurrence to her diminished appetite.

    a. State the physical and psychologic manifestations of stress that the nurse should take note of when assessing Alice.

    b. Discuss how the nurse can help Alice cope with stress and its consequences in a healthy manner.

    c. Alice expresses interest in attempting to stop smoking. "I felt so much better when I stopped the first time. That was over 2 years ago, and now here I am back at it again." Describe an approach the nurse could use to help Alice achieve a desired change in health behavior that is long lasting.

13. Laura is a 28-year-old pregnant woman at 8 weeks of gestation. This is her first pregnancy. During the health history interview she reveals that she smokes at least 2 packs of cigarettes each day. When discussing this practice with the nurse, Laura states, "My friends smoked when they were pregnant and their babies are okay. In fact, two of them had pregnancies that were a little shorter than expected and they had nice small babies." Describe how the nurse should respond to Laura's comments.

14. As a nurse working in a prenatal health clinic you must be alert to cues indicative of battery committed against women when they are pregnant.

    a. Identify the body parts of pregnant women targeted during a battering episode.

    b. Carol, a 24-year-old married woman, comes to the clinic to confirm her belief that she is pregnant. During the assessment phase of the visit, you note cues that lead you to suspect that Carol is being abused by her husband. Discuss the approach you would take to confirm your suspicion that Carol is being abused.

    c. Carol admits to you that her husband "beats her sometimes and it has been increasing." Now she is afraid it will get worse since she "was not supposed to get pregnant." Discuss the nursing actions that you could take to help Carol.

    d. List the possible reasons why Carol, now that she is pregnant, is experiencing an escalation of battering/abuse from her husband.

    e. Discuss how Carol's pregnancy could be adversely affected by the abuse she is experiencing.

    f. Describe the activities in which the nurse can become involved in order to prevent the escalating incidence of violence against women.

4 Reproductive System Concerns

I. LEARNING KEY TERMS

FILL IN THE BLANKS: Insert the term that corresponds to each of the following descriptions related to menstrual problems.

1. _____ Absence of menstrual flow.

2. _____ Cessation of menstruation related to a problem in the central hypothalamic–pituitary axis.

3. _____ Syndrome characterized by the interrelation of disordered eating, absence of menstrual flow, and premature osteoporosis.

4. _____ Painful menstruation; one of the most common gynecologic problems for women during their childbearing years.

5. _____ Type of painful menstruation associated with ovulatory cycles; it has a biochemical basis arising from the release of prostaglandins.

6. _____ Type of painful menstruation that occurs later in life, typically after age 25, and is associated with pelvic pathology.

7. _____ A cluster of physical and psychologic symptoms that begins in the luteal phase of the menstrual cycle and is followed by a symptom-free follicular phase.

8. _____ Diagnostic term for a disorder that affects a smaller percentage of women who suffer from severe PMS with an emphasis on symptoms related to mood disturbances.

9. _____ A menstrual disorder that is characterized by the presence and growth of endometrial tissue outside of the uterus.

10. _____ Infrequent menstrual periods.

11. _____ Scanty menstruation at normal intervals.

12. _____ Excessive bleeding during menstruation.

13. _____ Bleeding between menstrual periods.

14. _____ Any form of uterine bleeding that is irregular in amount, duration, or timing and is not related to regular menstrual bleeding; it can have organic causes such as systemic or reproductive tract disease.

15. _____ Uterine bleeding which is usually hormonally related; it often occurs around menarche or menopause.

FILL IN THE BLANKS: Insert the term that corresponds to each of the following descriptions related to infection.

16. _____ Infections or infectious disease syndromes primarily transmitted by sexual contact.

17. _____ The physical barrier promoted for the prevention of sexual transmission of human immunodeficiency virus (HIV) and other sexually transmitted infections (STIs).

18. _____ Bacterial infection that is the most common and fastest spreading STI in American women. This infection is often silent and highly destructive to the female reproductive tract.

19. _____ The oldest communicable disease in the United States. Because it is a reportable communicable disease, health care providers are legally responsible for reporting all cases to health authorities.

20. _____ One of the earliest sexually transmitted infections (STIs). It is caused by *Treponema pallidum,* a spirochete. During the primary stage a characteristic lesion called a _____ appears 5 to 90 days after infection. During the second stage, a widespread _____ appears on the palms and soles along with generalized _____. _____ (broad, painless, pink-gray, wartlike infectious lesions) may develop on the vulva, perineum, or anus.

21. _____ Infectious process that most commonly involves the uterine tubes, uterus, and more rarely, ovaries and peritoneal surfaces.

22. _____ Infection previously named genital or venereal warts. It is now the most common viral STI seen in ambulatory health care settings.

23. _____ A viral infection that is transmitted sexually and is characterized by painful recurrent ulcers.

24. _____ Viral infection acquired primarily through a fecal-oral route by ingestion of contaminated food and fluids and through person-to-person contact.

25. _____ Viral infection involving the liver that is transmitted parenterally, perinatally, and through intimate contact. A vaccine is available to protect infants, children, and adults.

26. _____ The most common blood-borne infection in the United States. It is a disease of the liver that is transmitted parenterally and through intimate contact. No vaccine is available to provide protection against this infection.

27. _____ A retrovirus that is transmitted primarily through exchange of body fluids. _____ Severe depression of the cellular immune system associated with this infection.

28. _____ Vaginal infection formerly called *nonspecific vaginitis, Haemophilus vaginitis*, or *Gardnerella*; it is the most common type of vaginitis and is characterized by a profuse, thin, and white, gray, or milky discharge that has a characteristic "fishy" odor.

29. _____ Yeast infection that is the second most common type of vaginal infection in the United States. It is characterized by a thick, white, lumpy discharge.

30. _____ A vaginal infection caused by an anaerobic one-celled protozoan with characteristic flagella. The typically copious discharge is yellowish green, frothy, mucopurulent, and malodorous. It is almost always sexually transmitted.

31. _____ A normal vaginal flora that is present in 9% to 23% of healthy pregnant women. It is associated with poor pregnancy outcomes. Vertical transmission to the newborn during birth has been implicated as an important factor in perinatal and neonatal morbidity and mortality.

II. REVIEWING KEY CONCEPTS

MATCHING: Match the description with the appropriate breast disorder.

1. _____ Lumpiness with or without tenderness in both breasts; nipple discharge may occur.

2. _____ Fatty unilateral breast tumor that is soft, nontender, and mobile with discrete borders; no nipple discharge occurs.

3. _____ Unilateral, firm, nontender, discrete benign breast mass; it increases in size during pregnancy but decreases in size with aging.

4. _____ Rare, benign condition that develops in the terminal nipple ducts and is usually too small to palpate; a unilateral spontaneous serous, serosanguineous, or bloody nipple discharge can also occur.

5. _____ Spontaneous, bilateral milky sticky breast discharge unrelated to malignancy.

6. _____ Inflammatory process in the breast characterized by a thick, sticky, white or colored discharge. Burning pain and itching may be experienced. A mass may be palpated behind the nipple.

a. Fibroadenoma

b. Fibrocystic changes

c. Mammary duct ectasia

d. Lipoma

e. Galactorrhea

f. Intraductal papilloma

7. Cite several common risk factors for sexually transmitted diseases.

8. Describe one implementation measure for each of the following Standard Precautions categories.

   Hand hygiene

   Use of personal protective equipment (PPE)

   Respiratory hygiene and cough etiquette

   Safe injection practices

9. Heterosexual transmission is the most common means of infecting women with HIV.

   a. What behaviors increase a woman's risk for HIV infection?

   b. List the clinical manifestations that may be exhibited during seroconversion to HIV positivity.

10. Breast cancer is a major health problem facing women in the United States. Nurses are often responsible for educating women about breast cancer.

    a. Outline the information the nurse should give women about the risk factors associated with breast cancer.

b. List the clinical manifestations that are strongly suggestive of breast cancer.

11. Describe how each of the following approaches are used in the diagnosis and care of women with breast cancer.

    a. Lumpectomy

    b. Mastectomy

    c. Breast reconstruction

    d. Radiation

    e. Adjuvant therapy

    f. Chemotherapy

    g. Testing for BRCA1 and BRCA2 genes

    h. Mammography

    i. Sonography

    j. Biopsy (fine needle; core needle; needle localization)

12. Which of the following women is at greatest risk for developing hypogonadotropic amenorrhea?
    a. 48-year-old woman experiencing perimenopausal changes
    b. 13-year-old figure skater
    c. 18-year-old softball player
    d. 30-year-old (G3 P3003) breastfeeding woman

13. Pharmacologic preparations can be used to treat primary dysmenorrhea. Which preparation would be least effective in relieving the symptoms of primary dysmenorrhea?
    a. Oral contraceptive pill (OCP)
    b. Naproxen sodium (Anaprox)
    c. Acetaminophen (Tylenol)
    d. Ibuprofen (Motrin)

14. Women experiencing PMS should be advised to avoid use of which of the following?
    a. Chamomile tea
    b. Coffee
    c. Whole-grain cereals
    d. Parsley to season food

15. The nurse counseling a 30-year-old woman regarding effective measures to use to relieve the discomfort associated with dysmenorrhea could suggest which of the following? (Circle all that apply.)
    a. Decrease intake of fruits, especially peaches and watermelon.
    b. Use back massages and heat application to abdomen to enhance relaxation and circulation.
    c. Avoid exercise just before and during menstruation when discomfort is at its peak.
    d. Add vegetables such as asparagus to the diet.
    e. Perform effleurage and guided imagery for relaxation and distraction.
    f. Limit intake of salty and fatty foods.

16. A 28-year-old woman has been diagnosed with endometriosis. She has been placed on a course of treatment with danazol (Danocrine). The woman exhibits understanding of this treatment when she says which of the following? (Circle all that apply.)
    a. "Because this medication stops ovulation, I do not need to use birth control."
    b. "I will experience more frequent and heavier menstrual periods when I take this medication."
    c. "I should follow a low-fat diet because this medication can increase the level of cholesterol in my blood."
    d. "I can experience a decrease in my breast size, oily skin, and hair growth on my face as a result of taking this medication."
    e. "I will need to spray this medication into my nose twice a day."
    f. "I may need to use a lubricant during intercourse to reduce discomfort."

17. A 55-year-old woman tells the nurse that she has started to experience pain when she and her husband have intercourse. The nurse would record that this woman is experiencing:
    a. dyspareunia.
    b. dysmenorrhea.
    c. dysuria.
    d. dyspnea.

18. Infections of the female midreproductive tract, such as chlamydia, are dangerous primarily because these infections:
    a. are asymptomatic.
    b. cause infertility.
    c. lead to PID.
    d. are difficult to treat effectively.

19. A finding associated with HPV infection would include which of the following?
    a. White, curd-like, adherent discharge
    b. Soft papillary swelling occurring singly or in clusters
    c. Vesicles progressing to pustules and then to ulcers
    d. Yellow to green frothy malodorous discharge

20. A recommended medication effective in the treatment of vulvovaginal candidiases would be which of the following?
    a. Metronidazole (Flagyl)
    b. Miconazole (Monistat)
    c. Ampicillin
    d. Acyclovir

21. A woman is determined to be Group B streptococcus (GBS) positive at the onset of her labor. The nurse should prepare this woman for which of the following?
    a. Cesarean birth
    b. Intravenous administration of an antibiotic during labor
    c. Transplacental infection of her newborn with GBS
    d. Application of acyclovir to her labial lesions

22. When providing a woman recovering from primary herpes with information regarding the recurrence of herpes infection of the genital tract, the nurse would tell her which of the following?
    a. Fever and flulike symptoms will precede each recurrent infection.
    b. Little can be done to control the recurrence of infection.
    c. Cortisone-based ointments should be used to decrease discomfort.
    d. Itching and tingling often occur before the appearance of vesicles.

23. When teaching women about breast cancer, the nurse should emphasize which of the following facts? (Circle all that apply.)
    a. The incidence of breast cancer is highest among African-American women.
    b. One in ten American women will develop breast cancer in her lifetime.
    c. The mortality rate from breast cancer decreases with early detection.
    d. Most women diagnosed with breast cancer report a family history of breast cancer.
    e. Maintaining a normal weight and reducing alcohol intake could have an effect on reducing a woman's chances of developing breast cancer.
    f. The majority of breast lumps found by women are not malignant.

24. When providing discharge instructions to a woman who had a modified right radical mastectomy, the nurse should emphasize the importance of which of the following?
    a. Reporting any tingling or numbness in her incisional site or right arm immediately
    b. Telling health care providers not to take a blood pressure or draw blood from her right arm
    c. Learning how to use her left arm to write and accomplish the activities of daily living such as brushing her hair
    d. Wearing clothing that snugly supports her right arm

25. A 26-year-old woman has just been diagnosed with fibrocystic change in her breasts. Which of the following nursing diagnoses would be a priority for this woman?
    a. Acute pain related to cyclical enlargement of breast cysts or lumps
    b. Risk for infection related to altered integrity of the areola associated with accumulation of thick, sticky discharge from nipples

    c. Anxiety related to anticipated surgery to remove the cysts in her breasts
    d. Fear related to high risk for breast cancer

26. When assessing a woman with a diagnosis of fibroadenoma, the nurse would expect to find which of the following characteristics?
    a. Bilateral tender lumps behind the nipple
    b. Milky discharge from one or both nipples
    c. Soft and nonmoveable lumps
    d. Well-delineated, firm moveable lump in one breast

27. A 40-year-old woman at risk for breast cancer has elected chemoprevention as an approach to reduce her risk. She will be receiving tamoxifen (Nolvadex). The nurse will recognize that this woman understood instructions given to her regarding this medication if she makes which of the following statements?
    a. "This medication helps prevent breast cancer by helping my body use estrogen efficiently."
    b. "I may need to wear a sweater to keep me warm when I experience chills that can occur when I am taking this medication."
    c. "I can take this medication on an empty stomach or with food."
    d. "I should use an oral contraceptive pill to ensure that I do not get pregnant."

28. Herbal preparations can be used as part of the treatment for a variety of menstrual disorders. Which of the following herbs would be beneficial for a woman experiencing menorrhagia?
    a. Ginger
    b. Shepherd's purse
    c. Black cohosh root
    d. Black haw

III. THINKING CRITICALLY

1. Marie is a 16-year-old gymnast who has been training vigorously for a placement on the U.S. Olympic team. She has been experiencing amenorrhea, and the development of her secondary sexual characteristics has been limited. Marie expresses concern because her nonathletic friends have all been menstruating for at least 1 year and have well-developed breasts. After a health assessment, Marie was diagnosed with hypogonadotropic amenorrhea.

   a. State the risk factors and assessment findings for this disorder that Marie most likely exhibited during the assessment process.

   b. State one nursing diagnosis reflective of Marie's concern.

   c. Outline a typical care management plan for Marie that will address the issues associated with hypogonadotropic amenorrhea.

   d. At Marie's all female high school there is a large athletic department that emphasizes participation and excellence in a wide variety of sports. As the school nurse, you are concerned that there are other students like Marie who may be exhibiting signs of the female athlete triad. The nurse has decided to institute an education program aimed at prevention and early detection of the triad.

      (1) What is the meaning of the female athlete triad?

      (2) Which sports should the nurse emphasize with her program?

      (3) What measures should this nurse include in her program as a means of prevention and early detection of the female athlete triad?

2. Mary, a 17-year-old who experienced menarche at age 16, comes to the women's health clinic for a routine checkup. She complains to the nurse that her last few periods have been very painful. "I have missed a few days of school because of it. What can I do to reduce the pain that I feel during my periods?" Physical examination and testing reveal normal structure and function of Mary's reproductive system. A medical diagnosis of primary dysmenorrhea is made.

   a. What questions should the nurse ask Mary to get a full description of her pain?

   b. What should the nurse tell Mary about the likely cause for the type of pain she is experiencing?

   c. Identify appropriate relief measures for primary dysmenorrhea that the nurse could suggest to Mary.

   d. What alternative therapies could the nurse suggest to Mary to help relieve her discomfort?

3. Susan experiences physical and psychologic signs and symptoms associated with PMS during every ovulatory menstrual cycle.

   a. List the signs and symptoms most likely described by Susan that led to the diagnosis of PMS.

b. Identify one nursing diagnosis that may be appropriate for Susan when she is experiencing the signs and symptoms of PMS.

c. Describe the approach the nurse would use in helping Susan deal with this menstrual disorder.

d. What symptoms would Susan describe that would indicate she is also experiencing PMDD?

4. Lisa is 26 years old and has been diagnosed recently with endometriosis.

   a. List the signs and symptoms Lisa most likely exhibited that led to this medical diagnosis.

   b. Lisa asks, "What is happening to my body as a result of this disease?" Describe the nurse's response.

   c. Lisa asks about her treatment options. "Are there medications I can take to make me feel better?" Describe the action/effect and potential side effects for each of the following pharmacologic approaches to treatment.

   Oral contraceptive pills

   Gonadotropin-releasing hormone agonists

   Androgenic synthetic steroids

   d. Identify support measures the nurse can suggest to assist Lisa to cope with the effects of endometriosis.

5. Terry, a 20-year-old woman, comes to a women's health clinic for her first visit.

   a. During the health history interview, it is imperative that the nurse practitioner determine Terry's risk for contracting an STI, including HIV. Write one question for each of the following risk categories.

Sexual risk

Drug use–related risk

Blood-related risk

HIV concerns

b. Terry asks the nurse about measures she could use to protect herself from STIs. Cite the major points that the nurse practitioner should emphasize when teaching Terry about prevention measures.

c. Terry tells the nurse that she does not know if she could ever tell a partner that he must wear a condom. Describe the approach the nurse can take to enhance Terry's assertiveness and communication skills.

6. Martha is 4 weeks pregnant. As part of her prenatal assessment, it was discovered that she was HIV positive. Identify the measures that can be used to reduce the risk of transmission of HIV from Martha to her baby.

7. Suzanne, a 20-year-old woman, is admitted for suspected severe, acute PID.

a. Identify the risk factors for PID that the nurse would be looking for in Suzanne's health history.

b. A complete physical examination is performed to determine whether the criteria for PID are met. Specify the criteria that Suzanne's health care provider would be alert for during the examination.

c. Suzanne is hospitalized when the diagnosis of PID secondary to chlamydial infection is confirmed. Intravenous antibiotics will be used as the primary medical treatment followed by oral antibiotics at the time of discharge. State three priority nursing diagnoses that are likely to be present during the acute stage of Suzanne's infection and treatment.

d. Outline a nursing management plan for Suzanne in terms of each of the following:

Position and activity

Comfort measures

Support measures

Health education in preparation for discharge

e. List the recommendations for Suzanne's self-care during the recovery phase.

f. Identify the reproductive health risks that Suzanne may face as a result of the pelvic infection she experienced.

8. Laura has just been diagnosed with gonorrhea, a sexually transmitted disease.

a. Laura, who is very upset by the diagnosis, states, "This is just awful. What kind of sex life can I have now?" Cite a nursing diagnosis that reflects Laura's concern.

b. Outline a management plan that will assist Laura in taking control of her self-care and prevent future infections.

9. Cheryl, a 27-year-old woman, is being treated for HPV. A primary diagnosis identified for Cheryl is "pain related to lesions on the vulva and around the anus secondary to HPV infection." State the measures the nurse could suggest to Cheryl to reduce the pain from the condylomata and enhance their healing.

10. Mary, a 20-year-old woman, has just been diagnosed with a primary herpes simplex 2 infection. In addition to the typical systemic symptoms, Mary exhibits multiple painful genital lesions.

    a. Relief of pain and healing without the development of a secondary infection are two expected outcomes for care. Identify several measures that the nurse can suggest to Mary in an effort to help her achieve the expected outcomes of care.

    b. Mary asks the nurse if there is anything she can do so that this infection does not return. Discuss what the nurse should tell Mary about the recurrence of HSV-2 infection and the influence of self-care measures.

11. Sonya is concerned that she has been exposed to HIV and has come to the women's health clinic for testing.

    a. During the health history the nurse questions Sonya about behaviors that could have placed her at risk for HIV transmission. Cite the behaviors that the nurse would be looking for.

    b. Explain the testing procedure that will most likely be followed to determine Sonya's HIV status.

    c. Outline the counseling protocol that should guide the nurse when caring for Sonya before and after the test.

    d. Sonya's test result is negative. Discuss the instructions the nurse should give Sonya regarding guidelines she should follow to reduce her risk for the transmission of HIV with future sexual partners.

12. Mary Anne comes to the women's health clinic complaining that her breasts feel lumpy.

    a. Outline the assessment process that should be used to determine the basis for Mary Anne's complaint.

    b. A diagnosis of fibrocystic breast changes is made. Describe the signs and symptoms Mary Anne most likely exhibited to support this diagnosis.

    c. State one nursing diagnosis that the nurse would identify as a priority when preparing a plan of care for Mary Anne.

d. Identify measures the nurse could suggest to Mary Anne for lessening the symptoms she experiences related to fibrocystic changes.

13. Molly, a 50-year-old woman, found a lump in her left breast during a breast self-examination. She comes to the women's health clinic for help.

   a. Describe the diagnostic protocol that should be followed to determine the basis for the lump Molly found in her breast.

   b. Molly elects to have a simple mastectomy based on the information provided by her health care providers and in consultation with her husband. Identify two priority postoperative nursing diagnoses and outline the nursing care management for the postoperative phase of Molly's treatment.

   Nursing diagnoses

   Postoperative phase care measures

   c. Molly will be discharged within 48 hours after her surgery. Describe the instructions that the nurse should give Molly to prepare her for self-care at home.

   d. Discuss support measures the nurse should use to address the concerns that Molly and her husband will most likely experience and express.

14. As a nurse working in a woman's health clinic, you have been given the task of developing a breast cancer screening program. You plan to emphasize the importance of women engaging in a self-management program regarding breast health. Describe the types of obstacles you are likely to encounter from women as they attempt to implement their program and the measures you will implement to overcome the obstacles.

5 Infertility, Contraception, and Abortion

I. LEARNING KEY TERMS

FILL IN THE BLANKS: Insert the term that corresponds to each of the following descriptions related to alterations in fertility.

1. _____ Diagnosis made when a couple has not achieved pregnancy after 1 year of regular, unprotected intercourse when the woman is less than 35 years of age or after 6 months when the woman is older than 35.

2. _____ Term used to describe the chances of achieving pregnancy and subsequent live birth within one menstrual cycle.

3. _____ Fertility treatments in which both eggs and sperm are handled.

4. _____ Assisted reproductive therapy that involves collection of a woman's eggs, then fertilizing them in the laboratory with sperm, and transferring the resultant embryo into her uterus.

5. _____ Assisted reproductive therapy that involves selection of one sperm cell that is injected directly into the egg to achieve fertilization; it is used with in vitro fertilization (IVF).

6. _____ Assisted reproductive therapy that involves retrieval of oocytes from the ovary, placing them in a catheter with washed motile sperm, and immediately transferring the gametes into the fimbriated end of the uterine tube. Fertilization occurs in the uterine tube.

7. _____ Assisted reproductive therapy that involves placing ova after IVF into one uterine tube during the zygote stage.

8. _____ Assisted reproductive therapy that involves using sperm from a person other than the male partner to inseminate the female partner.

9. _____ Assisted reproductive therapy that involves transferring embryo(s) from one couple into the uterus of another woman who has contracted with the couple to carry the baby to term. This woman has no genetic connection with the child.

10. _____ Assisted reproductive therapy that involves inseminating a woman with the semen from the infertile woman's partner; she then carries the baby until birth.

11. _____ Assisted reproductive therapy that involves penetrating the zona pellucida chemically or manually to create an opening for the dividing embryo to hatch and to implant into the uterine wall.

12. _____ Assisted reproductive therapy that involves donating eggs by an IVF procedure; the eggs are then inseminated and transferred into the recipient's uterus, which has been hormonally prepared with estrogen-progesterone therapy.

13. _____ Assisted reproductive therapy that involves transferring another woman's embryo into the uterus of an infertile woman at the appropriate time.

14. _____ Using the sperm of her partner to inseminate the woman.

15. _____ Procedure used to freeze embryos for later implantation.

16. _____ Early genetic testing designed to eliminate embryos with serious genetic diseases before placing them into the uterus through one of the assisted reproductive therapies and to avoid future termination of the pregnancy for genetic reasons.

17. _____ Basic test for male infertility; detects ability of sperm to fertilize an ovum.

18. _____ Examination of uterine cavity and tubes using radiopaque contrast material instilled through the cervix. It is often used to determine tubal patency and to release a blockage if present.

19. _____ Test used to detect the timing of lutein hormone surge before ovulation.

35

20. _____ Test performed to evaluate tubal patency, uterine cavity, and myometrium; it will not disrupt a fertilized ovum.

FILL IN THE BLANKS: Insert the term that corresponds to each of the following descriptions regarding methods to prevent or plan pregnancy.

21. _____ Intentional prevention of pregnancy during sexual intercourse.

22. _____ Device and/or practice used to decrease the risk of conceiving or bearing offspring.

23. _____ Conscious decision regarding when to conceive or to avoid pregnancy throughout the reproductive years.

24. _____ Term that refers to the percentage of contraceptive users expected to have an unplanned pregnancy during the first year of using a birth control method even when they use the method consistently and correctly.

25. _____ The most effective reversible contraceptive methods used to prevent pregnancy. They include contraceptive implants and intrauterine contraception.

26. _____ Contraceptive method that requires the male partner to withdraw his penis from the woman's vagina before ejaculation.

27. _____ Group of contraceptive methods that rely on avoidance of intercourse during fertile days.

28. _____ Method that combines the charting of signs and symptoms of the menstrual cycle with the use of abstinence or other contraceptive methods during fertile periods.

29. _____ Method based on the number of days in each cycle counting from the first day of menses. The fertile period is determined after accurately recording lengths of menstrual cycles for 6 months.

30. _____ A modified form of the calendar rhythm method that has a "fixed" number of days of fertility for each cycle; cycle beads can be used to track fertility, with day 1 of the menstrual flow as the first day to begin counting.

31. _____ Method based on variations in a woman's lowest body temperature, which is determined after waking and before getting out of bed.

32. _____ Method that requires the woman to recognize and interpret the cyclical changes in the amount and consistency of cervical mucus that characterize her own unique pattern of changes.

33. _____ Term that refers to the stretchiness of cervical mucus.

34. _____ Method that uses the physiologic and psychologic changes that occur during each phase of the menstrual cycle to determine the occurrence of ovulation and the fertile period.

35. _____ Method that requires the woman to ask herself two questions every day: (1) "Did I note secretions today?" and (2) "Did I note secretions yesterday?" An answer of "yes" requires the use of a backup method of birth control or avoidance of coitus.

36. _____ Temporary method of birth control that is based on the suppression of ovulation, which occurs with breastfeeding.

37. _____ Chemical that destroys or limits the mobility of sperm. When inserted into the vagina it acts as both a chemical and physical barrier to sperm. It is also an effective lubricant.

38. _____ Thin, stretchable sheath that covers the penis or is inserted into the vagina.

39. _____ Shallow, dome-shaped rubber device with a flexible rim that covers the cervix.

40. _____ A soft natural rubber dome with a firm but pliable rim that fits snugly around the base of the cervix close to the junction of the cervix and vaginal fornices.

41. _____ A small round polyurethane device that contains a spermicide. It fits over the cervix and has a woven polyester loop to facilitate its removal.

42. _____ Birth control method that is taken orally; it contains a combination of estrogen and progesterone that inhibits the maturation of follicles and ovulation.

43. _____ Combined estrogen-progesterone birth control method that involves application of the hormones to the skin of the lower abdomen, upper outer arms, buttocks, or upper torso where the hormones are absorbed; it is applied once a week for 3 weeks.

44. _____ Combined estrogen-progesterone birth control method that involves insertion of the hormones into the vagina for 3 weeks.

45. _____ Form of hormonal contraception in which a single-rod implant containing progestin is inserted subdermally into the inner aspect of the upper arm. The two-rod system is called _____.

46. _____ Form of emergency contraception that involves administration of a single progestin-only pill, which should be taken as soon as possible after but within 72 hours of unprotected intercourse or birth control mishap to prevent unintended pregnancy. _____ Form of emergency contraception that involves taking two progestin-only pills together or 12 hours apart.

47. _____ Small, T-shaped object inserted into the uterine cavity. It can be loaded with copper or a progestational agent.

48. _____ Surgical procedures intended to render the person infertile. _____ Method used to render a female infertile. _____ Method that is the easiest and most commonly used method for males; it involves ligating and then severing the vas deferens of each testicle.

49. _____ Purposeful interruption of a pregnancy before 20 weeks of gestation. If it is performed at the woman's request, it is termed an _____. If it is performed for reasons of maternal or fetal health or disease, it is termed a _____.

II. REVIEWING KEY CONCEPTS

1. A woman is a little uncomfortable about checking her cervical mucus and asks the nurse what she could possibly find out about doing this assessment. State the useful purpose of self-evaluation of cervical mucus.

2. Cite four factors that can contribute to a woman's decision to seek an induced abortion.

3. Joyce has chosen the diaphragm as her method of contraception. Which of the following actions would indicate that Joyce is using the diaphragm effectively? (Circle all that apply.)
   a. Joyce came to be refitted after healing was complete following the term vaginal birth of her son.
   b. Joyce applies a spermicide only to the rim of the diaphragm just before insertion because she dislikes the stickiness of the spermicide.
   c. Joyce empties her bladder before inserting the diaphragm.
   d. Joyce inserts the diaphragm about 3 to 4 hours before intercourse to increase spontaneity.
   e. Joyce applies more spermicide for each act of intercourse.
   f. Joyce removes the diaphragm within 1 hour of intercourse.
   g. After removal, Joyce washes the diaphragm with warm water and an antiseptic-type soap, dries it, and then applies baby powder.
   h. Joyce always uses the diaphragm during her menstrual periods.

4. A woman must assess herself for signs that ovulation is occurring. Which of the following is a sign associated with ovulation?
   a. Reduction in level of LH in the urine 12 to 24 hours before ovulation
   b. Spinnbarkeit
   c. Drop in BBT during the luteal phase of her menstrual cycle
   d. Increase in amount and thickness of cervical mucus

5. A single, young adult woman received instructions from the nurse regarding the use of an oral contraceptive. The woman would demonstrate a need for further instruction if she does which of the following?
   a. Stops asking her sexual partners to use condoms with spermicide
   b. States that her menstrual periods should be shorter with decreased blood loss
   c. Takes a pill every morning
   d. Uses a barrier method of birth control if she misses two or more pills

6. The most common, and for some women the most distressing, side effect of progestin-only contraceptives such as the minipill would be which of the following?
   a. Irregular vaginal bleeding
   b. Headache
   c. Nervousness
   d. Nausea

7. Women using Depo-Provera should be carefully screened for which of the following possible adverse reactions to its use?
   a. Diabetes mellitus—type 2
   b. Reproductive tract infection
   c. Decrease in bone mineral density
   d. Weight loss

8. A woman has had a ParaGard T380A IUD inserted. The nurse should recognize that the woman needs further teaching if she makes which of the following statements? (Circle all that apply.)
   a. "I should check the string before each menstrual period."
   b. "The IUD remains effective for 10 years."
   c. "It is normal to experience an increase in bleeding and cramping within the first year after it has been inserted."
   d. "My IUD works by releasing progesterone."
   e. "I should avoid using NSAIDs like Motrin if I have cramping."
   f. "I must use safer sex measures including maintaining a monogamous relationship to prevent infections in my uterus."

9. A woman experiencing infertility will begin taking clomiphene citrate (Clomid). In order to ensure she takes this medication safely and effectively, the nurse should do which of the following?
   a. Teach the patient's husband how to give his wife an IM injection.
   b. Show the woman how to spray the medication into one of her nostrils, emphasizing that she use a different nostril for each dose.
   c. Tell her to inject one dose of human chorionic gonadotropin subcutaneously the day after she takes the last does of the clomiphene citrate.
   d. Tell her to begin taking a 150 mg tablet daily on the 5th day of menstruation.

III. THINKING CRITICALLY

1. Mark and his wife, Mary, are undergoing testing for impaired fertility.

   a. Describe the nursing support measures that should be used when working with this couple.

   b. Mark must provide a specimen of semen for analysis. Describe the procedure he should follow to ensure accuracy of the test.

   c. State the semen characteristics that will be assessed.

   d. Mark and Mary tell the nurse that they would like to solve their problem by getting pregnant using non-medical measures if possible and ask the nurse about the use of alternative measures including the use of herbs to promote fertility. What types of measures could the nurse suggest they try?

2. Assisted reproductive therapies (ARTs) are being developed and perfected, creating a variety of ethical, legal, financial, and psychosocial concerns. Discuss the issues and concerns engendered by these technologies.

3. Kathy, an 18-year-old, has come to Planned Parenthood for information on birth control methods and assistance with making her choice. She tells the nurse that she is planning to become sexually active with her boyfriend of 6 months and is worried about getting pregnant. "I know I should know more about all of this, but I just don't."

   a. State the nursing diagnosis that reflects Kathy's concern.

   b. Outline the approach the nurse should use to help Kathy make an informed decision in choosing contraception that is right for her.

4. June plans to use a combination estrogen-progestin oral contraceptive.

   a. Describe the mode of action for this type of contraception.

   b. List the advantages of using oral contraception.

   c. Using the acronym ACHES, identify the signs and symptoms that would require June to stop taking the pill and notify her health care provider.

      A

      C

      H

      E

      S

   d. Specify the instructions the nurse should give June about taking the pill to ensure maximum effectiveness.

5. Anita has just had a levonorgestrel intrauterine system (IUD) inserted as her contraceptive method of choice. Specify the instructions that the nurse should give Anita before she leaves the women's health clinic after the insertion.

6. Judy (6-4-0-2-4) and Allen, both age 36, are contemplating sterilization now that their family is complete. They are seeking counseling regarding this decision.

   a. Describe the approach a nurse should use in helping Judy and Allen make the right decision for them.

   b. They decide that Allen will have a vasectomy. Discuss the preoperative and postoperative care and instructions required by Allen.

7. Anne and her husband, Ian, will be using the symptothermal method of fertility awareness.

   a. List the assessment components of this method that would indicate that ovulation is occurring and a period of fertility is present requiring abstinence or protected intercourse if pregnancy is not desired.

   b. Outline the points the nurse should emphasize when teaching Anne and Ian to ensure that they will accurately:

   Measure BBT

   Assess urine for LH

   Evaluate cervical mucus characteristics

   c. State the effectiveness of the symptothermal fertility awareness method of contraception.

8. Edna is a 20-year-old unmarried woman. She is 9 weeks pregnant and is unsure about what to do. She comes to the women's health clinic and asks for the nurse's help in making her decision, stating, "I just cannot support a baby right now. I am alone and trying to finish my education. What can I do?"

   a. Cite the nursing diagnosis reflective of Edna's current dilemma.

   b. Describe the approach the nurse should take in helping Edna make a decision that is right for her.

   c. Edna elects to have an abortion. A vacuum aspiration will be performed in the morning. Edna asks what will happen to her as part of the abortion procedure. Describe how the nurse should respond to Edna's question.

   d. Identify the nursing measures related to the physical care and emotional support that Edna will require as part of this procedure.

   e. Outline the discharge instructions that Edna should receive.

9. Felicia is 7 weeks pregnant and is scheduled for a medically induced abortion using methotrexate and misoprostol. What should the nurse tell Felicia about how these drugs work, the method of their administration, and what adverse reactions she could experience?

10. Marlee comes to the women's health clinic to report that she had unprotected intercourse last night. She is worried about getting pregnant because she is at midcycle and has already noticed signs of ovulation. Marlee tells the nurse that she hardly knows her partner and that her emotions just got the best of her. She is very anxious and asks the nurse what her options are. Describe the approach this nurse should use to assist Marlee with her concerns.

6 Genetics, Conception, and Fetal Development

I. LEARNING KEY TERMS

FILL IN THE BLANKS: Insert the term that corresponds to each of the following descriptions related to conception and fetal development.

1. _____ Union of a single egg and sperm. It marks the beginning of a pregnancy.

2. _____ Male and female germ cell. The male germ cell is a _____ and the female germ cell is an _____.

3. _____ Process whereby gametes are formed and mature. For the male, the process is called _____ and for the female, the process is called _____.

4. _____ Process of penetration of the membrane surrounding the ovum by a sperm. It takes place in the _____ of the uterine tube. The membrane becomes impenetrable to other sperm, a process termed _____. The _____ number of chromosomes is restored when this union of sperm and ovum occurs.

5. _____ The first cell of the new individual. Within 3 days it becomes a 16-cell solid ball of cells called a _____. This developing structure becomes known as the _____ when a cavity becomes recognizable within it. The outer layer of cells surrounding this cavity is called the _____.

6. _____ Attachment process whereby the blastocyst burrows into the endometrium. _____ or fingerlike projections develop out of the trophoblast and extend into the blood filled spaces of the uterine lining. The uterine lining is now called the _____. The portion of this lining directly under the blastocyst is called the _____ and the portion of this lining that covers the blastocyst is called the _____.

7. _____ The term that refers to the developing baby from day 15 until about 8 weeks after conception.

8. _____ The term that refers to the developing baby from 9 weeks of gestation to the end of pregnancy.

9. _____ Membranes that surround the developing baby and the fluid. The _____ is the outer layer of these membranes and becomes the covering of the fetal side of the placenta. The _____ is the inner layer.

10. _____ Fluid that surrounds the developing baby in utero.

11. _____ Structure that connects the developing baby to the placenta. It contains three vessels, namely two _____ and one _____. _____ The connective tissue that prevents compression of the blood vessels ensuring continued nourishment of the developing baby.

12. _____ Structure composed of 15 to 20 lobes called cotyledons. It produces _____ essential to maintain the pregnancy, supplies the _____ and _____ needed by the developing baby for survival and growth, and removes _____ and _____.

13. _____ Capability of fetus to survive outside the uterus.

14. _____ Surface-active phospholipid that needs to be present in fetal/newborn lungs to facilitate breathing after birth. A _____ ratio can be performed using amniotic fluid as one means of determining the degree to which this phospholipid is present in fetal lungs.

15. _____ Special circulatory pathway that allows fetal blood to bypass the lungs.

16. _____ Shunt that allows most of the fetal blood to bypass the liver and pass into the inferior vena cava.

17. _____ Opening between the fetal atria.

18. _____ Formation of blood.

19. _____ Maternal perception of fetal movement that occurs sometime between 16 and 20 weeks of gestation.

20. _____ Dark green to black tarry substance that contains fetal waste products. It accumulates in the fetal intestines.

21. _____ Twins that are formed from two zygotes. They are also called twins _____.

22. _____ Twins that are formed from one fertilized ovum that then divides. They are also called twins _____.

MATCHING: Match the description with the appropriate genetic concept.

23. _____ The hereditary material carried in the nucleus of each somatic (body) cell; it determines an individual's characteristics.

24. _____ The process by which germ cells divide, producing gametes that each contain 23 chromosomes.

25. _____ Failure of a pair of chromosomes to separate.

26. _____ Basic physical units of inheritance that are passed from parents to offspring and contain the information needed to specify traits.

27. _____ Abnormality in chromosome number; the numeric deviation is not an exact multiple of the haploid number of chromosomes.

28. _____ Cells that contain half of the genetic material of a normal somatic cell.

29. _____ Union of a normal gamete with a gamete containing an extra chromosome resulting in a cell with 47 chromosomes.

30. _____ X, Y

31. _____ Genes at corresponding loci on homologous chromosomes that code for different forms or variations of the same trait.

32. _____ Process whereby body (somatic) cells replicate to yield two cells with the same genetic makeup as the parent cell.

33. _____ Term that denotes the correct number of chromosomes.

34. _____ The complete set of genetic inheritance in the nucleus of each human cell.

35. _____ Process by which genetic material is transferred from one chromosome to another different chromosome.

36. _____ Threadlike packages of genes and other DNA in the nucleus of a cell.

37. _____ Abnormality in chromosome number in which the deviation is an exact multiple of the haploid number of chromosomes.

38. _____ Somatic cell containing the full number of 46 chromosomes.

a. Mitosis

b. Meiosis

c. Haploid

d. Diploid

e. Teratogen

f. Human genome

g. Chromosome

h. Genes

i. Sex chromosomes

j. DNA

k. Aneuploidy

l. Trisomy

m. Nondisjunction

n. Monosomy

o. Translocation

p. Mutation

q. Alleles

r. Euploidy

s. Polyploidy

t. Mosaicism

39. _____ Union of a normal gamete with a gamete missing a chromosome, resulting in a cell with only 45 chromosomes.

40. _____ A spontaneous and permanent change in normal gene structure.

41. _____ A mixture of cells, some with the normal number of chromosomes and others either missing a chromosome or containing an extra chromosome.

42. _____ Environmental substance or exposure that results in functional or structural disability of the embryo/fetus.

FILL IN THE BLANKS: Insert the term that corresponds to each of the following descriptions related to genetics.

43. _____ Analysis of human DNA, ribonucleic acid (RNA), chromosomes, or proteins to detect abnormalities related to an inherited condition.

44. _____ Direct examination of the DNA and RNA that make up a gene.

45. _____ Examination of the markers that are co-inherited with a gene that causes a genetic condition.

46. _____ Examination of the protein products of genes.

47. _____ Examination of chromosomes.

48. _____ Genetic testing that is used to clarify the genetic status of asymptomatic family members. _____ Genetic testing used to detect a disorder that is certain to appear if the defective gene is present and the individual lives long enough. _____ Genetic testing used to detect susceptibility to a disorder if the defective gene is present.

49. _____ Test used to identify individuals who have a gene mutation for a genetic condition but do not show symptoms of the condition because it is a condition that is inherited in an autosomal recessive form.

50. _____ Use of genetic information to individualize drug therapy.

51. _____ Therapy used to correct defective genes that are responsible for disease development; the most common technique is to insert a normal gene in a location within the genome to replace a gene that is non-functional.

52. _____ Matched chromosomes.

53. _____ Term that denotes an individual with two copies of the same allele for a given trait. If the two alleles are different, the person is said to be _____ for the trait.

54. _____ The genetic makeup of an individual; an individual's entire genetic makeup or all the genes that the person can pass on to future generations.

55. _____ Observable expression of an individual's genetic makeup.

56. _____ Pictorial analysis of the number, form, and size of an individual's chromosomes.

57. _____ Pattern of inheritance involving a combination of genetic and environmental factors.

58. _____ Pattern of inheritance in which a single gene controls a particular trait, disorder, or defect.

59. _____ Genetic disorder in which only one copy of a variant allele is needed for phenotypic expression.

60. _____ Genetic disorder in which both genes of a pair must be abnormal for the disorder to be expressed.

61. _____ Disorder reflecting absent or defective enzymes leading to abnormal metabolism.

II. REVIEWING KEY CONCEPTS

1. Each of the following structures plays a critical role in fetal growth and development. List the functions of each of the structures listed below.

   a. Yolk sac

b. Amniotic membranes and fluid

c. Umbilical cord

d. Placenta

2. Identify the tissues or organs that develop from each of the following primary germ layers.

Ectoderm

Mesoderm

Endoderm

3. Angela has come for her first prenatal visit. Identify the questions the nurse should ask during the health history interview to determine whether factors are present that would place Angela at risk for giving birth to a baby with an inheritable disorder.

4. Couples referred for genetic counseling receive an estimation of risk for the genetic disorder of concern. Explain the difference between an estimate of occurrence risk and an estimation of recurrence risk.

5. Explain the ethical issues that must be considered regarding the Human Genome Project.

6. Based on genetic testing of a newborn, a diagnosis of achondroplasia (dwarfism) was made. The parents ask the nurse if this could happen to future children. Because this is an example of autosomal dominant inheritance, the nurse would tell the parents:
   a. "For each pregnancy, there is a 50–50 chance the child will be affected by dwarfism."
   b. "This will not happen again because the dwarfism was caused by the harmful genetic effects of the infection you had during pregnancy."
   c. "For each pregnancy, there is a 25% chance the child will be a carrier of the defective gene but unaffected by the disorder."
   d. "Because you already have had an affected child, there is a decreased chance for this to happen in future pregnancies."

7. A female carries the gene for hemophilia on one of her X chromosomes. Now that she is pregnant, she asks the nurse how this might affect her baby. The nurse should tell her:
   a. "A female baby has a 50% chance of being a carrier."
   b. "Hemophilia is always expressed if a male inherits the defective gene."
   c. "Female babies are never affected by this disorder."
   d. "A male baby can be a carrier or have hemophilia."

8. A pregnant woman carries a single gene for cystic fibrosis. The father of her baby does not. Which of the following is true concerning the genetic pattern of cystic fibrosis as it applies to this family?
   a. The pregnant woman has cystic fibrosis herself.
   b. There is a 50% chance her baby will have the disorder.
   c. There is a 25% chance her baby will be a carrier.
   d. There is no chance her baby will be affected by the disorder.

9. When teaching a class of pregnant women about fetal development, the nurse would include which of the following statements? (Circle all that apply.)
   a. "The sex of your baby is determined by the ninth week of pregnancy."
   b. "The baby's heart begins to pump blood during the tenth week of your pregnancy."
   c. "You should be able to feel your baby move by week 16 to 20 of pregnancy."
   d. "We will begin to hear your baby's heartbeat using an ultrasound stethoscope by the eighteenth week of your pregnancy."
   e. "Your baby will be able to suck, swallow, and hiccup while in your uterus."
   f. "By the twenty-fourth week of your pregnancy, you will notice your baby responding to sounds in the environment such as your voice and music."

III. THINKING CRITICALLY

1. Imagine that you are a nurse-midwife working in partnership with an obstetrician. Formulate a response to each of the following concerns or questions directed to you from some of your prenatal patients.

a. June (2 months pregnant), Mary (5 months pregnant), and Alice (7 months pregnant) all ask for descriptions of their fetuses at the present time.

June

Mary

Alice

b. Jessica states that a friend told her that babies born after about 35 weeks have a better chance to survive because they can breathe easier. She asks if this is true.

c. Beth, who is 1 month pregnant, states that she heard that women who are pregnant experience quickening. She wants to know what that could mean and if it hurts.

d. Susan, who is 6 months pregnant, states that she read in a magazine that a fetus can actually hear and see. She feels that this is totally unbelievable.

e. Alexa is 2 months pregnant. She asks how the sex of her baby was determined and whether a sonogram could tell whether she is having a boy or a girl.

f. Karen is pregnant for the first time. She reveals that she has a history of twins in her family. She wants to know what causes twin pregnancies to occur and what the difference is between identical and fraternal twins.

2. Mr. and Mrs. G., a Jewish couple, are newly married and are planning for pregnancy. They express to the nurse their concern that Mrs. G. has a history of Tay-Sachs disease in her family. Mr. G. has never investigated his family history.

a. Describe the nurse's role in the process of assisting Mr. and Mrs. G. to determine their genetic risk.

b. Both Mr. and Mrs. G. are found to be carriers of the disorder. Discuss the estimation of risk and interpretation of risk as it applies to the couple for giving birth to a child who is normal, is a carrier, or is affected by the disorder.

c. Outline the nurse's role in the education and emotional support of the couple now that a diagnosis and estimation of risk have been made.

7 Anatomy and Physiology of Pregnancy

I. LEARNING KEY CONCEPTS

FILL IN THE BLANKS: Insert the term that corresponds to each of the following descriptions related to pregnancy.

1. _____ Pregnancy.

2. _____ The number of pregnancies in which the fetus or fetuses have reached 20 weeks of gestation, not the number of fetuses (e.g., twins) born. The numeric designation is not affected by whether the fetus is born alive or is stillborn (i.e., showing no signs of life at birth).

3. _____ A woman who is pregnant.

4. _____ A woman who has never been pregnant.

5. _____ A woman who has not completed a pregnancy with a fetus or fetuses beyond 20 weeks of gestation.

6. _____ A woman who is pregnant for the first time.

7. _____ A woman who has completed one pregnancy with a fetus or fetuses who have reached 20 weeks of gestation or more.

8. _____ A woman who has had two or more pregnancies.

9. _____ A woman who has completed two or more pregnancies to 20 weeks of gestation or more.

10. _____ Capacity to live outside the uterus; there are no clear limits of gestational age or weight.

11. _____ Designation given to a pregnancy that has reached 20 weeks of gestation but ends before completion of 37 weeks of gestation.

12. _____ Designation given to a pregnancy from the beginning of week 38 of gestation to the end of the week 42 of gestation.

13. _____ Designation given to a pregnancy that goes beyond 42 weeks of gestation. The designation _____ may also be given to refer to such a pregnancy.

14. _____ The biologic marker on which pregnancy tests are based. Its presence in urine or serum results in a positive pregnancy test result.

15. _____ Pregnancy-related changes felt by the woman.

16. _____ Pregnancy-related changes that can be observed by an examiner.

17. _____ Signs that can be attributed only to the presence of the fetus.

18. _____ Uterine contractions that can be felt through the abdominal wall soon after the fourth month of pregnancy.

19. _____ A rushing or blowing sound of maternal blood flow through the uterine arteries to the placenta that is synchronous with the maternal pulse.

20. _____ Sound of fetal blood coursing through the umbilical cord; it is synchronous with the fetal heart rate.

21. _____ Fetal movements first felt by the pregnant woman at 16 to 18 weeks of gestation.

22. _____ Change in blood pressure as a result of compression of abdominal blood vessels and decrease in cardiac output when a woman lies down on her back.

23. _____ Severe itching of the skin that occurs during pregnancy as a result of retention and accumulation of bile in the liver.

24. _____ Nonfood cravings for substances such as ice, clay, and laundry starch.

MATCHING: Match the assessment finding with the appropriate descriptive term.

25. _____ Menstrual bleeding no longer occurs.

26. _____ Fundal height decreased, fetal head in pelvic inlet.

27. _____ Cervix and vagina violet-bluish in color.

28. _____ Swelling of ankles and feet at the end of the day.

29. _____ Cervical tip softened.

30. _____ Lower uterine segment is soft and compressible.

31. _____ Fetal head rebounds with gentle upward tapping through the vagina.

32. _____ White or slightly gray mucoid vaginal discharge with faint, musty odor.

33. _____ Enlarged sebaceous glands in areola on both breasts.

34. _____ Plug of mucus fills endocervical canal.

35. _____ Pink stretch marks or depressed streaks on breasts and abdomen.

36. _____ Thick, creamy yellowish fluid expressed from nipples.

37. _____ Cheeks, nose, and forehead blotchy, brownish hyperpigmentation.

38. _____ Pigmented line extending up abdominal midline to the top of the fundus.

39. _____ Varicosities around the anus.

40. _____ Heartburn experienced after supper.

41. _____ Lumbosacral curve accentuated.

42. _____ Paresthesia and pain in right hand radiating to elbow.

43. _____ Spotting following cervical palpation or intercourse.

44. _____ Hematocrit decreased to 36% and hemoglobin to 11 g/dl.

45. _____ Vascular spiders on neck and thorax.

46. _____ Palms pinkish red, mottled.

47. _____ Abdominal wall muscles separated.

48. _____ Red raised nodule on gums; bleeds after brushing teeth.

a. Colostrum

b. Operculum

c. Amenorrhea

d. Angiomas

e. Pyrosis

f. Friability

g. Striae gravidarum

h. Physiologic anemia

i. Linea nigra

j. Ballottement

k. Chadwick's sign

l. Diastasis recti abdominis

m. Lordosis

n. Leukorrhea

o. Chloasma (melasma)

p. Lightening

q. Hemorrhoids

r. Palmar erythema

s. Goodell's sign

t. Physiologic/dependent edema

u. Hegar's sign

v. Montgomery tubercles

w. Carpal tunnel syndrome

x. Epulis (gingival granuloma gravidarum)

II. REVIEWING KEY CONCEPTS

1. Describe the obstetric history for each of the following women, using the 5-digit system.
   a. Nancy is pregnant. Her first pregnancy resulted in a stillbirth at 36 weeks of gestation and her second pregnancy resulted in the birth of her daughter at 42 weeks of gestation.

   4-digit

   5-digit

   b. Marsha is 6 weeks pregnant. Her previous pregnancies resulted in the live birth of a daughter at 40 weeks of gestation, the live birth of a son at 38 weeks of gestation, and a spontaneous abortion at 10 weeks of gestation.

   4-digit

   5-digit

   c. Linda is experiencing her fourth pregnancy. Her first pregnancy ended in a spontaneous abortion at 12 weeks, the second resulted in the live birth of twin boys at 32 weeks, and the third resulted in the live birth of a daughter at 39 weeks.

   4-digit

   5-digit

2. When assessing the pregnant woman, the nurse should keep in mind that baseline vital sign values will change as she progresses through her pregnancy. Describe how each of the following would change:

   a. Blood pressure (BP)

   b. Heart rate and patterns

   c. Respiratory rate and patterns

   d. Body temperature

3. Calculate the mean arterial pressure (MAP) for each of the following BP readings:

   a. 120/76

   b. 114/64

   c. 110/80

   d. 150/90

4. Specify the expected changes that occur in the following laboratory tests as a result of physiologic adaptations to pregnancy:

   a. CBC: hematocrit, hemoglobin, white blood cell count

   b. Clotting activity

   c. Acid/base balance

   d. Urinalysis

5. Explain the expected adaptations in elimination that occur during pregnancy. Include in your answer the basis for the changes that occur.

   Renal

   Bowel

6. A pregnant woman at 10 weeks of gestation exhibits the following signs of pregnancy during a routine prenatal checkup. Which ones would be categorized as probable signs of pregnancy? (Circle all that apply.)
   a. hCG in the urine
   b. Breast tenderness
   c. Ballottement
   d. Fetal heart sounds
   e. Hegar's sign
   f. Amenorrhea

7. A pregnant woman with four children reports the following obstetric history: a stillbirth at 32 weeks of gestation, triplets (2 sons and a daughter) born via cesarean section at 30 weeks of gestation, a spontaneous abortion at 8 weeks of gestation, and a daughter born vaginally at 39 weeks of gestation. Which of the following accurately expresses this woman's current obstetric history using the 5-digit system?
   a. 5-1-4-1-4
   b. 4-1-3-1-4
   c. 5-2-2-0-3
   d. 5-1-2-1-4

8. An essential component of prenatal health assessment of pregnant women is the determination of vital signs. Which of the following would be an expected change in vital sign findings as a result of pregnancy?
   a. Increase in systolic blood pressure by 30 mm Hg or more after assuming a supine position
   b. Increase in diastolic BP by 5 to 10 mm Hg beginning in the first trimester
   c. Chest breathing replaces abdominal breathing with upward displacement of the diaphragm
   d. Gradual decrease in baseline pulse rate of approximately 20 beats per minute

9. During an examination of a pregnant woman the nurse notes that her cervix is soft on its tip. The nurse would document this finding as:
   a. friability.
   b. Goodell's sign.
   c. Chadwick's sign.
   d. Hegar's sign.

III. THINKING CRITICALLY

1. Describe how the nurse should respond to each of the following patient concerns and questions.

   a. Tina is 14 weeks pregnant. She calls the prenatal clinic to report that she noticed slight, painless spotting this morning. She reveals that she did have intercourse with her partner the night before.

   b. Lisa suspects she is pregnant because her menstrual period is already 3 weeks late. She asks her friend, who is a nurse, how to use the pregnancy test that she just bought so that she obtains the most accurate results.

   c. Joan is 3 months pregnant. She tells the nurse that she is worried because a friend told her that vaginal and bladder infections are more common during pregnancy. She wants to know if this could be true and if so, why.

d. Tammy, who is 20 weeks pregnant, tells the nurse that she has noted some "problems" with her breasts: there are "little pimples" near her nipples and her breasts feel "lumpy and bumpy" and "leak a little" when she performs a breast self-examination (BSE).

e. Tamara is concerned because she read in a book about pregnancy that a pregnant woman's position could affect her circulation, especially to the baby. She asks what positions are good for her circulation now that she is pregnant.

f. Beth, a pregnant woman, calls to tell the nurse that she had a nosebleed this morning and has noticed occasional feelings of fullness in her ears. She asks if these occurrences are anything to worry about.

g. Karen is 7 months pregnant and works as a secretary full time. She asks the nurse if she should take a "water pill" that a friend gave her because she has noticed that her ankles "swell up" at the end of the day.

h. Jan is in her third trimester of pregnancy. She tells the nurse that her posture seems to have changed and that she occasionally experiences low back pain.

i. Monica, who is 36 weeks pregnant with her first baby, calls the clinic stating that she knows the baby is coming because she felt some uterine contractions before getting out of bed in the morning. Monica confirms that they seem to have decreased in intensity and frequency since she has gotten out of bed and walked around.

2. Accurate blood pressure readings are critical if significant changes in the cardiovascular system are to be detected as a woman adapts to pregnancy during the prenatal period. Write a protocol for blood pressure assessment that can be used by nurses working in a prenatal clinic to ensure accuracy of the results obtained during blood pressure assessment.

8 Nursing Care of the Family During Pregnancy

I. LEARNING KEY TERMS

FILL IN THE BLANKS: Insert the term that corresponds to each of the following descriptions.

1. _____ Rule used to determine the estimated day of birth by subtracting _____ months from, adding _____ days to, and one year to the first day of the _____. Alternatively, add _____ days to the first day of the _____ and count forward _____ months.

2. _____ The three 3-month periods into which pregnancy is divided.

3. _____ Measurement performed beginning in the second trimester as one indicator of the progress of fetal growth.

4. _____ Tasks accomplished by women and men as they adapt to the changes of pregnancy; these tasks include _____ _____, _____, _____, _____, and _____.

5. _____ Rapid unpredictable changes in mood.

6. _____ Having conflicting feelings about the pregnancy at the same time.

7. As a pregnant woman establishes a relationship with her fetus, she progresses through three phases. In phase one, she accepts the _____ and needs to be able to state _____. In phase two, the woman accepts the _____ and as a _____. She can now say _____. Finally, in phase three, the woman prepares realistically for the _____ and _____. She expresses the thought, _____.

8. _____ Change in blood pressure that can occur when a pregnant woman lies on her back for an examination of her abdomen. The _____ and the _____ are compressed by the weight of the abdominal contents, including the uterus.

9. _____ Change in blood pressure that can occur if a pregnant woman changes her position rapidly from supine to upright.

10. _____ and _____ Techniques used to assess fetal health status.

11. _____ Cultural expectations regarding the specific ways the male is to behave during pregnancy including the importance of respecting taboos associated with pregnancy and giving birth.

12. _____ Pregnancy-related phenomenon in which men experience pregnancy-like symptoms, such as nausea, weight gain, and other physical symptoms.

13. _____ Cultural directives that tell a woman what to do during pregnancy. _____ Cultural directives that tell a woman what not to do during pregnancy; they establish _____.

14. _____ Professionally trained woman who provides physical, emotional, and informational support to women and their partners during labor and birth and in the postpartum period.

15. _____ Tool that can be used by expectant couples to explore their childbirth options and choose those that are most important to them; it serves as a tentative guide because the reality of what is feasible may change as the actual labor and birth progress.

II. REVIEWING KEY CONCEPTS

1. Calculate the expected date of birth (EDB) for each of the following pregnant women using Nägele's rule.

   a. Diane's last menses began on May 5, 2013, and its last day occurred on May 10, 2013.

b. Sara had intercourse on February 4, 2013. She has not had a menstrual period since the one that began on January 19, 2013, and ended 5 days later.

c. Beth's last period began on July 4, 2013, and ended on July 10, 2013. She noted that her basal body temperature (BBT) began to rise on July 28, 2013.

2. Cultural beliefs and practices are important influencing factors during the prenatal period.

a. Describe how cultural beliefs can affect a woman's participation in prenatal care as it is defined by the Western biomedical model of care.

b. Identify one prescription and one proscription for each of the following areas:

Emotional responses

Clothing

Physical activity and rest

Sexual activity

Nutrition

3. Outline the assessment measures that should be used and the data that should be collected during each component of the initial prenatal visit and the follow-up prenatal visits.

INITIAL PRENATAL VISIT

Health History Interview

Physical Examination

Laboratory and Diagnostic Testing

FOLLOW-UP PRENATAL VISITS

Updating History Interview

Physical Examination

Fetal Assessment

Laboratory and Diagnostic Testing

4. Nurses responsible for the care management of pregnant women must be alert for warning signs of potential complications that women could develop as pregnancy progresses from trimester to trimester.

a. List the clinical manifestations (warning signs) for each of the following potential complications of pregnancy.

Hyperemesis gravidarum

Infection

Miscarriage

Hypertension conditions including preeclampsia

Premature rupture of the membranes (PROM)

Placental disorders (placenta previa; abruptio placentae)

Fetal jeopardy

b. Describe the approach a nurse should take when discussing potential complications with a pregnant woman and her family.

5. Create a protocol for fundal measurement that will facilitate accuracy.

6. Prevention of injury is an important goal for nurses as they teach pregnant women about how to care for themselves during pregnancy.

a. Describe three principles of body mechanics that a pregnant woman should be taught to prevent injury.

b. Identify five safety guidelines that the nurse should include in a pamphlet titled "Safety During Pregnancy" that will be distributed to pregnant women during a prenatal visit.

7. During the third trimester, parents often make a decision concerning the method they will use to feed their newborn. Identify factors that may influence a woman to choose bottle feeding rather than breast-feeding. How would you overcome this reluctance during a prenatal breastfeeding class?

8. Men experience pregnancy in many different ways. Three phases have been identified as characterizing the developmental tasks experienced by expectant fathers. Briefly, discuss each phase and how the nurse can help the father to progress through each phase.

Announcement Phase

Moratorium Phase

Focusing Phase

9. A nurse is assessing a pregnant woman during a prenatal visit. Several presumptive indicators of pregnancy are documented. Which of the following are presumptive indicators? (Circle all that apply.)
a. Nausea and vomiting
b. Quickening
c. Ballottement
d. Palpation of fetal movement by the nurse
e. Hegar's sign
f. Amenorrhea

10. A woman's last menstrual period (LMP) began on September 10, 2013, and it ended on September 15, 2013. Using Nägele's rule, the estimated date of birth would be:
a. June 17, 2014.
b. June 22, 2014.
c. August 17, 2014.
d. December 3, 2014.

11. A woman at 30 weeks of gestation assumes a supine position for a fundal measurement and Leopold's maneuvers. She begins to complain about feeling dizzy and nauseated. Her skin feels damp and cool. The nurse's first action would be to:
    a. assess the woman's respiratory rate and effort.
    b. provide the woman with an emesis basin.
    c. elevate the woman's legs 20 degrees from her hips.
    d. turn the woman on her side.

12. During an early bird prenatal class a nurse teaches a group of newly diagnosed pregnant women about their emotional reactions during pregnancy. Which of the following should the nurse discuss with the women? (Circle all that apply.)
    a. Sexual desire (libido) is usually increased during the second trimester of pregnancy.
    b. A referral for counseling should be sought if a woman experiences ambivalence in the first trimester.
    c. Rapid, unpredictable mood swings reflect gestational bipolar disorder.
    d. The need to seek safe passage and prepare for birth begins early in the third trimester.
    e. A woman's own mother will be her greatest source of emotional support during pregnancy.
    f. Attachment to the infant begins late in the third trimester when she begins preparing for birth by attending childbirth preparation classes

13. The nurse evaluates a pregnant woman's knowledge about prevention of urinary tract infections at the prenatal visit following a class on infection prevention that the woman attended. The nurse would recognize that the woman needs further instruction when she tells the nurse about which one of the following measures that she now uses to prevent urinary tract infections? (Circle all that apply.)
    a. "I drink about 1 quart of fluid a day."
    b. "I have stopped using bubble baths and bath oils."
    c. "I have started wearing panty hose and underpants with a cotton crotch."
    d. "I have yogurt for lunch or as an evening snack."
    e. "I should stop having intercourse with my partner since it increases my risk for urinary tract infections."
    f. "If I drink cranberry juice during breakfast and dinner I will not get a bladder infection."

14. Doulas are becoming important members of a laboring woman's health care team. Which of the following activities should be expected as part of the doula's role responsibilities?
    a. Monitoring hydration of the laboring woman, including adjusting IV flow rates
    b. Interpreting electronic fetal monitoring tracings to determine the well-being of the maternal-fetal unit
    c. Eliminating the need for the husband/partner to be present during labor and birth
    d. Providing continuous support throughout labor and birth, including explanations of labor progress

15. A pregnant woman is concerned about what she should do if she notices signs of preterm labor such as uterine contractions. After reviewing the signs of preterm labor with the woman, the nurse reviews measures the patient should implement should the signs occur. The nurse should discuss which of the following measures with the woman? (Circle all that apply.)
    a. Empty bladder
    b. Drink 3 to 4 glasses of water to ensure adequate hydration
    c. Assume a supine position
    d. Assess contractions for 2 or more hours
    e. Report contractions that occur every 10 minutes or more often for 1 hour
    f. Recognize that uterine contractions may be perceived as a tightening in her abdomen or as a backache

III. THINKING CRITICALLY

1. A health history interview of the pregnant woman by the nurse is included as part of the initial prenatal visit.

   a. State the purpose of the health history interview.

   b. Write two questions for each component that is included in the initial health history interview. Questions should be clear, concise, and understandable. Most of the questions should be open ended to elicit the most complete response from the patient.

c. Write four questions that should be included in the interview when updating the health history during follow-up visits.

2. Imagine that you are a nurse working in a prenatal clinic. You have been assigned to be the primary nurse for Martha, an 18-year-old who has come to the clinic for confirmation of pregnancy. She tells you that she knows she is pregnant because she has already missed three periods and a home pregnancy test that she did last week was positive. Martha states that she has had very little contact with the health care system, and the only reason she came today is because her boyfriend insisted that she "make sure" she is really pregnant. Describe the approach that you would take regarding data collection and nursing interventions appropriate for this woman.

3. Terry is a primigravida in her first trimester of pregnancy. She is accompanied by her husband, Tim, to her second prenatal visit. Answer each of the following questions asked by Terry and Tim:

   a. "At the last visit I was told that my estimated date of birth is December 25, 2014. Can I really count on my baby being born on Christmas Day?"

   b. "Before I became pregnant my friend told me I should be doing Kegel exercises. I was too embarrassed to ask her about them. What are they and is it safe for me to do them while I am pregnant?"

   c. "What effect will pregnancy have on our sex life? We are willing to abstain during pregnancy if we have to keep our baby safe."

   d. "This morning sickness I am experiencing is driving me crazy. I become nauseated in the morning and again late in the afternoon. Occasionally I vomit or have the dry heaves. Will this last for my entire pregnancy? Is there anything I can do to feel better?"

4. Tara is 2 months pregnant. She tells the nurse, at the prenatal clinic, that she is used to being active and exercises every day. Now that she is pregnant she wonders if she should reduce or stop her exercise routine. Discuss what information the nurse's response to Tara should include.

5. Write one nursing diagnosis for each of the following situations. State one expected outcome, and list appropriate nursing measures for the nursing diagnosis you identified.

    a. Beth is 6 weeks pregnant. During the health history interview, she tells you that she has limited her intake of fluids and tries to hold her urine as long as she can because, "I just hate having to go to the bathroom so frequently."

        Nursing diagnosis   Expected outcome   Nursing measures

    b. Doris, who is 23 weeks pregnant, tells you that she is beginning to experience more frequent lower back pain. You note that when she walked into the examining room her posture exhibited a moderate degree of lordosis and neck flexion. She was wearing shoes with 2-inch narrow heels.

        Nursing diagnosis   Expected outcome   Nursing measures

    c. Lisa, a primigravida at 32 weeks of gestation, comes for a prenatal visit accompanied by her partner, the father of the baby. They both express anxiety about the impending birth of the baby and how they will handle the experience of labor. Lisa is especially concerned about how she will survive the pain, and her partner is primarily concerned about how he will help Lisa cope with labor and make sure she and the baby are safe.

        Nursing diagnosis   Expected outcome   Nursing measures

6. Jane is a primigravida in her second trimester of pregnancy. Answer each of the following questions asked by Jane during a prenatal visit.

    a. "Why do you measure my abdomen every time I come in for a checkup?"

    b. "I am going to start changing the way that I dress now that I am beginning to show. Do you have any suggestions I could follow, especially since I have a limited amount of money to spend?"

    c. "What can I do about gas and constipation? I never had much of a problem before I was pregnant."

    d. "Since yesterday I have started to feel itchy all over. Do you think I am coming down with some sort of infection?"

e. "I will be flying out to Chicago to visit my father in 1 month. Is airline travel safe for me when I am 5 months pregnant?"

7. While a nurse is measuring a pregnant woman's fundus, the woman becomes pale and diaphoretic. The woman, who is at 23 weeks of gestation, states that she feels dizzy and lightheaded.

   a. State the most likely explanation for the assessment findings exhibited by this woman.

   b. Describe what the nurse's immediate action should be.

8. Kelly is a primigravida in her third trimester of pregnancy. Answer each of the following questions asked by Kelly during a prenatal visit.

   a. "My husband and I have decided to breastfeed our baby but friends told me it is very difficult if my nipples do not come out. Is there any way I can tell now if my nipples are okay for breastfeeding?"

   b. "My ankles are swollen by the time I get home from work late in the afternoon [Kelly teaches second grade]. I have been trying to drink about 3 liters of fluid every day. Should I reduce the amount of liquid I am drinking or ask my doctor for a water pill?"

   c. "I woke up last night with a terrible cramp in my leg. It finally went away but my husband and I just did not know what to do. What if this happens again tonight?"

9. Marge, a pregnant woman (2-0-0-1-0) beginning her third trimester, expresses concern about preterm birth. "I already had one miscarriage, and my sister's baby died after being born too early. I am so worried that this will happen to me."

   a. Identify one nursing diagnosis with an expected outcome that reflects Marge's concern.

   b. Indicate what the nurse can teach Marge about the signs of preterm labor.

   c. Describe the actions Marge should take if she experiences signs of preterm labor.

10. Carol is 4 months pregnant and is beginning to "show." She asks the nurse what she should expect as a reaction from her 13-year-old daughter and 3-year-old son. Describe the response the nurse would make.

11. Your neighbor, Jane, is in her second month of pregnancy. Knowing that you are a nurse, her husband, Tom, confides to you, "I just can't figure out Jane. One minute she is happy and the next minute she is crying for no reason at all! I do not know how I will be able to cope with this for 7 more months."

    a. Write a nursing diagnosis and expected outcome that reflects Tom's concern.

    b. Discuss how you would respond to his concern.

12. Jennifer (2-1-0-0-1) and her husband, Dan, are beginning their third trimester of a low risk pregnancy. As you work with them on their birth plan, they tell you that they are having trouble making a decision about their choice of a birth setting. They experienced a delivery room birth with their first child. Jennifer states, "My first pregnancy was perfectly normal, just like this one, but the birth was disappointing, so medically focused with monitors, IVs, and staying in bed." They ask you for your advice about the different birth settings they have heard and read about, namely labor, delivery, recovery, and postpartum (LDRP) rooms at their local hospital, the birthing center a few miles from their home, and even their own home. Describe the approach that you would take to guide Jennifer and Dan in their decision regarding a birth setting.

13. Nancy, a pregnant woman (3-2-0-0-2) at 26 weeks of gestation, asks the nurse about doulas. "My friend had a doula and she said that she was amazing. My first two birth experiences were difficult—my husband and I really needed someone to help us. Do you think a doula could be that person?"

    a. Explain the role of the doula so that Nancy will have the information she will need to make an informed decision.

    b. Nancy decides to try a doula for her upcoming labor. Identify what you would tell Nancy about finding a doula.

    c. Specify questions that Nancy should ask when she is making a choice about the doula she will hire for her labor.

14. Tony and Andrea are considering the possibility of giving birth to their second baby at home. They have been receiving prenatal care from a certified nurse-midwife who has experience with home birth. Their 5-year-old son and both sets of grandparents want to be present for the birth.

   a. Discuss the decision-making process that Tony and Andrea should follow to ensure that they make an informed decision that is right for them and their family.

   b. Tony and Andrea decide that home birth is an ideal choice for them. Outline the preparation measures you would recommend to Tony and Andrea to ensure a safe and positive experience for everyone.

9 Maternal and Fetal Nutrition

I. LEARNING KEY TERMS

FILL IN THE BLANKS: Insert the term that corresponds to each of the following descriptions.

1. _____ Birth weight of 2500 g or less.

2. _____ Nutrient, the adequate intake of which is important for decreasing risk for _____ or failures in the closure of the neural tube. An intake of _____ daily is recommended for all women capable of becoming pregnant.

3. _____ Nutritional recommendations from the Food and Nutrition Board of the National Academy of Sciences.

4. _____ Method used to evaluate the appropriateness of weight for height. If the calculated value is less than 18.5, the person is considered to be _____. If the calculated value is between 18.5 and 24.9, the person is considered to be _____. If the calculated value is between 25 and 29.9, the person is considered to be _____ and if greater than 30 the person is considered to be _____.

5. _____ Presence of ketones in the urine as a result of catabolism of fat stores; it has been found to correlate with the occurrence of preterm labor.

6. _____ Normal adaptation that occurs during pregnancy when the plasma volume increases more rapidly than RBC mass.

7. _____ Inability to digest milk sugar because of the absence of the lactase enzyme in the small intestine.

8. _____ Practice of consuming nonfood substances or excessive amounts of food stuffs low in nutritional value.

9. _____ Urge to consume specific types of foods such as ice cream, pickles, and pizza during pregnancy.

10. _____ Guide that can be used to make daily food choices during pregnancy and lactation, just as during other stages of the life cycle.

11. _____ A discomfort most commonly experienced in the first trimester of pregnancy; it usually causes only mild-to-moderate nutritional problems but may be a source of substantial discomfort.

12. _____ Severe and persistent vomiting during pregnancy causing weight loss, dehydration, and electrolyte abnormalities.

13. _____ Discomfort of pregnancy characterized by infrequent and difficult passage of hard, dry stool.

14. _____ Discomfort of pregnancy that is usually caused by reflux of gastric contents into the esophagus.

II. REVIEWING KEY CONCEPTS

1. Indicate the importance of each of the following nutrients for healthy maternal adaptation to pregnancy and optimum fetal growth and development. Indicate three food/fluid sources for each of the nutrients.

Nutrient	Importance for Pregnancy	Major Food Sources
Protein		
Iron		
Calcium		
Sodium		
Zinc		
Fat-soluble vitamins		
Water-soluble vitamins		

2. When assessing pregnant women, it is critical that nurses are alert for factors that could place women at nutritional risk so that early intervention can be implemented. Name five such indicators or risk factors of which the nurse should be aware.

3. Cite the pregnancy-related risks associated with the following nutritional problems.

   a. Underweight women

   b. Inappropriate weight gain during pregnancy (inadequate; excessive)

   c. Obese women

4. At her first prenatal visit, Marie, a 20-year-old primigravida, reports that she has been a strict vegetarian for the past 3 years. Identify two major guidelines that the nurse should follow when planning menus with Marie.

5. Evaluation of nutritional status is an essential part of a thorough physical assessment of pregnant women. Cite four signs of good nutrition and four signs of inadequate nutrition that the nurse should observe for during the assessment of a pregnant woman.

6. Calculate the BMI for each of the following women, and then determine the recommended weight gain and pattern for each woman based on her BMI.

Woman	BMI Meaning	Weight Gain (total; pattern)
a. June: 5 feet 3 inches, 120 pounds		
b. Alice: 5 feet 6 inches, 180 pounds		
c. Ann: 5 feet 5 inches, 95 pounds		

7. A nurse teaching a pregnant woman about the importance of iron in her diet would tell her to avoid consuming which of the following foods at the same time as her iron supplement because they will decrease iron absorption? (Circle all that apply.)
   a. Tomatoes
   b. Spinach
   c. Meat
   d. Eggs
   e. Milk
   f. Bran

8. A 30-year-old pregnant woman with a BMI of 31 asks the nurse about recommendations for diet and weight gain during pregnancy. Which of the following would the nurse tell this woman?
   a. Counsel her to begin a lifestyle change for weight reduction
   b. Recommend a total weight gain goal of 4 kg during pregnancy
   c. Set a weight gain goal of 0.3 kg per week during the second and third trimesters
   d. Limit her third trimester calorie increase to no more than 600 Kcal more than prepregnant needs

9. A 25-year-old pregnant woman is at 10 weeks of gestation. Her BMI is calculated to be 24. Which one of the following is recommended in terms of weight gain during pregnancy?
   a. Total weight gain of 18 kg
   b. First trimester weight gain of 1 to 2 kg
   c. Weight gain of 0.4 kg each week for 40 weeks
   d. Weight gain of 3 kg per month during the second and third trimesters

10. A pregnant woman at 6 weeks of gestation tells her nurse-midwife that she has been experiencing nausea with occasional vomiting every day. The nurse could recommend which of the following as an effective relief measure?
   a. Eat starchy foods such as buttered popcorn or peanut butter with crackers in the morning before getting out of bed.
   b. Avoid eating before going to bed at night.
   c. Alter eating patterns to a schedule of small meals every 2 to 3 hours.
   d. Skip a meal if nausea is experienced.

11. A woman demonstrates an understanding of the importance of increasing her intake of foods high in folic acid (100 mcg or more) when she includes which of the following foods in her diet? (Circle all that apply.)
    a. Seafood
    b. Legumes
    c. Eggs
    d. Liver (beef)
    e. Asparagus
    f. Oranges

III. THINKING CRITICALLY

1. Nutrition and weight gain are important areas of consideration for nurses who care for pregnant women. In addition, weight gain is often a source of stress and body image alteration for the pregnant woman. Discuss the approach you would use in each of the following situations.

   a. Kelly (5' 8" and 120 pounds) complains to you that her physician recommended a weight gain of approximately 30 pounds during her pregnancy. She states, "Babies only weigh about 7 pounds when they are born. Why do I have to gain much more than that?"

   b. Kate (5' 4" and 125 pounds) has just found out that she is pregnant. She states, "I am so glad to be pregnant. I love to eat, and now I can start eating for two. It will be great not to have to watch the scale or what I eat."

   c. June tells you that she does not have to worry about her nutrient intake during her pregnancy. "I take plenty of vitamins—everything from A to Z."

   d. Mary, a primigravida beginning her second month of pregnancy, asks you why she needs to increase her intake of so many nutrients during pregnancy and states, "I work every weekday and rely on fast foods to get through the week, though I try to eat better over the weekends."

   e. Sara (BMI = 28.7) is 1 month pregnant. She asks you for dietary guidance, including a weight reduction diet because she does not want to gain too much weight with this pregnancy.

   f. Beth is 2 months pregnant. She states, "I have cut down on my water intake. I do get a little thirsty, but it's worth it since I don't have to urinate so often."

   g. Hedy is 2 months pregnant and has come for her second prenatal visit. During a discussion about nutritional needs during pregnancy she states, "I know I will never get enough calcium because I get sick when I drink milk."

h. Lara is 36 weeks pregnant. She states that she would like to breastfeed her baby but is concerned about getting back into shape and losing weight after the baby is born. "My friends told me that I will lose weight more slowly since I will not be able to start on a weight reduction diet as long as I am breastfeeding."

i. Jean intends to breastfeed her infant until she returns to work in 6 months. She asks you what guidelines she should follow so that she makes good breast milk for her baby.

2. Yvonne's hemoglobin is 13 g/dL and her hematocrit is 37% at the onset of her pregnancy. She asks the nurse if she will have to take iron during her pregnancy if she tries to follow a good diet. "My friend took iron when she was pregnant and it made her sick to her stomach." Discuss the appropriate response by the nurse.

3. Identify three nursing measures appropriate for each of the following nursing diagnoses:

a. Imbalanced nutrition: less than body requirements related to inadequate intake associated with moderate nausea and vomiting (morning sickness) associated with pregnancy

b. Constipation related to decreased intestinal motility associated with increased progesterone levels during pregnancy

c. Pain related to reflux of gastric contents into esophagus following dinner

4. Gloria is an 18-year-old Native-American woman (5' 6" and 98 pounds) who has just been diagnosed as being 8 weeks pregnant. In her discussions with you at her first prenatal visit, she expresses a lack of knowledge regarding the nutritional requirements of pregnancy and an interest in learning about what to eat because she wants to have a healthy baby.

a. Outline the approach that you would use to help Gloria learn about and meet the nutritional requirements of her pregnancy.

b. Plan a 1-day menu that incorporates Gloria's nutritional needs and reflects the traditions of her culture.

10 Assessment of High Risk Pregnancy

I. LEARNING KEY TERMS

FILL IN THE BLANKS: Insert the term that corresponds to each of the following descriptions.

1. _____ A pregnancy in which the life or health of the mother or her fetus is jeopardized by a disorder coincidental with or unique to pregnancy.

2. _____ Assessment of fetal activity by the mother is a simple yet valuable method for monitoring the condition of the fetus. _____ Term used to refer to the cessation of fetal movements entirely for 12 hours.

3. _____ Diagnostic test that involves the use of sound having a frequency higher than that detectable by humans to examine structures inside the body. During pregnancy, it can be done by using either the _____ or _____ approach.

4. _____ Noninvasive study of blood flow in the fetus and placenta with ultrasound.

5. _____ Noninvasive dynamic assessment of the fetus and its environment that is based on acute and chronic markers of fetal disease. It uses both real-time _____ and external _____. This test includes assessment of five variables, namely _____, _____, _____, _____, and _____.

6. _____ Noninvasive radiologic technique used for obstetric and gynecologic diagnosis by providing excellent pictures of soft tissue without the use of ionizing radiation.

7. _____ Prenatal diagnostic test that is performed to obtain amniotic fluid to examine the fetal cells it contains.

8. _____ Prenatal diagnostic test that provides direct access to the fetal circulation during the second and third trimesters.

9. _____ Procedure that involves the removal of a small tissue specimen from the fetal portion of the placenta. Because this tissue originates from the zygote, it reflects the genetic makeup of the fetus and is performed between 10 and 13 weeks of gestation.

10. _____ Test used as a screening tool for neural tube defects in pregnancy. The test is ideally performed between 16 and 18 weeks of gestation.

11. _____ Test used to screen for Down syndrome. It is performed between 16 and 18 weeks of gestation. The levels of three markers, namely _____, _____, and _____, in combination with maternal _____ are used to determine risk. _____ Test used to screen for Down syndrome that adds an additional marker, namely _____; it increases accuracy of the test, especially in women less than 35 years of age.

12. _____ Screening test for Rh incompatibility by examining the serum of Rh negative women for Rh antibodies.

13. _____ Test based on the fact that the heart rate of a healthy fetus with an intact central nervous system will usually accelerate in response to its own movement.

14. _____ Test that determines fetal response to the stimulation of vibration and sound; the expected response is acceleration of the fetal heart rate.

15. _____ Test used to identify the jeopardized fetus that is stable at rest but shows evidence of compromise when exposed to the stress of uterine contractions. If the resultant hypoxia of the fetus is sufficient, a deceleration of the FHR will result. Two methods used for this test are the _____ test and the _____ test.

II. REVIEWING KEY CONCEPTS

1. Identify factors that would place the pregnant woman and fetus/neonate at risk, for each of the following categories:

   Biophysical factors

   Psychosocial factors

   Sociodemographic factors

   Environmental factors

2. Discuss the role of the nurse when caring for high-risk pregnant women who are required to undergo antepartal assessment testing to determine fetal well-being.

3. State two risk factors for each of the following pregnancy-related problems:

   Polyhydramnios

   Intrauterine growth restriction

   Oligohydramnios

   Chromosomal abnormalities

4. A 34-year-old woman at 36 weeks of gestation has been scheduled for a biophysical profile. She asks the nurse why the test needs to be performed. The nurse would tell her that the test:
   a. determines how well her baby will breathe after it is born.
   b. evaluates the response of her baby's heart to uterine contractions.
   c. measures her baby's head size and length.
   d. observes her baby's activities in utero to ensure that her baby is getting enough oxygen.

5. As part of preparing a 24-year-old woman at 42 weeks of gestation for a nonstress test, the nurse would:
   a. tell the woman to fast for 8 hours before the test.
   b. explain that the test will evaluate how well her baby is moving inside her uterus.
   c. show her how to indicate when her baby moves.
   d. attach a spiral electrode to the presenting part to determine FHR patterns.

6. A 40-year-old woman at 18 weeks of gestation is having a triple marker test performed. She is obese, and her health history reveals that she is Rh negative. The primary purpose of this test is to screen for:
   a. spina bifida.
   b. Down syndrome.
   c. gestational diabetes.
   d. Rh antibodies.

7. During a contraction stress test, four contractions lasting 45 to 55 seconds were recorded in a 10-minute period. A late deceleration was noted during the third contraction. The nurse conducting the test would document that the result is:
   a. negative.
   b. positive.
   c. suspicious.
   d. unsatisfactory.

8. A pregnant woman is scheduled for a transvaginal ultrasound test to establish gestational age. In preparing this woman for the test, the nurse would:
   a. place the woman in a supine position with her hips elevated on a folded pillow.
   b. instruct her to come for the test with a full bladder.
   c. administer an analgesic 30 minutes before the test.
   d. lubricate the vaginal probe with transmission gel.

III. THINKING CRITICALLY

1. Annie is a primigravida who is at 10 weeks of gestation. Her prenatal history reveals that she was treated for pelvic inflammatory disease 2 years ago. She describes irregular menstrual cycles and is therefore unsure about the first day of her last menstrual period. Annie is scheduled for a transvaginal ultrasound.

   a. Cite the likely reasons for the performance of this test.

   b. Describe how the nurse should prepare Annie for this test.

2. Latisha, a pregnant woman at 20 weeks of gestation, is scheduled for a series of transabdominal ultrasounds to monitor the growth of her fetus. Describe the nursing role as it applies to Latisha and transabdominal ultrasound examinations.

3. Mary is at 42 weeks of gestation. Her physician has ordered a biophysical profile (BPP). She is very upset and tells the nurse, "All my doctor told me is that this test will see if my baby is okay. I do not know what is going to happen and if it will be painful to me or harmful for my baby."

   a. State a nursing diagnosis that reflects this situation.

   b. Describe how the nurse should respond to Mary's concerns.

   c. Mary receives a score of 8 for the BPP. List the factors that were evaluated to obtain this score and specify the meaning of Mary's test result of 8.

4. Jan, age 42, is 18 weeks pregnant. Because of her age, Jan's fetus is at risk for genetic anomalies. Jan's blood type is A negative and her partner's, the father of her baby, is B positive. Her primary health care provider has suggested an amniocentesis. Describe the nurse's role in terms of each of the following:

   a. Preparing Jan for the amniocentesis

   b. Supporting Jan during the procedure

c. Providing Jan with postprocedure care and instructions

5. Susan, who has diabetes and is in week 36 of pregnancy, has been scheduled for a nonstress test.

a. Discuss what you would tell Susan about the purpose of this test and what will be learned about her baby's well-being.

b. Describe how you would prepare Susan for this test.

c. Discuss how you would conduct the test.

d. Indicate the criteria you would use to determine whether the result of the test was:

Reactive

Nonreactive

6. Beth is scheduled for a contraction stress test following a nonreactive result on a nonstress test. Nipple stimulation will be used to stimulate the required contractions.

a. Discuss what you would tell Beth about the purpose of this test and what will be learned about the well-being of her fetus.

b. Describe how you would prepare Beth for the test.

c. Indicate how you would conduct the test.

d. State how you would conduct the test differently if exogenous oxytocin (Pitocin) is used instead of nipple stimulation.

e. Indicate the criteria you would use to determine whether the result of the test was:

Negative

Positive

Suspicious or equivocal

Equivocal-hyperstimulatory

Unsatisfactory

11 High Risk Perinatal Care: Preexisting Conditions

I. LEARNING KEY TERMS

FILL IN THE BLANKS: Insert the term that corresponds to each of the following descriptions related to diabetes mellitus.

1. _____ A group of metabolic diseases characterized by hyperglycemia resulting from defects in insulin secretion, insulin action, or both.

2. _____ Accumulation of excessive glucose in the blood.

3. _____ A normal blood glucose level.

4. _____ Blood glucose level that is too low.

5. _____ Excretion of large volumes of urine.

6. _____ Excessive thirst.

7. _____ Excessive eating.

8. _____ Excretion of unusable glucose into the urine.

9. _____ Accumulation of ketones in the blood resulting from hyperglycemia and leading to metabolic acidosis. _____ Term used to refer to spillage of ketones into the urine.

10. _____ Classification of diabetes mellitus primarily caused by pancreatic islet β-cell destruction and prone to ketoacidosis; persons with this form of diabetes usually have an absolute insulin deficiency.

11. _____ Most prevalent classification of diabetes mellitus; persons with this form of diabetes have insulin resistance and usually relative (rather than absolute) insulin deficiency.

12. _____ Label given to diabetes mellitus that existed before pregnancy.

13. _____ Any degree of glucose intolerance with its onset or first recognition occurring during pregnancy.

14. _____ Blood test that provides a measurement of glycemic control over time, specifically over the previous 4 to 6 weeks.

15. _____ Excessive fetal growth; birth weight greater than 4000 to 4500 g.

16. _____ Excessive amniotic fluid.

17. _____ Device persons with diabetes mellitus can use to measure blood glucose levels.

FILL IN THE BLANKS: Insert the term that corresponds to each of the following descriptions related to selected preexisting medical disorders during pregnancy.

18. _____ Inability of the heart to maintain a sufficient cardiac output. Physiologic stress on the heart is greatest between week _____ and _____ of gestation because the cardiac output is at its peak. Risk for this complication is also higher during _____ and the first _____ to _____ hours after birth.

19. _____ Classification system for cardiovascular disorders developed by the New York Heart Association. Class I implies _____. Class II implies _____. Class III implies _____. Class IV implies _____.

20. _____ Cardiac disorder characterized by the development of congestive heart failure in the last month of pregnancy or within 5 postpartum months, lack of another cause for heart failure, and the absence of heart disease before the last month of pregnancy; etiology for the disorder may be related to genetic predisposition, autoimmunity, and viral infections.

21. _____ Damage of the heart valves and the chordae tendineae cordis as a result of an infection originating from an inadequately treated group A β-hemolytic streptococcal infection of the throat.

72

22. _____ Narrowing of the valve between the left atrium and the left ventricle of the heart by stiffening of the valve leaflets, which obstructs blood flow from the atrium to the ventricles. _____ Narrowing of the aortic valve.

23. _____ Acute ischemic event involving cardiac muscle.

24. _____ Inflammation of the innermost lining of the heart caused by invasion of bacteria.

25. _____ Common, usually benign, cardiac condition that involves the protrusion of the leaflets of the mitral valve back into the left atrium during ventricular systole, allowing some backflow of blood.

26. _____ A hemoglobin level of less than 11 g/dL in the first and third trimester and less than 10.5 gm/dL in the second trimester; it is mainly a result of an _____ deficiency.

27. _____ Disease caused by the presence of abnormal hemoglobin in the blood. It is a recessive, hereditary, familial hemolytic anemia that affects those of African-American or Mediterranean ancestry.

28. _____ Relatively common anemia in which an insufficient amount of globin is produced to fill red blood cells.

29. _____ Acute respiratory illness caused by allergens, irritants, marked changes in ambient temperature, certain medications, or exercise. In response to stimuli, there is widespread but reversible narrowing of the hyperactive airways making it difficult to breathe.

30. _____ Common autosomal recessive genetic disorder in which the exocrine glands produce excessive viscous secretions, causing problems with both respiratory and digestive functions.

31. _____ Generalized itching during pregnancy without the presence of a rash.

32. _____ Integumentary condition during pregnancy characterized by itching and urticarial papules and plaques most often appearing during the mid-to late third trimester.

33. _____ Liver disorder unique to pregnancy that is characterized by generalized pruritus, usually beginning during the third trimester, most severely affecting the palms and soles, and is worse at night.

34. _____ Disorder of the brain causing recurrent seizures; it is the most common neurologic disorder accompanying pregnancy.

35. _____ Patchy demyelinization of the spinal cord and CNS; may be viral in origin.

36. _____ Acute idiopathic facial paralysis that can occur during pregnancy, especially in the third trimester and puerperium.

37. _____ Chronic, multisystem, inflammatory disease characterized by autoimmune antibody production that affects the skin, joints, kidneys, lungs, central nervous system (CNS), liver, and other body organs.

38. _____ Sensorimotor disorder characterized by discomfort of the legs and an urge to move them, usually when at rest or during periods of inactivity.

II. REVIEWING KEY CONCEPTS

1. Identify the major maternal and fetal/neonatal risks and complications associated with diabetic pregnancies. Indicate the underlying pathophysiologic basis for each of the complications you identify.

2. Explain the current recommendations for screening for and diagnosing of gestational diabetes mellitus developed by the Expert Committee on the Diagnosis and Classification of Diabetes Mellitus.

3. State how hyperthyroidism and hypothyroidism can affect reproductive well-being and pregnancy.

4. Identify the maternal and fetal complications that are more common among pregnant women who have cardiac problems.

5. State how the 4 Ps Plus Screening Tool could be used during pregnancy and the information it is designed to gather.

6. A pregestational diabetic woman at 20 weeks of gestation exhibits the following: thirst, nausea and vomiting, abdominal pain, drowsiness, and increased urination. Her skin is flushed and dry and her breathing is rapid with a fruity odor. A priority nursing action when caring for this woman would be to:
   a. provide the woman with a simple carbohydrate immediately.
   b. request an order for an antiemetic.
   c. assist the woman into a lateral position to rest.
   d. administer insulin according to the woman's blood glucose level.

7. During her pregnancy, a woman with pregestational diabetes has been monitoring her blood glucose level several times a day. Which of the following levels would require further assessment?
   a. 85 mg/dL—before breakfast
   b. 90 mg/dL—before lunch
   c. 135 mg/dL—2 hours after supper
   d. 126 mg/dL—1 hour after breakfast

8. A nurse is working with a pregestational diabetic woman to plan the diet she will follow during pregnancy. Which of the following nutritional guidelines should be used to ensure a euglycemic state and appropriate weight gain? (Circle all that apply.)
   a. Substantial bedtime snack composed of complex carbohydrates with some protein and fat

   b. Average calories per day of 2200 during the first trimester and 2500 during the second and third trimesters
   c. Caloric distribution among three meals and one or two snacks
   d. Minimum of 45% carbohydrate daily
   e. Protein intake of at least 30% of the total kilocalories in a day
   f. Fat intake of 30% to 40% of the daily caloric intake

9. An obese pregnant woman with gestational diabetes is learning self-injection of insulin. While evaluating the woman's technique for self-injection, the nurse would recognize that the woman understood the instructions when she:
   a. washed her hands and put on a pair of clean gloves.
   b. shook the NPH insulin vial vigorously to fully mix the insulin.
   c. drew the NPH insulin into her syringe first.
   d. spread her skin taut and punctured the skin at a 90-degree angle.

10. When assessing a pregnant woman at 28 weeks of gestation who is diagnosed with mitral valve stenosis, the nurse must be alert for signs indicating cardiac decompensation. Signs of cardiac decompensation would include which of the following? (Circle all that apply.)
    a. Dry, hacking cough
    b. Increasing fatigue
    c. Wheezing with inspiration and expiration
    d. Bradycardia
    e. Progressive generalized edema
    f. Orthopnea with increasing dyspnea

11. A woman at 30 weeks of gestation with a class II cardiac disorder calls her primary health care provider's office and speaks to the nurse practitioner. She tells the nurse that she has been experiencing a frequent, moist cough for the past few days. In addition, she has been feeling more tired and is having difficulty completing her routine activities as a result of some difficulty with breathing. The nurse's best response would be:
    a. "Have someone bring you to the office so we can assess your cardiac status."
    b. "Try to get more rest during the day because this is a difficult time for your heart."
    c. "Take an extra diuretic tonight before you go to bed, since you may be developing some fluid in your lungs."
    d. "Ask your family to come over and do your housework for the next few days so you can rest."

12. A pregnant woman with a cardiac disorder will begin anticoagulant therapy to prevent clot formation. In preparing this woman for this treatment measure, the nurse would expect to teach the woman about self-administration of which of the following medications?
    a. Furosemide
    b. Propranolol
    c. Heparin
    d. Warfarin

13. At a previous antepartal visit, the nurse taught a pregnant woman diagnosed with a class II cardiac disorder about measures to use to lower her risk for cardiac decompensation. This woman would demonstrate need for further instruction if she tells the nurse she will use which of the following measures?
    a. Increase roughage in her diet
    b. Remain on bed rest, getting out of bed only to go to the bathroom
    c. Sleep 10 hours every night and take a short nap after meals
    d. Will call the nurse immediately if she experiences any pain or swelling in her legs

III. THINKING CRITICALLY

1. Mary is a 24-year-old woman with diabetes. When Mary informed her gynecologist that she and her husband are trying to get pregnant, she was referred to her endocrinologist for preconception counseling. Mary tells the nurse that she just cannot understand why this is necessary. "I have had diabetes since I was 12 years old, and I have not had many problems. All I want to do is get pregnant!" Discuss how the nurse should respond to Mary's comments.

2. Luann is a 25-year-old nulliparous woman in her first trimester of pregnancy (6th week of gestation). She has had type 1 diabetes since she was 15 years old. Recently, she has been experiencing some nausea and is eating less as a result. She took her usual dose of regular and NPH insulin before eating a very light breakfast of tea and a piece of toast. Just before her midmorning snack at work, she began to experience nervousness and weakness. She felt dizzy and became diaphoretic and pale.

    a. Identify the problem that Luann is experiencing. Indicate the basis for her symptoms.

    b. State the action that Luann should take.

3. Judy's first pregnancy has just been confirmed. She also has Type 1 diabetes.

    a. As a result of her high risk status, a variety of additional assessment measures are emphasized during her prenatal period to evaluate her status and that of her fetus. Identify these additional assessment measures and their relevance in a diabetic pregnancy.

    b. Discuss the stressors that might confront Judy and her family as a result of her status as a diabetic woman who is pregnant.

c. Indicate the activity and exercise recommendations that Judy should be given.

d. Outline the nursing interventions and health teaching for self-management in terms of nutrition, blood glucose monitoring, and insulin requirements at each stage of Judy's pregnancy.

Antepartum

Intrapartum

Postpartum

e. Judy expresses a desire to breastfeed her baby and wonders if this is a good idea for her and her baby. What should the nurse tell Judy about breastfeeding?

f. Discuss the birth control options that would be best for Judy and her partner.

4. Elena (2-1-0-0-1) is a 32-year-old Hispanic-American woman in week 28 of her pregnancy. She is obese. Her mother, who is 59, was recently diagnosed with type 2 diabetes. Elena's first pregnancy resulted in the birth of a 10 pound 6 ounce daughter who is now 2 years old. A 1-hour, 50-g glucose tolerance test last week revealed a glucose level of 152 mg/dL. A 3-hour glucose tolerance test was done yesterday with the following results: Fasting—108 mg/dL, 1 hr—195 mg/dL, 2 hr—170 mg/dL, 3 hr—140 mg/dL.

a. Identify the complication of pregnancy Elena is exhibiting. State the rationale for your answer.

b. List the risk factors for this health problem that are present in Elena's assessment data.

c. Describe the pathophysiology involved in creating Elena's problem.

d. Identify the maternal and fetal/neonatal risks and complications that are possible in this situation.

e. Outline the ongoing assessment measures necessitated by Elena's health problem.

f. State two nursing diagnoses for Elena and her fetus.

g. Describe how Elena should be advised to maintain euglycemia for the remainder of her pregnancy. Explain to her why euglycemia is so important.

h. Before discharge after the birth of her second daughter, Elena asks the nurse whether the health problem she experienced during this pregnancy will continue now that she has had her baby. She also wonders if it will happen with her next pregnancy because she wants to get pregnant again soon so she can "try for a son." Discuss the response the nurse should give to Elena's concerns.

5. Linda, age 26, had rheumatic fever as a child and subsequently developed mitral valve stenosis. She is presently 6 weeks pregnant. She is classified as class II according to the New York Heart Association functional classification of heart disease. This is the first pregnancy for Linda and her husband, Sam.

a. Discuss a recommended therapeutic plan for Linda that will reduce her risk for cardiac decompensation in terms of each of the following:

Rest/sleep/activity patterns

Prevention of infection

Nutrition

Bowel elimination

b. Identify physiologic and psychosocial factors that could increase the stress placed on Linda's heart during her pregnancy.

Physiologic factors   Psychosocial factors

   c. List the subjective symptoms that the nurse should teach Linda and her family to look for as indicators of possible cardiac decompensation.

   d. List the objective signs that could indicate that Linda is experiencing signs of cardiac decompensation and heart failure.

   e. Linda is admitted to the labor unit. Her cardiac condition is still classified as class II. Outline the nursing measures designed to assess Linda and promote optimum cardiac function during labor and birth.

   f. Linda should be observed carefully during the postpartum period because cardiac risk continues. Indicate the physiologic events after birth that place Linda at risk for cardiac decompensation.

   g. Discuss the measures the nurse can use to reduce the stress placed on Linda's heart during the postpartum period.

   h. Linda indicates that she wishes to breastfeed her infant. Describe the nurse's response.

   i. Identify the important factors to be considered when preparing Linda's discharge plan.

6. Allison is a pregnant woman with a cardiac disorder. As part of her medical regimen, her primary health care provider substituted subcutaneous heparin for the oral warfarin sodium (Coumadin) she had been taking before pregnancy.

   a. Allison states, "I cannot give myself a shot! Why can't I just take the medication orally?" Discuss how you would respond as to the purpose of heparin and why it must be used instead of the Coumadin she is used to taking.

   b. Indicate the information that the nurse should give Allison to ensure safe use of the heparin.

7. Jean is a primigravida at 4 weeks of gestation. She has been an epileptic for several years and her seizures have been controlled with phenytoin (Dilantin). Jean expresses concern regarding how her medication use will affect her pregnancy and her baby. She wants to stop taking the Dilantin. Describe the approach you would take in addressing Jean's concern and the course of action she is contemplating.

8. Imagine that you are an advanced practice nurse who specializes in the treatment of men and women who are alcohol and drug dependent. You have been asked to establish a treatment program specifically designed for pregnant women. Outline the approach you would take to ensure that the program you establish takes into consideration the unique characteristics and needs of women in general and pregnant women in particular who abuse alcohol and drugs.

12 High Risk Perinatal Care: Gestational Conditions

I. LEARNING KEY TERMS

FILL IN THE BLANKS: Insert the term that corresponds to each of the following descriptions of gestational conditions during pregnancy.

1. _____ A systolic BP greater than 140 mm Hg or a diastolic BP greater than 90 mm Hg recorded on two separate occasions at least 4 to 6 hours apart but within a maximum of a 1-week period.

2. _____ Development of hypertension after week 20 of pregnancy in a previously normotensive woman without proteinuria.

3. _____ Pregnancy-specific syndrome in which hypertension and proteinuria develop after 20 weeks of gestation in a woman who previously had neither condition. It is a vasospastic disorder usually categorized as mild or severe for purposes of management.

4. _____ Presence of a BP of 160/110 mm Hg or greater on 2 or more occasions at least 6 hours apart and 5 g or more of protein in a 24-hour urine specimen. Other signs and symptoms reflective of multisystem organ involvement are also present.

5. _____ Onset of seizure activity or coma in the woman with preeclampsia, with no history of preexisting pathology, that can result in seizure activity.

6. _____ Hypertension present before pregnancy or develops before 20 weeks of gestation.

7. _____ Process that diminishes the diameter of blood vessels, which results in poor tissue perfusion in organ systems, increased peripheral resistance and blood pressure, and increased cellular permeability. Protein and fluid loss occurs and plasma volume is reduced.

8. _____ Laboratory diagnosis for a variant of severe preeclampsia that involves hepatic dysfunction; it is characterized by _____, _____, and _____.

9. _____ Protein concentration of 30 mg/dL or more ($\geq 1+$ with dipstick) in at least two random urine specimens collected at least 6 hours apart. In a 24-hour urine specimen, it is a concentration of ≥ 300 mg/24 hours.

10. _____ Increased amount of urine produced to reduce fluid retention.

11. _____ Excessive vomiting during pregnancy that leads to significant weight loss along with dehydration, electrolyte imbalance, nutritional deficiency, and ketonuria.

12. _____ Pregnancy that ends as a result of natural causes before 20 weeks of gestation or less than 500 g birthweight. It is termed _____ if it occurs before 12 weeks of gestation and _____ if it occurs between 12 and 20 weeks of gestation.

13. _____ Pregnancy in which the fetus has died but the products of conception are retained in utero for up to several weeks.

14. _____ Three or more consecutive pregnancy losses before 20 weeks of gestation.

15. _____ Passive and painless dilation of the cervix during the second trimester.

16. _____ Procedure that involves placement of a suture around the cervix beneath the mucosa to constrict the internal os of the cervix.

17. _____ Pregnancy in which the fertilized ovum is implanted outside the uterine cavity, most often in the ampulla of the uterine tube.

18. _____ Group of pregnancy-related trophoblastic proliferative disorders without a viable fetus that are caused by abnormal fertilization. It includes _____, _____, and _____.

19. _____ Disorder that results when an egg without an active nucleus has been fertilized.

20. _____ Disorder that results when two sperm fertilize an apparently normal ovum.

21. _____ Implantation of the placenta in the lower uterine segment totally covering the internal cervical os.

22. _____ Implantation of the placenta in the lower uterine segment without reaching the os.

23. _____ Detachment of part or all of the placenta from its implantation site.

24. _____ Condition in which the fetal vessels lie over the cervical os. _____ Variation of vasa previa in which the cord vessels begin to branch at the membranes and then course into the placenta. _____ A second variation of vasa previa in which the placenta is divided into two or more lobes rather than remaining as a single mass. Fetal vessels run between the lobes and collect at the periphery, eventually uniting to form the vessels of the umbilical cord.

25. _____ Marginal insertion of the cord into the placenta, which also increases the risk for fetal hemorrhage.

26. _____ Pathologic form of clotting that is diffuse and consumes large amounts of clotting factors, causing widespread external or internal bleeding or both.

27. _____ Persistent presence of bacteria within the urinary tract of women who have no symptoms.

28. _____ Bladder infection characterized by dysuria, urgency, and frequency, along with lower abdominal or suprapubic pain.

29. _____ Renal infection that is a common serious medical complication of pregnancy and the second most common nondelivery reason for hospitalization.

30. _____ The most common nonobstetric surgical emergency during pregnancy.

31. _____ Presence of gallstones in the gallbladder.

32. _____ Inflammation of the gallbladder.

II. REVEWING KEY CONCEPTS

1. State the principles you would follow to ensure the accuracy of BP measurement during pregnancy.

2. Describe the assessment technique used to determine whether the following findings are present in women with preeclampsia. (Note: You may wish to review this information in a physical assessment textbook for a complete explanation of each technique.)

   a. Hyperreflexia and ankle clonus

   b. Proteinuria

   c. Pitting edema

MATCHING: Match the client description with the appropriate diagnosis.

3. _____ At 30 weeks of gestation, a woman's BP is consistently above 140/90; her latest urinalysis indicated a protein level of 2+ on dipstick; biceps and patellar reflexes are 2+.

4. _____ At 24 weeks of gestation, a normotensive woman's BP rose from a pre-pregnant baseline of 118/70 to 148/92. No other problematic signs and symptoms including proteinuria were noted.

5. _____ A 34-year-old pregnant woman has had a consistently high BP ranging from 148/92 to 160/98 since she was 28 years old. Her weight gain has followed normal patterns, and urinalysis remains normal as well.

6. _____ At 32 weeks of gestation, a woman, with hypertension since 28 weeks, hyperactive DTRs with clonus, and proteinuria of 4+, has a convulsion.

7. _____ A pregnant woman has been hypertensive since her twenty-fourth week of pregnancy. Urinalysis indicates a protein content of 3+. Further testing reveals a platelet count of 95,000 and elevated AST and ALT levels; she has begun to experience nausea with some vomiting and epigastric pain.

a. Eclampsia

b. Chronic hypertension

c. Gestational hypertension

d. HELLP syndrome

e. Preeclampsia

MATCHING: Match the medication description with the appropriate medication.

8. _____ Drug of choice in the prevention and treatment of seizure activity (eclampsia) caused by severe preeclampsia.

9. _____ Intravenous antihypertensive agent for the treatment of hypertension that occurs with severe preeclampsia.

10. _____ Antihypertensive agent of choice for the treatment of chronic hypertension during pregnancy.

11. _____ Antiemetic medication that is recommended to treat hyperemesis gravidarum.

12. _____ Synthetic prostaglandin E$_1$ analog administered orally or vaginally as part of the medical management of a miscarriage.

13. _____ Antimetabolite and folic acid antagonist that is used to destroy rapidly dividing cells; it is used for the medical management of an unruptured ectopic pregnancy.

14. _____ Prostaglandin derivative that can be administered intramuscularly to contract the uterus and treat excessive bleeding following evacuating the products of conception when a miscarriage has occurred.

15. _____ Antihypertensive medication that can be used in the postpartum period to treat persistent hypertension in women diagnosed with severe gestational hypertension or severe preeclampsia.

a. pyridoxine

b. methotrexate

c. magnesium sulfate

d. methyldopa

e. nifedipine

f. carboprost tromethamine

g. hydralazine

h. misoprostol

16. When measuring the BP to ensure consistency and to facilitate early detection of BP changes consistent with gestational hypertension, the nurse should:
    a. place the woman in a supine position.
    b. allow the woman to rest for at least 15 minutes before measuring her BP.
    c. use the same arm for each BP measurement.
    d. use a proper sized cuff that covers at least 50% of her upper arm.

17. When caring for a woman with mild preeclampsia, it is critical that during assessment the nurse is alert for signs of progress to severe preeclampsia. Progress to severe preeclampsia would be indicated by which one of the following assessment findings?
    a. Proteinuria of 3+ or greater
    b. Platelet level of 200,000/mm³
    c. Deep tendon reflexes 2+, ankle clonus is absent
    d. BP of 154/94 and 156/100, 6 hours apart

18. A woman's preeclampsia has advanced to the severe stage. She is admitted to the hospital and her primary health care provider has ordered an infusion of magnesium sulfate be started. In fulfilling this order the nurse would implement which of the following? (Circle all that apply.)
    a. Prepare a loading dose of 2 g of magnesium sulfate in 200 ml of 5% glucose in water to be given over 15 minutes.
    b. Prepare the maintenance solution by mixing 40 g of magnesium sulfate in 1000 ml of lactated Ringer's solution.
    c. Monitor maternal vital signs, fetal heart rate (FHR) patterns, and uterine contractions every 2 hours.
    d. Expect the maintenance dose to be approximately 2 g/hour.
    e. Report a respiratory rate of 14 breaths or less per minute to the primary health care provider immediately.
    f. Recognize that urinary output should be at least 25–30 ml per hour.

19. The primary expected outcome for care associated with the administration of magnesium sulfate would be met if the woman exhibits which of the following?
    a. Exhibits a decrease in both systolic and diastolic BP
    b. Experiences no seizures
    c. States that she feels more relaxed and calm
    d. Urinates more frequently, resulting in a decrease in pathologic edema

20. A woman has been diagnosed with mild preeclampsia and will be treated at home. The nurse, in teaching this woman about her treatment regimen for mild preeclampsia, would tell her to do which of the following? (Circle all that apply.)
    a. Check her respirations before and after taking her oral dose of magnesium sulfate

b. Place a dipstick into a clean-catch sample of her urine to test for protein
    c. Reduce her fluid intake to four to five 8-ounce glasses each day
    d. Do gentle exercises such as hand and feet circles and gently tensing and relaxing arm and leg muscles
    e. Avoid excessively salty foods
    f. Maintain strict bed rest in a quiet dimly lighted room with minimal stimuli

21. A woman has just been admitted with a diagnosis of hyperemesis gravidarum. She has been unable to retain any oral intake and as a result has lost weight and is exhibiting signs of dehydration with electrolyte imbalance and acetonuria. The care management of this woman would include which of the following?
    a. Administering labetalol to control nausea and vomiting
    b. Assessing the woman's urine for ketones
    c. Avoiding oral hygiene until the woman is able to tolerate oral fluids
    d. Providing small frequent meals consisting of bland foods and warm fluids together once the woman begins to respond to treatment

22. A primigravida at 10 weeks of gestation reports slight vaginal spotting without passage of tissue and mild uterine cramping. When examined, no cervical dilation is noted. The nurse caring for this woman would:
    a. anticipate that the woman will be sent home and placed on bed rest with instructions to avoid stress and orgasm.
    b. prepare the woman for a dilation and curettage.
    c. inform the woman that frequent blood tests will be required to check the level of estrogen.
    d. tell the woman that the doctor will most likely perform a cerclage to help her maintain her pregnancy.

23. A woman is admitted through the emergency room with a medical diagnosis of ruptured ectopic pregnancy. The primary nursing diagnosis at this time would be:
    a. acute pain related to irritation of the peritoneum with blood.
    b. risk for infection related to tissue trauma.
    c. deficient fluid volume related to blood loss associated with rupture of the uterine tube.
    d. anticipatory grieving related to unexpected pregnancy outcome.

24. A woman diagnosed with an ectopic pregnancy is given an intramuscular injection of methotrexate. The nurse would tell the woman which of the following?
    a. Methotrexate is an analgesic that will relieve the dull abdominal pain she is experiencing.

b. She should avoid alcohol until her primary care provider tells her the treatment is complete.

c. Follow-up blood tests will be required every other month for 6 months after the injection of the methotrexate.

d. She should continue to take her prenatal vitamin and folic acid to enhance healing.

25. A pregnant woman at 32 weeks of gestation comes to the emergency room because she has begun to experience bright red vaginal bleeding. She reports that she is experiencing no pain. The admission nurse suspects:

a. abruptio placentae.

b. disseminated intravascular coagulation.

c. placenta previa.

d. preterm labor.

26. A pregnant woman, at 38 weeks of gestation diagnosed with marginal placenta previa, has just given birth to a healthy newborn male. The nurse recognizes that the immediate focus for the care of this woman would be:

a. preventing hemorrhage.

b. relieving pain.

c. preventing infection.

d. fostering attachment of the woman with her new son.

III. THINKING CRITICALLY

1. Jean (1-0-0-0-0) is at 30 weeks of gestation and has been diagnosed with mild preeclampsia. The treatment plan includes home care with limited activity consisting of bed rest with bathroom privileges and out of bed twice a day for meals, appropriate nutrition, and stress reduction. She and her husband are very anxious about the diagnosis and are also concerned about how they will manage the care of their active 3-year-old adopted daughter, Anne.

a. What factors could be present in Jean's history that would increase her risk for developing preeclampsia?

b. Indicate the clinical manifestations that would be present to indicate this diagnosis.

c. Describe how you would help this couple organize their home care routine.

d. Specify what you would teach them with regard to assessment of Jean's status in terms of each of the following:

BP

Protein in urine

Fetal well-being

Signs of a worsening condition

e. Describe the instructions you would give Jean regarding her nutrient and fluid intake.

f. Discuss the measures Jean can use to cope with the boredom and alteration in circulation and muscle tone that accompany bed rest.

g. Limited activity can lead to a nursing diagnosis of constipation related to changes in bowel function associated with pregnancy and limited activity. Cite two measures that Jean can use to enhance bowel elimination and prevent constipation.

2. Ellen, a pregnant woman at 37 weeks of gestation, is admitted to the hospital with a diagnosis of severe preeclampsia.

a. Indicate the signs and symptoms that would be present to indicate this diagnosis.

b. Specify the precautionary measures that should be taken to protect Ellen and her fetus from injury.

c. Ellen's physician orders magnesium sulfate to be infused at 4 g in 20 minutes as a loading dose, and then a maintenance intravenous infusion of 2 g/hr.

   • Identify the guidelines that must be followed when preparing and administering the magnesium sulfate infusion.

   • Explain the expected therapeutic effect of magnesium sulfate to Ellen and her family.

d. List the maternal-fetal assessments that should be accomplished on a regular basis during the infusion of magnesium sulfate.

   • Identify the progressive signs of magnesium sulfate toxicity.

   • State the interventions that must be instituted immediately if magnesium sulfate toxicity occurs.

e. Despite all prevention efforts, Ellen has a convulsion.

- Specify the nursing measures that should be implemented at the onset of the convulsion and immediately afterward.

- List the problems that can occur as a result of the convulsion that Ellen experienced.

f. Ellen successfully gave birth vaginally despite her high risk status. Describe Ellen's care management during the first 48 hours of her postpartum recovery period.

3. Marie, an 18-year-old obese primigravida at 9 weeks of gestation, is diagnosed with hyperemesis gravidarum. She is unmarried and lives at home with her parents. Marie is admitted to the high risk antepartal unit. During the admission interview, Marie confides to the nurse that her parents have been very unhappy about her pregnancy. She now is worried that she may have made the wrong decision to continue with her pregnancy and raise her baby as a single parent.

a. Identify the etiologic factors that may have contributed to Marie's current health problem.

b. List the physiologic and psychologic factors that the nurse should be alert for when assessing Marie upon her admission.

c. State one nursing diagnosis related to Marie's current health status.

d. Outline the nursing care measures appropriate for Marie while hospitalized.

e. Once stabilized, Marie is discharged to home care. She is able to tolerate oral food and fluid intake. Explain the important care measures that the nurse should discuss with Marie and her family before she goes home.

4. Andrea is admitted to the hospital, where a diagnosis of acute ruptured ectopic pregnancy in her fallopian tube is made.

a. State the risk factors associated with ectopic pregnancy.

b. Describe the findings that were most likely experienced and exhibited by Andrea as her ectopic pregnancy progressed and then ruptured.

c. Identify the other health care problems that share the same or similar clinical manifestations as ectopic pregnancy.

d. State the major care management problem at this time. Support your answer.

e. Outline the nursing measures Andrea will require during the preoperative and postoperative period.

5. Janet is 10 weeks pregnant. She comes to the clinic and states that she has been experiencing slight bleeding with mild cramping for about 4 hours. No tissue has been passed and pelvic examination reveals that the cervical os is closed.

a. Indicate the most likely basis for Janet's signs and symptoms.

b. Outline the expected care management of Janet's problem.

6. Denise, a primigravida, calls the clinic. She is crying while she tells the nurse that she has noted "a lot of bleeding" and that she is sure she is losing her baby.

a. Write several questions the nurse should ask Denise to obtain a more definitive picture of the bleeding she is experiencing.

b. Based on the data collected, Denise is admitted to the hospital for further evaluation. A medical diagnosis of incomplete abortion is made. Describe the assessment findings that would indicate the diagnosis of incomplete abortion.

c. State the nursing diagnosis that would take priority at this time.

d. Outline the nursing measures that would be appropriate for the priority nursing diagnosis you identified and for the expected medical management of Denise's health problem.

e. Specify the instructions that Denise should receive before her discharge from the hospital.

f. List the nursing measures appropriate for the following nursing diagnosis: Anticipatory grieving related to unexpected outcome of pregnancy.

7. Mary has been diagnosed with hydatidiform mole (complete).

a. Identify the typical signs and symptoms Mary would most likely exhibit to establish this diagnosis.

b. Specify the posttreatment instructions that the nurse must stress when discussing follow-up management with Mary.

c. Name the major concern associated with complete hydatidiform mole and indicate the signs that would indicate that it is occurring.

8. Two pregnant women are admitted to the labor unit with vaginal bleeding. Sara is at 29 weeks of gestation and is diagnosed with marginal placenta previa. Jane is at 34 weeks of gestation and is diagnosed with a moderate (grade II) premature separation of the placenta (abruptio placentae).

a. Compare the clinical picture each of these women is likely to exhibit during assessment.

        Sara   Jane

b. Identify one priority nursing diagnosis for both Sara and Jane.

c. Contrast the care management approach required by each of the women as it relates to their diagnosis and the typical medical management.

        Sara   Jane

d. Indicate the considerations that must be given top priority following birth for each of these women.

        Sara   Jane

9. Trauma continues to be a common complication during pregnancy that may require obstetric critical care.

    a. Discuss the significance of this complication using statistical data to describe the scope of the problem in terms of incidence, timing during pregnancy, and forms of trauma.

    b. Indicate the effects trauma can have on pregnancy.

    c. Describe the potential impact of trauma on the fetus.

    d. Identify the priorities of care for the pregnant woman following trauma.

    e. Outline the major components of the assessment and care of a pregnant woman who has experienced trauma.

       Primary survey

       Secondary survey

    f. Explain how cardiopulmonary resuscitation (CPR) should be adapted for a pregnant woman.

13 Labor and Birth Processes

I. LEARNING KEY TERMS

FILL IN THE BLANKS: Insert the term that corresponds to each of the following descriptions.

1. _____, _____, _____, _____, and _____ The five factors or "Ps" of labor and birth.

2. _____ Membrane-filled spaces that are located where the membranous sutures that unite the bones in the fetal/neonatal skull intersect.

3. _____ Slight overlapping of the bones of the fetal skull that occurs during childbirth; it permits the skull to adapt to the various pelvic diameters.

4. _____ Part of the fetus that enters the pelvic inlet first. The three main types are _____ (head first), _____ (buttocks first), and _____.

5. _____ Part of the fetal body first felt by the examining finger during a vaginal examination. The three types are _____, _____, and _____.

6. _____ Relationship of the long axis (spine) of the fetus to the long axis (spine) of the mother. There are two types: _____, when the spines are parallel to each other, and _____, when the spines are at right angles or diagonal to each other.

7. _____ Relationship of the fetal body parts to one another. The most common type is one of general _____.

8. _____ Largest transverse diameter of the fetal skull. _____ Smallest anteroposterior diameter of the fetal skull to enter the maternal pelvis when the fetal head is in complete flexion.

9. _____ Relationship of a reference point on the fetal presenting part to the four quadrants of the maternal pelvis.

10. _____ Term that indicates that the largest transverse diameter of the presenting part has passed through the maternal pelvic brim or inlet into the true pelvis, reaching the level of the ischial spines.

11. _____ Relationship of the presenting part of the fetus to an imaginary line drawn between the maternal ischial spines; this is a measure of the degree of fetal descent through the birth canal.

12. _____ and _____ The two components of the maternal passageway or birth canal.

13. _____ Shortening and thinning of the cervix during the first stage of labor; it is expressed as a percentage.

14. _____ Enlargement or widening of the cervical opening (os) and the cervical canal, which occurs once labor has begun; degree of progress is expressed in centimeters (cm) from less than 1 cm to 10 cm.

15. _____ Descent of the fetal presenting part into the true pelvis approximately 2 weeks before term for the primigravida and after uterine contractions are established and true labor is in progress for the multipara.

16. _____ Primary powers of labor.

17. _____ Secondary powers of labor.

18. _____ Brownish or blood-tinged cervical mucus representing the passage of the mucous plug as the cervix ripens in preparation for labor.

19. _____ The seven turns and adjustments of the fetal head, to facilitate passage through the birth canal. In a vertex presentation these turns and adjustments include _____, _____, _____, _____, _____, _____, and finally birth by _____.

20. _____ Pushing method during the second stage of labor characterized by a closed glottis with prolonged bearing down.

21. _____ Process of moving the fetus, placenta, and membranes out of the uterus and through the birth canal.

22. _____ Maternal urge to bear down that occurs when the fetal presenting part reaches the perineal floor and stretching of the cervix and vagina occur; oxytocin is released.

23. The first stage of labor is considered to last from the onset of _____ to full _____ of the cervix. It is divided into three phases, namely _____, _____, and _____.

24. The second stage of labor lasts from the time the cervix is fully _____ to the _____.

25. The third stage of labor lasts from the _____ until the _____ is delivered.

26. The fourth stage of labor is the period of immediate _____ when _____ is reestablished.

27. _____, _____, _____, and _____ The four factors that affect fetal circulation during labor.

28. _____ Morphine-like chemicals produced naturally in the body, which raise the pain threshold and produce sedation.

II. REVIEWING KEY CONCEPTS

1. Describe how the five factors (the five Ps) affect the process of labor and birth.

2. A vaginal examination during labor reveals the following information: LOA, −1, 75%, 3 cm. An accurate interpretation of this data would include which of the following? (Circle all that apply.)
   a. Attitude: flexed
   b. Station: 3 cm below the ischial spines
   c. Presentation: cephalic
   d. Lie: longitudinal
   e. Effacement: 75% complete
   f. Dilation: 9 cm more to reach full dilation

3. Changes occur as a woman progresses through labor. Which of the following maternal adaptations would be expected during labor? (Circle all that apply.)
   a. Increase in both systolic and diastolic blood pressure during uterine contractions in the first stage of labor
   b. Decrease in white blood cell count
   c. Slight increase in heart rate during the first and second stages of labor
   d. Decrease in gastric motility leading to nausea and vomiting during the first stage of labor
   e. Hypoglycemia
   f. Proteinuria up to 1+

4. A nurse is instructing a group of primigravid women about the onset of labor. Which of the following signs could the women observe preceding the onset of their labors? (Circle all that apply.)
   a. Urinary frequency
   b. Weight gain of 2 kg
   c. Quickening
   d. Energy surge
   e. Bloody show
   f. Shortness of breath

III. THINKING CRITICALLY

1. As part of their care of the laboring woman, nurses perform vaginal examinations and interpret the results. State the meaning of each of the following vaginal examination findings.

Exam I	Exam II	Exam III	Exam IV
ROP	RMA	LST	OA
−1	0	+1	+3
50%	25%	75%	100%
3 cm	2 cm	6 cm	10 cm

2. Brooke is a primigravida at 36 weeks of gestation. During a prenatal visit at 34 weeks of gestation, she asks you the following questions regarding her approaching labor. Describe how you would respond.

   a. "What gets labor to start?"

   b. "Are there things I should watch for that would tell me my labor is getting closer to starting?"

   c. "My friend just had a baby and she told me the nurses kept helping her change her position and even encouraged her to walk! Isn't that dangerous for the baby and painful for the mom?"

   d. "How will my baby know to start breathing after it is born?"

14 Pain Management

I. LEARNING KEY TERMS

FILL IN THE BLANKS: Insert the term that corresponds to each of the following descriptions related to childbirth discomfort and its management.

1. _____ Decreased blood flow to the uterus during a contraction leading to an oxygen deficit.

2. _____ Pain that predominates during the first stage of labor; it results from cervical changes, distention of the lower uterine segment, and uterine ischemia.

3. _____ Pain that predominates during the second stage of labor; it results from stretching and distention of perineal tissues and the pelvic floor to allow passage of the fetus, from distention and traction on the peritoneum and utero-cervical supports during contractions, and from lacerations of soft tissues.

4. _____ Pain in labor and birth that originates in the uterus and radiates to the abdominal wall, lumbosacral area of the back, iliac crests, gluteal area, and down the thighs.

5. _____ Level of pain a person is willing to endure.

6. _____ Theory of pain based on the premise that pain sensations travel along sensory nerve pathways to the brain, but only a limited number of sensations or messages can travel through these nerve pathways at one time; by using distraction techniques (e.g., massage, music, focal points, imagery) the capacity of nerve pathways to transmit pain is reduced or completely blocked.

7. _____ Endogenous opioids secreted by the pituitary gland that act on the central and peripheral nervous systems to reduce pain; their level increases during pregnancy and birth, thereby enhancing a woman's ability to tolerate acute pain and reducing anxiety.

8. _____ Childbirth method, also known as the natural childbirth method or childbirth without fear, which is based on the theory that childbirth pain is socially conditioned and caused by a fear-tension-pain syndrome.

9. _____ Childbirth method, also known as the psychoprophylactic method, that conditions women to respond to uterine contractions with relaxation techniques and breathing patterns.

10. _____ Childbirth method, also known as husband-coached childbirth, that emphasizes working in harmony with the body using breath control, abdominal breathing, and general body relaxation; it stresses environmental factors such as darkness, solitude, and quiet to make childbirth a more natural experience.

11. _____ Childbirth method in which pregnant women (couples) learn how the birthing muscles work when the woman is in a state of relaxation; the woman will be relaxed, in control, and experience surges (contractions) while calm and relaxed, free of fear and tension.

12. _____ Childbirth method based on the belief that childbirth is not a medical event but a profound rite of passage; parents are taught the power of birthing-in awareness while mentors create a safe, nurturing class experience and assist parents to find their personal strength and wisdom and to develop a pain-coping mindset.

13. _____ Relaxed deep breath in through the nose and out through the mouth that begins each breathing pattern and ends each contraction.

14. _____ Paced breathing technique during which a woman breathes at approximately 6 to 8 breaths per minute (half the normal breathing rate).

15. _____ Paced breathing technique during which a woman breathes at approximately 32 to 40 breaths per minute (twice the normal breathing rate).

16. _____ Paced breathing technique during which a woman breathes at approximately 32 to 40 breaths per minute interspersed with blowing out of air in a ratio of 3:1 or 4:1; this technique enhances concentration.

17. _____ Undesirable reaction to a rapid-paced breathing pattern characterized by rapid deep respirations that lead to signs of respiratory alkalosis such as lightheadedness, dizziness, tingling of the fingers, or circumoral numbness. Breathing into a paper bag held tightly around the mouth will help to reestablish normal breathing.

18. _____ Light massage (stroking) of the abdomen or other body part in rhythm with breathing during contractions.

19. _____ Steady pressure against the sacrum using the fist or heel of the hand or a firm object to help the woman cope with the sensations of internal pressure and pain in the lower back.

20. _____ Bathing, showering, or whirlpool baths using warm water to promote comfort and relaxation during labor, stimulate the release of endorphin, close the gate on pain, promote circulation and oxygenation, and help to soften the perineum.

21. _____ Method that involves placement of two pairs of electrodes on either side of the woman's thoracic and sacral spine to provide continuous low-intensity electrical impulses that can be increased during a contraction, thereby stimulating the release of endorphins that provide relief from discomfort.

22. _____ Application of pressure, heat, or cold over the skin of specific points on the body termed tsubos, which have increased density of neuroreceptors and increased electrical conductivity.

23. _____ Insertion of fine needles into specific areas of the body to restore the flow of qi (energy) and decrease pain, which is thought to be obstructing the flow of energy.

24. _____ Relaxation technique that can be used for labor that is based on the theory that, if a person can recognize physical signals, certain internal physiologic events can be changed (i.e., whatever signs the woman has that are associated with her pain).

25. _____ Use of oils distilled from plants, flowers, herbs, and trees to promote health and to treat and balance the mind, body, and spirit.

26. _____ Injection of small amounts of sterile water by using a fine-gauge needle into four locations on the lower back to relieve back pain; effectiveness of this method may be related to the mechanism of counterirritation, gate control, or an increase in the level of endorphins.

27. _____ Technique based on the concept of energy fields within the body called prana; it involves the laying-on of hands by a specially trained person to redirect energy fields associated with pain.

II. REVIEWING KEY CONCEPTS

1. Describe the factors that could influence the following nursing diagnosis identified for a woman in labor: Acute pain related to the processes involved in labor and birth.

2. Explain the theoretic basis for using techniques such as massage, stroking, music, and imagery to reduce the sensation of pain during childbirth.

MATCHING: Match the description with the appropriate pharmacologic method for discomfort management during childbirth.

3. _____ Abolition of pain perception by interrupting nerve impulses going to the brain. Loss of sensation (partial or complete) and sometimes loss of consciousness occurs.

4. _____ Method used to repair a tear or hole in the dura mater around the spinal cord as a result of spinal anesthesia; the goal is to prevent or treat postdural puncture headaches (PDPH).

5. _____ Single-injection, subarachnoid anesthesia useful for pain control during birth but not for labor; it is often used for cesarean birth.

6. _____ Systemic analgesic such as nalbuphine and butorphanol that relieves pain without causing significant maternal or neonatal respiratory depression and is less likely to cause nausea and vomiting.

7. _____ Provides rapid perineal anesthesia for performing and repairing an episiotomy or lacerations.

8. _____ Gas mixed with oxygen to provide analgesia during the first and second stages of labor.

9. _____ Medication such as phenothiazines and benzodiazepines that can be used to relieve anxiety, to induce sleep, to augment the effectiveness of analgesics, and to reduce nausea and vomiting.

10. _____ Technique that can be used to block pain transmission without compromising motor ability because an opioid with or without a local anesthetic is injected intrathecally and into the peridural space; with this technique women are able to walk if they choose to do so.

11. _____ Drug that promptly reverses the effects of opioids, including maternal and neonatal CNS depression, especially respiratory depression.

12. _____ Use of a medication such as an opioid analgesic that is administered IM or IV for pain relief during labor.

13. _____ Alleviation of pain sensation or raising of the pain threshold without loss of consciousness.

14. _____ Relief from pain of uterine contractions and birth by injecting a local anesthetic agent, an opioid, or both into the peridural space.

15. _____ Anesthetic that relieves pain in the lower vagina, vulva, and perineum, making it useful if an episiotomy is to be performed or forceps- or vacuum-assistance is required to facilitate birth.

16. _____ Systemic analgesic such as meperidine or fentanyl that relieves pain and creates a feeling of well-being but can also result in respiratory depression (maternal and neonate), nausea, and vomiting.

a. Opioid agonist-antagonist analgesic

b. Anesthesia

c. Analgesia

d. Combined spinal-epidural analgesic

e. Epidural analgesia/anesthesia (block)

f. Autologous epidural blood patch

g. Local infiltration anesthesia

h. Spinal anesthesia (block)

i. Opioid antagonist

j. Nitrous oxide

k. Pudendal nerve block

l. Systemic analgesic

m. Sedative

n. Opioid agonist analgesic

17. Compare each of the following commonly used methods for nerve block analgesia and anesthesia. Indicate the effects, timing of administration, advantages and disadvantages, and nursing care management for each method in your comparison.

    Local perineal infiltration anesthesia

    Spinal anesthesia (block)

    Epidural anesthesia/analgesia (block)

    Combined spinal-epidural analgesia

    Epidural and intrathecal opioids

18. Systemic analgesics cross the placenta and affect the fetus.

    a. List three factors that influence the effect systemic analgesics have on the fetus.

    b. Identify the fetal effects of systemic analgesics.

19. Explain why the intravenous route is preferred to the intramuscular route for the administration of systemic analgesics during labor.

20. In her birth plan, a woman requests that she be allowed to use the new whirlpool bath during labor. When implementing this woman's request the nurse would do which of the following?
    a. Assist the woman to maintain a reclining position when in the tub.
    b. Tell the woman she will need to leave the tub as soon as her membranes rupture.
    c. Limit her to no longer than 1 hour in the tub.
    d. Wait to initiate the bath until the woman has entered the active phase of her labor.

21. The use of benzodiazepines can potentiate the action of analgesics and reduce nausea. When preparing to administer a benzodiazepine to a laboring woman, the nurse could expect to give which one of the following medications?
    a. diazepam (Valium)
    b. promethazine (Phenergan)
    c. butorphanol tartrate (Stadol)
    d. fentanyl (Sublimaze)

22. The nurse has just administered metoclopramide (Reglan) to a woman in labor. Which of the following would be an expected effect of this medication?
    a. Analgesia
    b. Nausea and vomiting
    c. Potentiation of opioid analgesics
    d. Respiratory depression

23. The doctor has ordered meperidine (Demerol) 25 mg IV q2-3 hr prn for pain associated with labor. In fulfilling this order, the nurse should consider which of the following?
    a. Abstinence syndrome will occur if the woman is opioid-dependent.
    b. Dosage of the analgesic is too high for IV administration, necessitating a new order.
    c. Maternal respiratory depression is more likely to occur when compared with morphine.
    d. The newborn should be observed for respiratory depression if birth occurs within 4 hours of the dose.

24. Following administration of fentanyl (Sublimaze) IV for labor pain, a woman's labor progresses more rapidly than expected. The physician orders that a stat dose of naloxone (Narcan) 1 mg be administered intravenously to the woman to reverse respiratory depression in the newborn after its birth. In fulfilling this order the nurse would:
    a. question the route because this medication should be administered orally.
    b. recognize that the dose is too low.
    c. monitor maternal condition for possible side effects.
    d. observe the woman for bradycardia and lethargy.

25. An anesthesiologist is preparing to begin a continuous epidural block using a combination local anesthetic and opioid analgesic as a pain relief measure for a laboring woman. Nursing measures related to this type of nerve block would include which of the following? (Circle all that apply.)
    a. Assist the woman into a modified Sims position or upright position with back curved for administration of the block.
    b. Alternate her position from side to side every hour.
    c. Assess the woman for headaches because they commonly occur in the postpartum period if an epidural is used for labor.
    d. Assist the woman to urinate every 2 hours during labor to prevent bladder distention.
    e. Prepare the woman for use of forceps- or vacuum-assisted birth because she will be unable to bear down.
    f. Assess blood pressure frequently because severe hypotension can occur.

26. Administering an opioid antagonist to a woman who is opioid dependent will result in the opioid abstinence syndrome. The nurse would recognize which of the following clinical manifestations as evidence that this syndrome is occurring? (Circle all that apply.)
    a. Yawning
    b. Piloerection
    c. Anorexia
    d. Coughing
    e. Dry skin, eyes, and nose
    f. Miosis

27. After induction of a spinal block in preparation for an elective cesarean birth, a woman's blood pressure decreases from 124/76 to 96/60. The nurse's initial action would be to do which of the following?
    a. Administer a vasopressor intravenously to raise the blood pressure.
    b. Change the woman's position from supine to lateral.
    c. Begin to administer oxygen by mask at 10 to 12 L/min.
    d. Notify the woman's health care provider.

III. THINKING CRITICALLY

1. A nurse working with a group of expectant fathers is asked if there really is "a physical reason for all the pain women say they feel when they are in labor." Describe the response that this nurse should give.

2. On admission to the labor unit in the latent phase of labor, Mr. and Mrs. T. (2-0-0-1-0) tell you that they are so glad they took Lamaze classes and did so much reading about childbirth. "We will not need any medication now that we know what to do. But most importantly our baby will be safe." Describe how you would respond if you were their primary nurse for childbirth.

3. Imagine you are the nurse manager of a labor and birth unit. Major renovations are being planned for your unit and your input is required. You and your staff nurses believe that water therapy, including the use of showers and whirlpool baths, is a beneficial nonpharmacologic method to relieve pain and discomfort and to enhance the progress of labor. Discuss the rationale you would use to convince planners that installation of a shower and a whirlpool bath into each birthing room is cost-effective.

4. Tara has been in labor for 4 hours. Her blood pressure had been stable, averaging 130/80 when assessed between contractions, and the FHR pattern consistently exhibited criteria of a reassuring pattern. A lumbar epidural block was initiated. Shortly afterward, during assessment of maternal vital signs and FHR, Tara's blood pressure decreased to 102/60 and the FHR pattern began to exhibit a decrease in rate and variability.

   a. State what Tara is experiencing. Support your answer and explain the physiologic basis for what is happening to Tara.

   b. List the immediate nursing actions.

5. Moira, a primigravida, has elected a continuous epidural block as her pharmacologic method of choice during childbirth.

   a. Identify the assessment procedures that should be used to determine Moira's readiness for the initiation of the epidural block.

   b. Describe the preparation methods that should be implemented.

   c. Describe two positions you could help Moira to assume for the induction of the epidural block.

   d. Outline the nursing care management interventions recommended while Moira is receiving the anesthesia to ensure her well-being and that of her fetus.

Fetal Assessment During Labor

I. LEARNING KEY TERMS

FILL IN THE BLANKS: Insert the term that corresponds to each of the following descriptions related to fetal assessment.

1. _____ Occurrence of five or more uterine contractions in 10 minutes averaged over a 30-minute window.

2. _____ Listening to fetal heart sounds at periodic intervals to assess fetal heart rate.

3. _____ Instrument used to assess the fetal heart rate through the transmission of ultrahigh-frequency sound waves reflecting movement of the fetal heart and the conversion of these sounds into an electronic signal that can be counted.

4. _____ Method used to continuously assess the FHR pattern. _____ _____ and _____ are the two modes used to accomplish this method of assessment.

5. _____ Device used in external monitoring to assess fetal heart rate and pattern.

6. _____ Device used in external monitoring to measure uterine activity transabdominally; it can determine the frequency, regularity, and approximate duration of uterine contractions but not their intensity.

7. _____ Device used in internal monitoring to obtain a continuous assessment of the fetal heart rate and pattern.

8. _____ Device used in internal monitoring to measure the frequency, duration, and intensity of uterine contractions as well as uterine resting tone.

9. _____ The interventions initiated when an abnormal FHR pattern is detected; these interventions involve providing supplemental oxygen, instituting maternal position changes, and increasing intravenous fluid administration.

10. _____ Assessment method that uses digital pressure or vibroacoustic stimulation to elicit an acceleration of the FHR of 15 beats/min for at least 15 seconds and/or to improve FHR variability.

11. _____ Abnormally small amount of amniotic fluid.

12. _____ Absence of amniotic fluid.

13. _____ Instillation of room temperature isotonic fluid into the uterine cavity when the volume of amniotic fluid is low for the purpose of adding fluid around the umbilical cord and thus preventing its compression during uterine contractions or fetal movement.

14. _____ Relaxation of the uterus achieved through the administration of drugs that inhibit uterine contractions.

II. REVIEWING KEY CONCEPTS

MATCHING: Match the definition with the appropriate term related to FHR pattern.

1. _____ Average of FHR during a 10-minute segment that excludes periodic or episodic changes, periods of marked variability, and segments of the baseline that differ by more than 25 beats per minute; it is assessed during the absence of uterine activity or between contractions.

2. _____ Expected irregular fluctuations in the baseline FHR are not detected.

3. _____ Persistent (10 minutes or longer) baseline FHR less than 110 beats/min.

4. _____ Visually apparent decrease in the FHR of 15 beats/min or more below the baseline, which lasts more than 2 minutes but less than 10 minutes.

5. _____ Changes from baseline patterns in FHR that occur with uterine contractions.

6. _____ Persistent (10 minutes or longer) baseline FHR greater than 160 beats/min.

7. _____ Irregular fluctuations or waves in the baseline FHR of 2 cycles per minute or greater.

8. _____ Visually apparent gradual decrease in and return to baseline FHR in response to transient fetal head compression during a uterine contraction; it is considered a normal and benign finding.

9. _____ Visually apparent gradual decrease in and return to baseline FHR in response to uteroplacental insufficiency resulting in a transient disruption of oxygen transfer to the fetus; lowest point occurs after the peak of the contraction and baseline rate is not usually regained until the uterine contraction is over.

10. _____ Visually abrupt decrease in FHR below baseline of 15 beats or more, lasting 15 seconds and returning to baseline in less than 2 minutes from the time of onset, which can occur at any time during a contraction as a result of umbilical cord compression.

11. _____ Visually apparent abrupt increase in the FHR of 15 beats/min or greater above the baseline, which lasts 15 seconds or more with return to baseline less than 2 minutes from the beginning of the increase.

12. _____ Changes from baseline patterns in FHR that are not associated with uterine contraction.

a. Acceleration

b. Early deceleration

c. Variability

d. Late deceleration

e. Variable deceleration

f. Tachycardia

g. Prolonged deceleration

h. Bradycardia

i. Baseline FHR

j. Absent or minimal variability

k. Periodic changes

l. Episodic changes

13. Describe the factors associated with a reduction in fetal oxygen supply.

14. It is critical that a nurse working on a labor unit be knowledgeable concerning the characteristics of normal (reassuring) and abnormal (nonreassuring) FHR patterns, and characteristics of normal and abnormal uterine activity. List the required information for each of the following:

    a. Characteristics of a normal (reassuring) FHR pattern

    b. Characteristics of abnormal (nonreassuring) FHR patterns

    c. Characteristics of normal uterine activity

15. Nurses caring for women in labor must review FHR tracings on a regular basis. Name several essential components that the nurse must evaluate each time the monitor tracing is observed.

16. Nurses caring for laboring women use a variety of methods to assess fetal health and well-being during labor. State the advantages and disadvantages of each of the following methods to assess FHR and pattern as well as uterine activity. Outline the nursing care measures required for each of the monitoring methods.

    a. External fetal monitoring

    b. Internal fetal monitoring

    c. Portable telemetry

17. State the legal responsibilities related to fetal monitoring for nurses who care for women during childbirth.

18. A laboring woman's uterine contractions are being internally monitored. When evaluating the monitor tracing, which of the following findings would be a source of concern and require further assessment?
    a. Frequency every 2½ to 3 minutes
    b. Duration of 80 to 85 seconds
    c. Intensity during a uterine contraction of 55 to 80 mm Hg
    d. Average resting pressure of 25 to 30 mm Hg

19. External electronic fetal monitoring will be used for a woman just admitted to the labor unit in active labor. Guidelines the nurse should follow when implementing this form of monitoring would be which of the following? (Circle all that apply.)
    a. Use Leopold maneuvers to determine correct placement of the ultrasound transducer.
    b. Assist woman to maintain a dorsal recumbent position to ensure accurate monitor tracings for evaluation.
    c. Reposition the tocotransducer, cleanse abdomen, and reapply gel when the fetus changes position.
    d. Tell the woman she can perform effleurage along the sides of her abdomen.
    e. Palpate the fundus to estimate the intensity of uterine contractions.

20. When evaluating the external fetal monitor tracing of a woman whose labor is being induced, the nurse identifies signs of persistent late deceleration patterns and begins intrauterine resuscitation interventions. Which of the following reflects that the appropriate interventions were implemented in the recommended order of priority?
    1. Increase rate of maintenance intravenous solution.
    2. Palpate uterus for tachysystole.
    3. Discontinue Pitocin infusion.
    4. Change maternal position to a lateral position; then elevate her legs if woman is hypotensive.
    5. Administer oxygen at 8 to 10 L/min with a tight face mask.
        a. 2, 1, 5, 4, 3
        b. 4, 1, 2, 3, 5
        c. 5, 3, 4, 1, 2
        d. 4, 5, 1, 2, 3

21. The nurse caring for women in labor should be aware of signs characterizing normal (reassuring) and abnormal (nonreassuring) FHR patterns. Which of the following would be nonreassuring signs? (Circle all that apply.)
    a. Moderate baseline variability
    b. Average baseline FHR of 100 beats/min
    c. Acceleration with fetal movement
    d. Late deceleration patterns approximately every 3 contractions
    e. FHR of 155 beats/min between contractions
    f. Early deceleration patterns

22. A laboring woman's temperature is elevated as a result of an upper respiratory infection. The FHR pattern that reflects maternal fever would be:
    a. diminished variability.
    b. variable decelerations.
    c. tachycardia.
    d. early decelerations.

23. A nulliparous woman is in the active phase of labor and her cervix has progressed to 6 cm dilation. The nurse caring for this woman evaluates the external monitor tracing and notes the following: decrease in FHR shortly after onset of several uterine contractions returning to baseline rate by the end of the contraction; shape is uniform. Based on these findings the nurse should do which of the following?
    a. Change the woman's position to her left side.
    b. Document the finding on the woman's chart.
    c. Notify the physician.
    d. Perform a vaginal examination to check for cord prolapse.

III. THINKING CRITICALLY

1. Darlene, a primigravida in active labor, has just been admitted to the labor unit. She becomes very anxious when external electronic monitoring equipment is set up. She tells the nurse that her father had a heart attack 2 months ago. "He was so sick they had to put him on a monitor too. Does this mean that my baby has a heart problem just like my father?" Describe the nurse's expected response.

2. Terry is a primigravida at 43 weeks of gestation. Her labor is being stimulated with oxytocin administered IV. Her contractions have been increasing in intensity with a frequency of every 2 to 2½ minutes and a duration of 80 to 85 seconds. She is currently in a supine position with a 30-degree elevation of her head. On observation of the monitor tracing, you note that during the last two contractions the FHR decreased after the contraction peaked and did not return to baseline until about 10 seconds into the rest period. A slight decrease in variability and baseline rate was observed.

    a. Identify the pattern described and the possible factors responsible for it.

    b. Describe the actions you would take. State the rationale for each action.

3. Taisha is a multiparous woman in active labor. Her membranes rupture and the nurse caring for her immediately evaluates the EFM tracing.

   a. What type of periodic FHR pattern would the nurse be alert for when evaluating the tracing? Explain the rationale for your answer.

   b. State the actions the nurse should take in order of priority if the pattern is noted.

4. Marianna is a primigravida in labor. On the labor and birth unit where she is a patient, intermittent auscultation (IA) with a Doppler device is used for low risk pregnant women during the latent phase and early active phases if the admission FHR monitor tracing reflects a reassuring FHR pattern. State the guidelines the nurse caring for Marianna should follow when using IA.

16 Nursing Care of the Family During Labor and Birth

I. LEARNING KEY TERMS

FILL IN THE BLANKS: Insert the term that corresponds to each of the following descriptions associated with stages of labor.

1. The first stage of labor begins with the onset of _____ and ends with complete cervical _____ and _____. A blood-tinged mucous discharge (bloody show) from the vagina usually indicates the passage of the _____.

2. During the latent phase of the first stage of labor the cervix dilates up to ___ cm in approximately ___ to ____ hours. Cervical dilation progresses from ___ to ____ cm in about ____ to ___ hours during the active phase of the first stage of labor. The duration of the transition phase is approximately ___ to ___ minutes and the cervix dilates from ____ to ____ cm.

3. The second stage of labor is the stage in which the _____. It begins with full cervical _____ and complete _____. It ends with the _____.

4. The third stage of labor lasts from the _____ until the _____. Detachment of the placenta from the wall of the uterus or separation is indicated by a firmly contracted _____; change in the shape of the uterus from _____ to _____; a sudden _____ from the introitus; apparent _____; and the finding of _____ and appearance of _____ at the introitus.

5. The fourth stage of labor is considered to be the first _____ after birth. During this stage, the mother and newborn recover from the physical process of childbirth and get to know each other.

MATCHING: Match the description with the appropriate term.

6. _____ Appearance of fetal intestinal contents in the amniotic fluid giving it a greenish color.

7. _____ Prolonged breath holding while bearing down (closed glottis pushing).

8. _____ Burning sensation of acute pain as vagina stretches and crowning occurs.

9. _____ Artificial rupture of membranes (AROM, ARM).

10. _____ Occurs when widest part of the head (biparietal diameter) distends the vulva just before birth.

11. _____ Incision into perineum to enlarge the vaginal outlet.

12. _____ Test to determine whether membranes have ruptured by assessing pH of the fluid.

13. _____ Technique used to control birth of fetal head in order to prevent fetal intracranial injury, protect maternal tissues, and reduce postpartum perineal pain.

14. _____ Method of breathing during bearing-down efforts characterized by a strong expiratory grunt or groan.

15. _____ Expulsion of placenta with shiny fetal side emerging first.

16. _____ Cord encircles the fetal neck.

a. Ritgen maneuver (modified)

b. Episiotomy

c. Oxytocic

d. Ferguson reflex

e. Shultz mechanism

f. Valsalva maneuver

g. Ring of fire

h. Crowning

i. Duncan mechanism

j. Amniotomy

k. Nuchal cord

l. Prolapse of umbilical cord

m. Nitrazine test

n. Leopold maneuvers

17. _____ Method used to palpate fetus through abdomen.

18. _____ Occurs when pressure of presenting part against pelvic floor stretch receptors results in a woman's perception of an urge to bear down.

19. _____ Frondlike crystalline pattern created by amniotic fluid when it is placed on a glass slide.

20. _____ Classification of medication that stimulates the uterus to contract (a uterotonic).

21. _____ Expulsion of placenta with roughened maternal surface emerging first.

22. _____ Application of a gentle yet steady pressure with hands pressed against the fundus to facilitate vaginal birth.

23. _____ Protrusion of umbilical cord in advance of the presenting part.

o. Ferning

p. Meconium staining

q. Open glottis pushing

r. Fundal pressure

FILL IN THE BLANKS: Insert the term that corresponds to each of the following descriptions related to the characteristics of the powers of labor.

24. _____ The primary powers of labor that act involuntarily to expel the fetus and the placenta from the uterus.

25. _____ "Building up" of a contraction from its onset.

26. _____ The peak of a contraction.

27. _____ "Letting down" of a contraction.

28. _____ How often uterine contractions occur; the time that elapses from the beginning of one contraction to the beginning of the next contraction.

29. _____ The strength of a contraction at its peak.

30. _____ The time that elapses between the onset and the end of a contraction.

31. _____ The tension of the uterine muscle between contractions.

32. _____ Period of rest between contractions.

33. _____ An involuntary urge to push in response to the Ferguson reflex.

II. REVIEWING KEY CONCEPTS

1. Laura (3-1-1-0-1) has just been admitted in the latent phase of the first stage of labor. As part of the admission procedure, you review her prenatal record and interview her regarding what she has observed regarding her labor and discuss her current health status.

    a. List the essential data you would need to obtain from her prenatal record to plan appropriate care for Laura.

    b. Identify the information required regarding the status of Laura's labor.

    c. State the information required regarding Laura's current health status.

2. A nurse caring for a laboring woman needs to be alert for signs indicative of obstetric emergencies during labor. State the signs reflecting each of the following emergencies:

    Abnormal (nonreassuring) fetal heart rate and pattern

Inadequate uterine relaxation

Vaginal bleeding

Infection

Prolapse of the cord

3. Identify two advantages for each of the following labor positions.

Semirecumbent

Lateral

Upright

Hands and knees

4. Outline the critical factors to be included in the physical assessment of the maternal-fetal unit during labor.

5. Indicate the laboratory and diagnostic tests that are recommended during labor. State the purpose for each.

6. Identify the factors that can influence the duration of the second stage of labor.

7. Describe the maternal positions recommended to enhance the effectiveness of a woman's bearing-down efforts during the second stage of labor. State the basis for each position's effectiveness in facilitating the descent and birth of the fetus.

8. Explain why the nurse should encourage a woman planning to breastfeed to begin breastfeeding during the fourth stage of labor.

9. Following spontaneous rupture of the membranes, a variable deceleration pattern appears on the monitor tracing and the umbilical cord is observed to be protruding slightly below the vaginal introitus. It is essential that the nurse caring for this woman perform which of the following measures to prevent fetal hypoxia? (Circle all that apply.)
   a. Elevate the woman's legs.
   b. Call someone to notify the woman's primary health care provider.
   c. Insert fingers into the vagina and push up against the presenting part.
   d. Administer oxygen at 8 to 10 L/min via a face mask.
   e. Place the woman in a modified Sims position.
   f. Wrap the cord with a compress saturated in cool tap water.

10. A primigravida calls the hospital and tells a nurse on the labor unit that she knows that she is in labor. The nurse's initial response would be which of the following?
   a. "Tell me what is happening to indicate to you that you are in labor."
   b. "How far do you live from the hospital?"
   c. "When is your expected date of birth?"
   d. "Have your membranes ruptured?"

11. A woman's amniotic membranes have apparently ruptured. The nurse assesses the fluid to determine its characteristics and confirm membrane rupture. Which of the following would be an expected assessment finding?
    a. pH 5.5
    b. Absence of ferning
    c. Pale straw-colored fluid with white flecks
    d. Strong odor

12. When admitting a primigravida to the labor unit, the nurse observes for signs that indicate that the woman is in true labor and should be admitted. The nurse would recognize which of the following as signs indicative of true labor? (Circle all that apply.)
    a. Woman reports that her contractions seem stronger since she walked from the car to her room on the labor unit.
    b. Cervix feels soft and is 50% effaced.
    c. Woman perceives pain to be in her back or abdomen above the level of the navel.
    d. Fetus is engaged in the pelvis at zero station.
    e. Cervix is in the posterior position.
    f. Woman continues to feel her contractions intensify following a backrub and with use of effleurage.

13. A vaginal examination is performed on a multiparous woman who is in labor. The results of the examination were documented as 4 cm, 75%, +2, LOE. Which of the following would be an accurate interpretation of this data?
    a. Woman is in the latent phase of the first stage of labor.
    b. Station is 2 cm above the ischial spines.
    c. Presentation is cephalic.
    d. Lie is transverse.

14. A physical care measure for a laboring woman that has been identified as unlikely to be beneficial and may even be harmful would be:
    a. allowing the laboring woman to drink fluids and eat light solids as tolerated.
    b. administering a Fleet enema at admission.
    c. ambulating periodically throughout labor as tolerated.
    d. using a whirlpool bath once active labor is established.

III. THINKING CRITICALLY

1. Alice, a primigravida, calls the labor unit. She tells the nurse that she thinks she is in labor. "I have had some pains for about 2 hours. Should my husband bring me to the hospital now?"

    a. Describe how the nurse should approach this situation.

    b. Write several questions the nurse could use to elicit the appropriate information required to determine the course of action required.

    c. Based on the data collected during the telephone interview, the nurse determines that Alice is in very early labor. Because she lives fairly close to the hospital, she is instructed to stay home until her labor progresses. Outline the instructions and recommendations for care Alice and her husband should be given.

2. Analyze the assessment findings documented for each of the following women.

Denise (2-0-0-1-0)	**Teresa (4-3-0-0-3)**	**Danielle (2-1-0-0-1)**
5 cm	9 cm	2 cm
moderate	very strong	mild
q4min	q2-3min	q6-8min
40-55 sec	65-75 sec	30-35 sec
0	+2	−1

   a. Identify the phase of labor being experienced by each woman.

   b. Describe the behavior and appearance you would expect to be exhibited by each woman.

   c. Specify the physical care and emotional support measures you would implement if you were caring for each of these women.

   d. Denise's husband, Sam, is her major support person during labor. The nurse observes that he is beginning to appear fatigued and "stressed" after being with Denise since her admission 5 hours ago. Describe the actions this nurse can take to support Sam and his efforts to care for Denise.

3. Describe the procedure that should be followed before auscultating the FHR or applying an ultrasound transducer to the abdomen of a laboring woman. Explain the rationale for utilizing this procedure.

4. Tonya, a woman in active labor, begins to cry during a vaginal examination to assess her status. "Why not watch the monitor to see how I am progressing instead of doing these vaginal exams? They really hurt and they are embarrassing!"

   a. Describe the response the nurse should make in regard to Tonya's concern.

   b. Discuss the measures the nurse could use to meet Tonya's safety and comfort needs during a vaginal examination.

5. Tasha is dilated 6 cm. Her coach comes to tell you that her "water just broke with a gush!" Identify each action you would take in this situation, in order of priority. State the rationale for the actions you have identified.

6. Sara, a 17-year-old primigravida, is admitted in the latent phase of labor. Her boyfriend, Dan, is with her as her only support. They appear committed to each other. During the admission interview, Sara tells you that they did not go to any classes because she was embarrassed about not being married. Both Sara and Dan appear very nervous and assessment indicates they know little about what is happening, what to expect, and how to work together with the process of labor. Identify the nursing diagnosis reflected in this data. State one expected outcome and list nursing measures appropriate for the diagnosis you identified.

   Nursing diagnosis   Expected outcome   Nursing measures

7. Identifying a laboring couple's cultural and religious beliefs and practices regarding childbirth is a critical factor in providing culturally sensitive care that enhances the couple's sense of control and eventual satisfaction with their childbirth experience.

   a. List the questions you would ask when assessing a couple's cultural and religious preferences for childbirth.

   b. Discuss the problems that can occur if the nurse does not consider the couple's cultural and religious preferences when planning and implementing care.

8. Cori (4-3-0-0-3) is in latent labor. She and her husband are being oriented to the birthing room. Their last birth occurred in a delivery room 10 years ago. Both Cori and her husband are amazed by the birthing room and the birthing bed that will allow her to give birth in an upright position. They are also informed that changes in bearing-down efforts now allow a woman to follow her own body feelings and even to vocalize with pushing. Both Cori and her husband state that with every other birth they put her legs in stirrups; she held her breath for as long as she could, and pushed quietly. "Everything turned out okay, so why should we change?" Describe the response the primary nurse caring for this couple should make to their concerns.

9. A nurse living in a rural area is called to her neighbor's home to assist his wife who is in labor. "Everything is happening so fast. She says she is ready to deliver!"

   a. Identify the measures the nurse can use to reassure and comfort the woman.

   b. Shortly after the nurse arrives, crowning begins. State what the nurse should do.

   c. Describe the action the nurse should take after the birth of the head.

   d. List the measures the nurse should use to prevent excessive neonatal heat loss after the birth.

   e. Identify the infection control measures that should be implemented during a home birth.

   f. Specify the measures the nurse should use to prevent excessive maternal blood loss or hemorrhage until the ambulance arrives.

   g. Outline the information the nurse should document regarding the childbirth.

10. Beth is in the descent phase of the second stage of labor. She is actively pushing/bearing down to facilitate birth. Indicate the criteria a nurse would use to evaluate the correctness of Beth's technique.

11. Imagine that you are participating in a panel discussion on childbirth practices. Your topic is "Episiotomy—is it needed to ensure the safety and well-being of the laboring woman and her fetus?" Outline the information you would include in your presentation.

12. Imagine that you are a staff nurse on a childbirth unit. Your hospital is instituting a change in policy that would allow the participation of children in the labor and birth process of their mother. You are asked to be a part of the committee that will formulate the guidelines regarding sibling participation during childbirth. Discuss the suggestions you would make to help ensure a positive outcome for parents, children, and health care providers.

13. Annie is a primipara in the fourth stage of labor following a long and difficult childbirth process.

    a. Identify the essential nursing assessment and care measures required to ensure Annie's safety and recovery during this stage of her labor.

    b. As she performs the first assessment, the nurse notes that Annie seems disinterested in her baby. She looks him over quickly and then asks the nurse to take him back to the nursery. Identify the factors that could be accounting for Annie's behavior.

    c. Discuss the nursing measures you would use to encourage future maternal-newborn interactions and facilitate the attachment process.

Labor and Birth Complications

I. LEARNING KEY TERMS

FILL IN THE BLANKS: Insert the term that corresponds to each of the following descriptions.

1. _____ Cervical changes and uterine contractions occurring between 20 and 37 weeks of pregnancy.

2. _____ Any birth that occurs before the completion of 37 weeks of pregnancy regardless of birth weight.

3. _____ Weight at the time of birth of 2500 g or less.

4. _____ Glycoproteins found in plasma and produced during fetal life; their reappearance in the cervical canal between 24 and 34 weeks of gestation could predict preterm labor.

5. _____ Characteristic of the cervix that could be a predictor for preterm labor.

6. _____ Spontaneous rupture of the amniotic sac and leakage of amniotic fluid beginning before the onset of labor at any gestational age.

7. _____ Spontaneous rupture of the amniotic sac and leakage of fluid before the completion of 37 weeks of gestation often associated with weakening of the membranes caused by inflammation, stress from uterine contractions, or other factors that cause increased intrauterine pressure.

8. _____ A bacterial infection of the amniotic cavity that is potentially life-threatening for the fetus and the woman.

9. _____ Long, difficult, or abnormal labor caused by various conditions associated with the five factors affecting labor.

10. _____ or _____ Abnormal uterine activity often experienced by an anxious first-time mother who is having painful and frequent contractions that are ineffective in causing cervical dilation and effacement to progress. It usually occurs in the latent phase of the first stage of labor.

11. _____ or _____ Abnormal uterine activity that usually occurs when a woman initially makes normal progress into the active phase of the first stage of labor and then uterine contractions become weak and inefficient or stop altogether.

12. _____ Abnormal labor caused by contractures of the pelvic diameters that reduce the capacity of the bony pelvis, including the inlet, midpelvis, outlet, or any combination of these planes.

13. _____ Abnormal labor caused by obstruction of the birth passage by an anatomic abnormality other than that involving the bony pelvis; the obstruction may result from placenta previa, leiomyomas (uterine fibroid tumors), ovarian tumors, or a full bladder or rectum.

14. _____ Abnormal labor caused by fetal anomalies, excessive fetal size, malpresentation, malposition, or multifetal pregnancy.

15. _____ or _____ Abnormal labor caused by excessive fetal size.

16. _____ The most common fetal malposition.

17. _____ The most common form of malpresentation.

18. _____ Gestation of twins, triplets, quadruplets, or more infants.

19. _____ Labor pattern defined as a latent phase that exceeds 20 hours in nulliparas and exceeds 14 hours in multiparas.

20. _____ Labor pattern defined as an active phase during which cervical dilation occurs at a rate of less than 1.2 cm/hr in nulliparas and less than 1.5 cm/hr in multiparas.

21. _____ Labor pattern defined as no progress in dilation for 2 hours or more in both nulliparas and multiparas.

22. _____ Labor pattern during which fetal progress through the birth canal occurs at a rate of less than 1 cm/hr in nulliparas and less than 2 cm/hr in multiparas.

23. _____ Labor pattern defined as no progress in fetal descent for one hour or more in a nulliparous labor and ½ hour or more for a multiparous labor.

24. _____ Labor pattern defined as no change in fetal progress through the birth canal during the deceleration phase and second stage of labor.

25. _____ Labor pattern that lasts less than 3 hours from the onset of contractions to the time of birth, often resulting from hypertonic uterine contractions that are tetanic in intensity.

26. _____ Attempt to turn the fetus from a breech or shoulder presentation to a vertex presentation for birth by exerting gentle, constant pressure on the abdomen.

27. _____ Observance of a woman and her fetus for a reasonable period of spontaneous active labor to assess the safety of a vaginal birth for both.

28. _____ Chemical or mechanical initiation of uterine contractions before their spontaneous onset for the purpose of bringing about the birth.

29. _____ Rating system used to evaluate the inducibility of the cervix.

30. _____ Artificial rupture of the membranes often used to induce labor when the cervix is ripe or to augment labor if the progress begins to slow.

31. _____ Stimulation of uterine contractions after labor has started spontaneously but progress is unsatisfactory. Common methods include infusion of oxytocin and rupture of membranes.

32. _____ Chemical, mechanical, and physical methods used to prepare the cervix for stimulation of labor by making it more inducible.

33. _____ Term applied to the occurrence of more than five contractions in 10 minutes averaged over a 30-minute window; it can occur in both spontaneous and stimulated labors.

34. _____ Birth method in which an instrument with two curved blades is used to assist the birth of the fetal head.

35. _____ or _____ Birth method involving the attachment of a vacuum cup to the fetal head, using negative pressure.

36. _____ Birth of the fetus through a transabdominal incision of the uterus.

37. _____ or _____ Pregnancy that extends beyond the end of week 42 of gestation. _____ Syndrome that can occur in a neonate born after pregnancy that extends beyond 42 weeks; the neonate exhibits dry, cracked, peeling skin, long nails, meconium staining of skin, nails, and umbilical cord, and loss of subcutaneous fat and muscle mass.

38. _____ Uncommon obstetric emergency in which the head of the fetus is born but the anterior shoulder cannot pass under the pubic arch. Two major causes are _____ or _____ maternal.

39. _____ Obstetric emergency in which the umbilical cord lies below the presenting part of the fetus; it may be occult (hidden) or more commonly frank (visible).

40. _____ or _____ Obstetric emergency in which a foreign substance present in the amniotic fluid enters the maternal circulation triggering a rapid, complex series of pathophysiologic events that lead to life-threatening maternal symptoms including acute hypoxia, hypotension, cardiovascular collapse, and coagulopathies.

II. REVIEWING KEY CONCEPTS

1. Compare and contrast spontaneous and indicated preterm birth.

2. Explain why bed rest may be more harmful than helpful as a component of preterm labor care management.

MATCHING: Match the description of medications used as part of the management of preterm labor with the appropriate medication.

3. _____ An antenatal glucocorticoid used to accelerate fetal lung maturity when there is risk for preterm birth.

4. _____ Beta$_2$-adrenergic receptor agonist often administered subcutaneously; it inhibits uterine activity and causes bronchodilation.

5. _____ A calcium channel blocker that relaxes smooth muscles including those of the contracting uterus; maternal hypotension is a major concern.

6. _____ Classification of drugs used to arrest labor after uterine contractions and cervical changes have occurred.

7. _____ A central nervous system (CNS) depressant used during preterm labor for its ability to relax smooth muscles including the uterus; it is administered intravenously.

8. _____ A prostaglandin synthesis inhibitor that relaxes uterine smooth muscle; it is administered orally.

a. tocolytic

b. betamethasone

c. terbutaline (Brethine)

d. magnesium sulfate

e. nifedipine (Procardia)

f. indomethacin (Indocin)

MATCHING: Match the description of medications used during the process of stimulating uterine contractions and cervical ripening with the medication listed.

9. _____ Tocolytic medication administered subcutaneously to suppress uterine tachysystole.

10. _____ Classification of medications that can be used to ripen the cervix, stimulate uterine contractions, or both.

11. _____ Cervical ripening agent in the form of a vaginal insert that is placed in the posterior fornix of the vagina.

12. _____ Cervical ripening agent in the form of a gel that is inserted into the cervical canal just below the internal os or into the posterior fornix.

13. _____ Pituitary hormone used to stimulate uterine contractions in the augmentation or induction of labor.

14. _____ Natural cervical dilator made from seaweed.

15. _____ Synthetic cervical dilator containing magnesium sulfate.

16. _____ Cervical ripening agent, used in the form of a tablet that is most commonly inserted intravaginally into the posterior fornix.

a. oxytocin (Pitocin)

b. misoprostol (Cytotec)

c. dinoprostone (Cervidil)

d. dinoprostone (Prepidil)

e. terbutaline (Brethine)

f. prostaglandin

g. laminaria tent

h. Lamisil

17. Describe each of the five factors that cause labor to be long, difficult, or abnormal. Explain how they interrelate.

18. Explain the treatment approach of therapeutic rest.

19. Angela (1-0-0-0-0) is experiencing hypertonic uterine dysfunction and Helena (3-1-0-1-1) is experiencing hypotonic uterine dysfunction. Compare and contrast each woman's labor in terms of causes/precipitating factors, maternal-fetal effects, change in pattern of progress, and care management.

    a. Angela—hypertonic uterine dysfunction

    b. Helena—hypotonic uterine dysfunction

20. Identify four indications for oxytocin induction and four contraindications to the use of oxytocin to stimulate the onset of labor.

    Indications

    Contraindications

21. When assessing a Caucasian pregnant woman, the nurse is alert for factors associated with spontaneous preterm labor. Which of the following factors, if exhibited by this woman, would increase her risk for spontaneous preterm labor? (Circle all that apply.)
    a. Caucasian race
    b. Obstetric history: 3-0-2-0-1
    c. Fibronectin found in cervical and vaginal mucous
    d. Exhibits leukorrhea
    e. Personal history of being born prematurely
    f. BMI of 22

22. Bed rest for prevention of preterm birth can result in which of the following effects? (Circle all that apply.)
    a. Bone demineralization with calcium loss
    b. Weight gain
    c. Fatigue
    d. Dysphoria and guilt
    e. Increase in cardiac output
    f. Emotional lability

23. A woman's labor is being suppressed using intravenous magnesium sulfate. Which of the following measures should be implemented during the infusion?
    a. Limit fluid intake to 2500 to 3000 ml per day.
    b. Discontinue infusion if maternal respirations are less than 12 breaths per minute.

    c. Ensure that indomethacin is available should toxicity occur.
    d. Assist woman to maintain a comfortable semirecumbent position when in bed.

24. The physician has ordered that dinoprostone (Cervidil) be administered to ripen a pregnant woman's cervix in preparation for an induction of her labor. In fulfilling this order, the nurse would do which of the following?
    a. Insert the Cervidil into the cervical canal just below the internal os.
    b. Tell the woman to remain in bed for at least 15 minutes.
    c. Observe the woman for signs of tachysystole.
    d. Begin induction using oxytocin (Pitocin) 8 hours after removal of the insert.

25. A nulliparous woman experiencing a postterm pregnancy is admitted for labor induction. Assessment reveals a Bishop score of 9. The nurse would:
    a. call the woman's primary health care provider to order a cervical ripening agent.
    b. mix 20 units of oxytocin (Pitocin) in 500 ml of 5% glucose in water.
    c. piggyback the Pitocin solution into the port nearest the drip chamber of the primary IV tubing.
    d. begin the infusion at a rate between 0.5 to 2 milliunits/min as determined by the induction protocol.

26. A woman's labor is being induced. The nurse assesses the woman's status and that of her fetus and the labor process just before an infusion increment of 2 milliunits/min. The nurse would discontinue the infusion and notify the woman's primary health care provider if which of the following had been noted during the assessment?
    a. Frequency of uterine contractions: every 1½ minutes
    b. Variability of FHR: present
    c. Deceleration patterns: early decelerations noted with several contractions
    d. Strong uterine contractions lasting 80 to 90 seconds each.

27. A laboring woman's vaginal examination reveals the following: 3 cm, 50%, LSA, 0. The nurse caring for this woman would:
    a. place the ultrasound transducer in the left lower quadrant of the woman's abdomen.
    b. recognize that passage of meconium would be a definitive sign of fetal distress.
    c. expect the progress of fetal descent to be slower than usual.
    d. assist the woman into a knee-chest position for each contraction.

28. A nurse is caring for a pregnant woman at 30 weeks of gestation in preterm labor. The woman's physician orders Betamethasone 12 mg for two doses with the first dose to be given at 11 AM. In implementing this order, the nurse would do which of the following?
    a. Consult with the physician because the dose is too high.
    b. Administer the medication orally.
    c. Schedule the second dose for 11 PM.
    d. Assess the woman for signs of hyperglycemia.

29. A nurse caring for a pregnant woman suspected of being in preterm labor would recognize which of the following as diagnostic of preterm labor?
    a. Cervical dilation of at least 2 cm
    b. Uterine contractions occurring every 15 minutes
    c. Spontaneous rupture of the membranes
    d. Presence of fetal fibronectin in cervical secretions

III. THINKING CRITICALLY

1. Imagine that you are a nurse-midwife working at an inner-city women's health clinic. You are concerned about the rate of preterm labor and birth among the pregnant women who come to your clinic for care. Outline a preterm labor and birth prevention program that you would implement at your clinic to reduce the rate of preterm labors and birth.

2. Sara, a primiparous woman (2-0-1-0-1) at 22 weeks of gestation, comes to the clinic for her scheduled prenatal visit. She is anxious because her last labor began at 26 weeks and she is worried that this will happen again. "I had no warning the last time. Is there anything I can do this time to have my baby later or at least know that labor is starting so I can let you know?"

    a. Identify the signs of preterm labor that the nurse-midwife should teach Sara.

    b. Explain how the nurse-midwife could help Sara implement a plan to reduce her risk for preterm labor.

    c. Sara calls the clinic 3 weeks later and tells her nurse-midwife that she has been having uterine contractions about every 8 minutes or so for the last hour. She is admitted for possible tocolytic therapy. Specify the criteria that Sara must meet before tocolysis can be safely initiated.

    d. Sara is started on a tocolysis regimen that involves the intravenous administration of magnesium sulfate. Outline the nursing care measures that must be implemented during the infusion to ensure the safety of Sara and her fetus.

    e. The nurse is preparing to give Sara a dose of betamethasone as ordered by the physician.

       1. State the purpose of this medication.

       2. Explain the protocol that the nurse should follow in fulfilling this order.

3. Debra has been experiencing signs of preterm labor. After a period of hospitalization, her labor was successfully suppressed and she was discharged to be cared for at home. Debra is receiving nifedipine (Procardia) 30 mg every 12 hours orally. She will palpate her uterine activity twice a day. Debra must also remain on bed rest with only bathroom privileges.

   a. State what the nurse should tell Debra about how the nifedipine works.

   b. Identify the side effects of terbutaline that the nurse should teach Debra before discharge.

   c. Describe the instructions that Debra should be given regarding palpating her uterus for contractions.

   d. Debra has 2 children who are 5 years old and 8 years old. Specify the suggestions you would give to help Debra and her children cope with the bed rest requirement ordered by Debra's primary health care provider.

4. Denise, a primigravida, has reached the second stage of her labor with her fetus at zero station and positioned LOP. She is experiencing intense low back pain. Denise did not attend any childbirth classes and is having difficulty pushing effectively. No anesthesia has been used.

   a. Identify the factors that can have a negative effect on the secondary powers of labor (bearing-down efforts).

   b. Describe how you would help Denise use her expulsive forces to facilitate the descent and birth of her baby.

   c. Specify the positions that would be recommended based on the position of the presenting part of Denise's fetus.

5. Anne, a primigravida, attended Lamaze classes with her husband, Mark. They were looking forward to working together during the labor and birth of their baby. Because of fetal distress with meconium staining, an emergency low-segment cesarean section with a transverse incision was performed after 18 hours of labor. Even though Anne and her son are in stable condition and she is glad that "everything turned out okay" for her son, she expresses a sense of failure, stating, "I could not manage to give birth to my son in the normal way and now I never will!"

   a. List the preoperative nursing measures that should have been implemented to prepare Anne physically and emotionally for the unexpected cesarean birth.

   b. Describe the major focus of care for Anne's newborn immediately after his birth related to his distress during labor.

c. Specify the assessment measures that are critical when Anne is in the recovery room following the birth of her son.

d. State the postoperative nursing care measures that Anne requires.

e. Identify the nursing diagnosis reflected in Anne's statement, "I could not manage to give birth to my son in the normal way and now I never will!" Specify the support measures the nurse could use to put her cesarean birth into perspective.

6. A vaginal examination reveals that Marie's fetus is RSA. Specify the considerations that the nurse should keep in mind when providing care for Marie.

7. Angela (2-0-0-1-0) is at 42 weeks of gestation and has been admitted for induction of her labor.

a. Assessment of Angela at admission included determination of her Bishop score. State the purpose of the Bishop score and identify the factors that are evaluated.

b. Angela's score was 5. Interpret this result in terms of the planned induction of her labor.

c. Angela's primary health care provider ordered that dinoprostone (Cervidil) be inserted. State the purpose of the Cervidil, method of application, and potential side effects that can occur.

d. Before induction of her labor, Angela's primary health provider performs an amniotomy.

  1. State the rationale for performing an amniotomy at this time.

  2. Specify the nursing responsibilities before, during, and after this procedure.

e. Indicate which of the following actions reflect appropriate care (A) for Angela during the induction of her labor with intravenous oxytocin. If the action is not appropriate (NA), state what the correct action would be.

1. _____ Assist Angela into a lateral or upright position.

2. _____ Apply an external electronic fetal monitor and evaluate the tracing every 30 minutes throughout labor.

3. _____ Explain to Angela what to expect and techniques used.

4. _____ Add 10 units of oxytocin (Pitocin) into 1000 ml of an isotonic electrolyte solution.

5. _____ Piggyback the oxytocin (Pitocin) solution to the proximal port (port nearest the venous insertion site) of the primary IV.

6. _____ Begin infusion at 4 milliunits/min.

7. _____ Increase oxytocin by 1 to 2 milliunits/min at 5- to 10-minute intervals after the initial dose until the desired pattern of contractions is achieved.

8. _____ Stop increasing the dosage and maintain level of oxytocin when strong contractions occur every 2 to 3 minutes, and last 80 to 90 seconds each.

9. _____ Monitor maternal blood pressure and pulse every 15 minutes and after every increment.

10. _____ Limit IV intake to 1500 ml/8 hours.

f. State the reportable conditions associated with oxytocin (Pitocin) induction for which the nurse must be alert when managing Angela's labor.

g. The nurse notes a uterine hyperstimulation pattern when evaluating Angela's monitor tracing. List the actions the nurse should take in order of priority.

8. Lora is a 37-year-old nulliparous woman beginning her forty-second week of pregnancy. She and her primary health care provider have decided on a conservative "watchful waiting" approach because both she and her fetus are not experiencing distress.

a. In helping Lora make this decision, the risks she and her fetus face as a result of a postterm pregnancy were explained. Identify the risks that Lora should have considered in making her decision.

b. State the clinical manifestations that Lora is likely to experience as her pregnancy continues.

c. Outline the typical care management measures that should be implemented to ensure the safety of Lora and her fetus.

d. Specify the instructions that the nurse should give to Lora regarding her self-care as she awaits the onset of labor.

9. Julia is in latent labor. Her BMI prior to pregnancy was 35 and she gained 80 pounds during her pregnancy. If you were the nurse caring for Julia, what considerations related to her BMI would you keep in mind as you manage her care?

18 Maternal Physiologic Changes

I. LEARNING KEY TERMS

FILL IN THE BLANKS: Insert the term that corresponds to each of the following descriptions.

1. _____ Profuse sweating that occurs after birth, especially at night, to rid the body of fluid retained during pregnancy.

2. _____ Uncomfortable uterine cramping that occurs during the early postpartum period as a result of periodic relaxation and vigorous contractions.

3. _____ Lactogenic hormone secreted by the pituitary gland of lactating women. _____ Pituitary hormone that is responsible for uterine contraction and the let-down reflex.

4. _____ Surgical incision of the perineum to facilitate birth.

5. _____ Failure of the uterine muscle to contract firmly. It is the most frequent cause of excessive postpartum bleeding.

6. _____ Anal varicosity.

7. _____ Return of the uterus to a nonpregnant state.

8. _____ Self-destruction of excess hypertrophied uterine tissue as a result of the decrease in estrogen and progesterone level following birth.

9. _____ and _____ Terms used interchangeably with postpartum to refer to the period of recovery after childbirth when reproductive organs return to their nonpregnant state; it lasts approximately 6 weeks though the time can vary from woman to woman.

10. _____ Separation of the abdominal wall muscles related to the effect of the enlargement of the uterus on the abdominal musculature.

11. _____ Postbirth uterine discharge or flow.

12. _____ Bright red, bloody uterine discharge that occurs for the first few days following birth; it consists primarily of blood, decidual tissue, trophoblastic debris, and sometimes small clots.

13. _____ Pink to brownish uterine discharge that begins about 3 to 4 days after birth; it consists of old blood, serum, leukocytes, and tissue debris.

14. _____ Yellowish white flow that begins about 10 days after birth and continues for 2 to 6 weeks; it consists of leukocytes, decidua, epithelial cells, mucus, serum, and bacteria.

15. _____ Term that describes distended, firm, tender, and warm breasts during the postpartum period.

16. _____ Failure of the uterus to return to a nonpregnant state. The most common causes for this failure are _____ and _____.

17. _____ Medication most commonly administered intravenously immediately after expulsion of the placenta to ensure that the uterus remains firm and well contracted.

18. _____ Coital discomfort or pain with intercourse.

19. _____ Exercises that help to strengthen perineal muscles and encourage healing.

20. _____ Yellowish fluid produced in the breasts before lactation.

21. _____ Increased production of urine that occurs in the postpartum period to rid the body of fluid retained during pregnancy.

22. _____ Stretch marks which can appear during pregnancy on the breasts, abdomen, and thighs.

II. REVIEWING KEY CONCEPTS

1. When caring for a woman following vaginal birth, it is of critical importance for the nurse to assess the woman's bladder for distention.

   a. Explain why bladder distention is more likely to occur during the immediate postpartum period.

   b. Identify the problems that can occur if the bladder is allowed to become distended.

2. Cite the factors that can interfere with bowel elimination in the postpartum period.

3. Explain why hypovolemic shock is less likely to occur in the postpartum woman experiencing a normal or average blood loss.

4. Indicate the factors that place a postpartum woman at increased risk for the development of thrombophlebitis.

5. Compare and contrast the characteristics of lochial bleeding and nonlochial bleeding.

6. A nurse has assessed a woman who gave birth vaginally 24 hours ago. Which of the following findings would require further assessment?
   a. Bright to dark red uterine discharge
   b. Midline episiotomy—approximated, moderate edema, slight erythema, absence of ecchymosis
   c. Protrusion of abdomen with sight separation of abdominal wall muscles
   d. Fundus firm at 1 cm above the umbilicus and to the right of midline

7. A woman, 24 hours after giving birth, complains to the nurse that her sleep was interrupted the night before because of sweating and the need to have her gown and bed linen changed. The nurse's first action would be to:
   a. assess this woman for additional clinical manifestations of infection.
   b. explain to the woman that the sweating represents her body's attempt to eliminate the fluid that was accumulated during pregnancy.
   c. notify her physician of the finding.
   d. document the finding as postpartum diaphoresis.

8. Which of the following women at 24 hours after giving birth is least likely to experience afterpains?
   a. Primipara who is breastfeeding her twins that were born at 38 weeks of gestation
   b. Multipara who is breastfeeding her 10-pound full-term baby girl
   c. Multipara who is bottle-feeding her 8-pound baby boy
   d. Primipara who is bottle-feeding her 7-pound baby girl

III. THINKING CRITICALLY

1. Describe how you would respond to each of the following typical questions/concerns of postpartum women.

   a. Mary is a primipara who is breastfeeding. "Why am I experiencing so many painful cramps in my uterus? I thought this happens only in women who have had babies before."

   b. Susan is being discharged after giving birth 20 hours ago. "For how many days should I be able to palpate my uterus to make sure it is firm?"

   c. June is a primipara. "My friend, who had a baby last year, said she had a flow for 6 weeks. Isn't that a long time to bleed after having a baby?"

   d. Jean is at 24 hours postpartum. "I cannot believe it—I look as if I am still pregnant! How can this be?"

   e. Marion is 1 day postpartum. "It seems like I am urinating all the time; do you think that I have a bladder infection?"

   f. Joan is a primipara who is breastfeeding her baby. "My friend told me that I cannot get pregnant as long as I continue to breastfeed. This is great because I do not like to use birth control."

   g. Alice, a primiparous, bottle-feeding women, is concerned. She states, "My mother told me that I should be getting a drug to dry up my breasts like she got after she gave birth. How will my breasts ever stop making milk and get back to normal?"

   h. Andrea, a primipara, is 1 day postpartum. While breastfeeding her baby she confides to the nurse that she does not know how long she will continue to breastfeed. "My husband and I have always had a satisfying sex life, but my friend told me that as long as I breastfeed, intercourse is painful."

19 Nursing Care of the Family During the Postpartum Period

I. LEARNING KEY TERMS

FILL IN THE BLANKS: Insert the term that corresponds to each of the following descriptions regarding the postpartum period.

1. _____ Nursing care management approach in which one nurse cares for both the mother and her infant. It is also called _____ or _____.

2. _____ Term used for the decreasing length of hospital stays of mothers and their babies after low risk vaginal births. Other terms used are _____ or _____.

3. _____ Classification of medications that stimulate contraction of the uterine smooth muscle.

4. _____ Failure of the uterine muscle to contract firmly. It is the most frequent cause for excessive bleeding following childbirth.

5. _____ Perineal treatment that involves sitting in warm water for approximately 20 minutes to soothe and cleanse the site and to increase blood flow, thereby enhancing healing.

6. _____ Menstrual-like cramps experienced by many women as the uterus contracts after childbirth.

7. _____ Dilation of the blood vessels supplying the intestines as a result of the rapid decease in intraabdominal pressure after birth. It causes blood to pool in the viscera and thereby contributes to the development of _____ when the woman who has recently given birth sits or stands, first ambulates, or takes a warm shower.

8. _____ Exercises that can assist women to regain muscle tone that is often lost when pelvic tissues are stretched and torn during pregnancy and birth.

9. _____ Swelling of breast tissue caused by increased blood and lymph supply to the breasts as the body begins the process of lactation.

10. _____ Vaccine that can be given to postpartum women whose antibody titer is less than 1:8 or whose EIA level is less than 0.8. It is used to prevent nonimmune women from contracting this TORCH infection during a subsequent pregnancy.

11. _____ Blood product that is administered to Rh-negative, antibody (Coombs')-negative women who give birth to Rh-positive newborns. It is administered at 28 weeks of gestation and again within 72 hours after birth.

12. _____ Telephone-based postpartum consultation service that can provide information and support; it is not a crisis intervention line to be used for emergencies.

II. REVIEWING KEY CONCEPTS

1. Explain to a woman who has just given birth why breastfeeding her newborn during the fourth stage of labor is beneficial to her and to her baby.

2. A postpartum woman at 6 hours after a vaginal birth is having difficulty voiding. List the measures that you would try to help this woman void spontaneously.

3. Identify the measures the nurse should teach a postpartum woman in an effort to prevent the development of thrombophlebitis.

4. Identify the measures you would teach a bottle-feeding mother to suppress lactation naturally and to relieve discomfort during breast engorgement.

5. State the two most important interventions that can be used to prevent excessive postpartum bleeding in the early postpartum period. Indicate the rationale for the effectiveness of each intervention you identified.

6. Identify the signs of potential psychosocial complications that may occur during the postpartum period.

7. The nurse is prepared to assess a postpartum woman's fundus. The nurse would tell the woman to:
   a. elevate the head of the bed.
   b. place her hands under her head.
   c. flex her knees.
   d. lie flat with legs extended and toes pointed.

8. The expected outcome for care when methylergonovine (Methergine), an oxytocic, is administered to a postpartum woman during the fourth stage of labor would be which of the following? The woman will:
   a. demonstrate expected lochial characteristics.
   b. achieve relief of pain associated with uterine cramping.
   c. remain free from infection.
   d. void spontaneously within 4 hours of birth.

9. A nurse is preparing to administer RhoGAM to a postpartum woman. Before implementing this care measure the nurse should:
   a. ensure that medication is given at least 24 hours after the birth.
   b. verify that the Coombs' test results are negative.
   c. make sure that the newborn is Rh negative.
   d. cancel the administration of the RhoGAM if it was given to the woman during her pregnancy at 28 weeks of gestation.

10. When teaching a postpartum woman with an episiotomy about using a sitz bath, the nurse should emphasize:
    a. using sterile equipment.
    b. filling the sitz bath basin with hot water (at least 42° C).
    c. taking a sitz bath once a day for 10 minutes.
    d. squeezing her buttocks together before sitting down, then relaxing them.

11. Prior to discharge at 2 days postpartum, the nurse evaluates a woman's level of knowledge regarding the care of her second degree perineal laceration. Which of the following statements if made by the woman would indicate the need for further instruction before she goes home? (Circle all that apply.)
    a. "I will wash my stitches at least once a day with mild soap and warm water."
    b. "I will change my pad every time I go to the bathroom—at least 4 times each day."
    c. "I will use my squeeze bottle filled with warm water to cleanse my stitches after I urinate."
    d. "I will take a sitz bath once a day before bed for about 10 minutes."
    e. "I will apply the anesthetic cream to my stitches at least 6 times per day."

12. When assessing postpartum women during the first 24 hours after birth, the nurse must be alert for signs that could indicate the development of postpartum physiologic complications. Which of the following signs would be of concern to the nurse? (Circle all that apply.)
    a. Temperature—38° C
    b. Fundus—midline, boggy
    c. Lochia—3/4 of pad saturated in 3 hours
    d. Anorexia
    e. Voids approximately 150 to 200 ml of urine for each of the first three voidings after birth.

III. THINKING CRITICALLY

1. Tara is a breastfeeding woman at 12 hours postpartum. She requests medication for pain. Describe the approach that you would take when fulfilling Tara's request.

2. When caring for a woman who gave birth 4 hours earlier, the nurse notes an excessive rubra flow and early signs of hypovolemic shock.

   a. State the criteria that the nurse should have used to determine that the flow is rubra and excessive and that the early signs of hypovolemic shock are being exhibited.

   b. Identify the nurse's priority action in response to these assessment findings.

   c. Identify additional interventions that a nurse may need to implement to ensure this woman's safety and to prevent the development of further complications.

3. Carrie is a postpartum woman awaiting discharge. Because her rubella titer indicates that she is not immune, a rubella vaccination has been ordered before discharge. State what you would tell Carrie with regard to this vaccination.

4. The physician has written the following order for a postpartum woman: "Administer RhoGAM (Rh immunoglobulin) if indicated." Describe the actions the nurse should take in fulfilling this order.

5. Susan, a postpartum breastfeeding woman, confides to the nurse, "My partner and I have always had a very satisfying sex life, even when I was pregnant. My sister told me that this will definitely change now that I have had a baby." Describe what the nurse should tell Susan regarding sexual changes and activity after birth.

6. Identify the priority nursing diagnosis as well as one expected outcome and appropriate nursing management for each of the following situations.

   a. Tina is 2 days postpartum. During a home visit the nurse notes that Tina's episiotomy is edematous and slightly reddened, with approximated wound edges and no drainage. A distinct odor is noted and there is a build up of secretions and the Hurricaine gel Tina uses for discomfort. During the interview Tina reveals that she is afraid to wash the area, "I rinse with a little water in my peri bottle in the morning and again at night. I also apply plenty of my gel."

   Nursing diagnosis   Expected outcome   Nursing management

   b. Erin, who gave birth 3 days ago, has not had a bowel movement since a day or two before labor. She tells the visiting nurse during the interview that she has been avoiding "fiber" foods for fear that the baby will get diarrhea. Her activity level is low. "My family is taking good care of me. I do not have to lift a finger! Besides I would prefer to wait until my 'bottom' is less sore before trying to have a bowel movement."

   Nursing diagnosis   Expected outcome   Nursing management

   c. Mary gave birth 24 hours ago. She complains of perineal discomfort. "My hemorrhoids and stitches are killing me, but I do not want to take any medication because it will get into my breast milk and hurt my baby."

   Nursing diagnosis   Expected outcome   Nursing management

7. Dawn gave birth 8 hours ago. Upon palpation, her fundus was found to be two fingerbreadths above the umbilicus and deviated to the right of midline. It was also assessed to be less firm than previously noted.

   a. State the most likely basis for these findings.

   b. Describe the action that the nurse should take based on these assessment findings.

8. Jill gave birth 3 hours ago. During labor, epidural anesthesia was used for pain relief. Jill's primary health care provider has written the following order: "Out of bed and ambulating when able." Discuss the approach the nurse should take in safely fulfilling this order.

9. Taisha and her husband, Raushaun, are expecting their first baby. They have been given the option by their nurse-midwife of early postpartum discharge but are unsure of what to do.

   a. Describe the approach the nurse-midwife could take to help this couple make a decision that is right for them.

   b. Taisha and Raushaun decide to take the option of early discharge within 12 hours of birth. Identify the criteria for discharge that Taisha and her newborn must meet before discharge from the hospital to home.

   c. Outline the essential content that must be taught before discharge. A home visit by a nurse is planned for Taisha's third postpartum day.

10. Cultural beliefs and practices must be considered when planning and implementing care in the postpartum period.

    a. Discuss the importance of using a culturally sensitive approach when providing care to postpartum women and their families.

    b. Kim, a Korean-American woman, has just given birth. Assessment reveals that she and her family are guided by beliefs and practices based on a balance of heat and cold. Describe how the nurse would adjust typical postpartum care in order to respect and accommodate Kim's cultural beliefs and practices.

    c. A Muslim woman has been admitted to the postpartum unit following the birth of her second son. Describe the approach you would use in managing this woman's care in a culturally sensitive manner.

11. Tamara delivered vaginally 2 hours ago. She has a midline episiotomy.

    a. Describe the position that Tamara should assume in order to facilitate palpation of her fundus.

    b. Identify the characteristics of Tamara's fundus that should be assessed.

    c. Describe the position Tamara should assume in order to facilitate the examination of her episiotomy.

d. Identify the characteristics that should be assessed to determine progress of healing and adequacy of Tamara's perineal self-care measures.

e. State the characteristics of Tamara's uterine flow that should be assessed.

12. Imagine that you are the nurse who cared for a woman during her labor and birth and her recovery during the fourth stage of labor. Outline the information that you would report to the mother-baby nurse when you transfer the new mother and her baby to her room on the postpartum unit.

13. Infection control measures should guide the practice of nurses working on a postpartum unit.

    a. Discuss the measures designed to prevent transmission of infection from person to person.

    b. Discuss measures a postpartum woman should be taught to reduce her risk of infection.

20 Transition to Parenthood

I. LEARNING KEY TERMS

FILL IN THE BLANKS: Insert the appropriate term for each of the following descriptions regarding parent-infant interaction and parenting.

1. _____ Process by which a parent comes to love and accept a child and a child comes to love and accept a parent. The term _____ is often used to refer to this process.

2. _____ Process that occurs as parents interact with their newborn and maintain close proximity as they identify the infant as an individual and claim him or her as a member of the family; parents will touch, talk to, make eye contact with, and explore their newborn.

3. _____ Infant behaviors and characteristics call forth a corresponding set of maternal behaviors and characteristics.

4. _____ Infant behaviors such as crying, smiling, and cooing that initiate the contact and bring the caregiver to the child.

5. _____ Infant behaviors such as rooting, grasping, and postural adjustments that maintain the contact.

6. _____ Process in which parents identify the new baby, first in terms of likeness to other family members, second in terms of differences, and third in terms of uniqueness.

7. _____ Position used for mutual gazing in which the parent's face and the infant's face are approximately 8 inches apart and are on the same plane.

8. _____ Newborns move in time with the structure of adult speech by waving their arms, lifting their heads, and kicking their legs, seemingly "dancing in tune" to a parent's voice.

9. _____ Personal biorhythm developed by the infant; parents facilitate this process by giving consistent loving care and using their infant's alert state to develop responsive behavior and thereby increase social interaction and opportunities for learning.

10. _____ Type of body movement or behavior that provides the observer with cues. The observer or receiver interprets those cues and responds to them.

11. _____ The "fit" between the infant's cues and the parents' response.

12. _____ Period from the decision to conceive through the first months of having a child.

13. _____ Phase of maternal adjustment that occurs during the first 24 hours (range of 1 to 2 days) when the woman focuses on herself and meeting basic needs with a reliance on others for comfort, rest, closeness, and nourishment. She is often talkative and desires to discuss her childbirth experience.

14. _____ Phase of maternal adjustment that begins on the second or third day postpartum and lasts for about 10 days to several weeks, during which the woman focuses on caring for her baby and becoming competent as a mother; she is eager to learn and to practice and may experience baby blues.

15. _____ Phase of maternal adjustment during which the woman reasserts her relationship with her partner and resumes sexual intimacy; individual roles are resolved.

16. _____ Process of transformation and growth of the mother identity during which the woman learns new skills and increases her confidence in herself as she meets new challenges in caring for her child(ren).

17. _____ Period surrounding the first day or two after giving birth, characterized by heightened joy and feelings of well-being.
_____ Period following birth that is characterized by emotional lability, depression, a let-down feeling, restlessness, fatigue, insomnia, anxiety, sadness, and anger. Lability peaks around the fifth day postpartum and subsides by the tenth day.

18. _____ Father's absorption, preoccupation, and interest in his infant.

19. _____ Contingent responses that occur within a specific time and are similar in form to a stimulus behavior.

II. REVIEWING KEY CONCEPTS

1. Attachment of the newborn to parents and family is critical for optimum growth and development.

   a. List conditions that must be present for the parent-newborn attachment process to begin favorably.

   b. Discuss how you would assess the progress of attachment between parents and their new baby.

   c. Indentify what nurses can do to facilitate the process of attachment in the immediate postbirth period.

2. Describe three parental tasks and responsibilities that are part of parental adjustment to a new baby.

3. Discuss how each of the following forms of parent-infant contact can facilitate attachment and promote the family as a focus of care.

   a. Early contact

   b. Extended contact

4. Describe how a mother's touching of her newborn progresses during the immediate postbirth period.

5. Describe how each of the following factors influences the manner in which parents respond to the birth of their child. State two nursing implications/actions related to each factor.

   Adolescent parents

   Parental age older than 35

   Lesbian couple

   Social support

   Culture

   Socioeconomic conditions

   Personal aspirations

   Sensory impairment

6. During the final phase of the claiming process of a newborn, which of the following might a mother say?
   a. "She has her grandfather's nose."
   b. "His ears lay nice and flat against his head, not like mine and his sister's, which stick out."
   c. "She gave me nothing but trouble during pregnancy, and now she is so stubborn she won't wake up to breastfeed."
   d. "He has such a sweet disposition and pleasant expression. I have never seen a baby quite like him before."

7. Which of the following nursing actions would be least effective in facilitating parent attachment to their new infant?
   a. Referring the couple to a lactation consultant to ensure continuing success with breastfeeding
   b. Keeping the baby in the nursery as much as possible for the first 24 hours after birth so the mother can rest
   c. Extending visiting hours for the woman's partner or significant other as they desire
   d. Providing guidance and support as the parents care for their baby's nutrition and hygiene needs

8. Which of the following behaviors illustrates engrossment?
   a. A father is sitting in a rocking chair, holding his new baby boy, touching his toes, and making eye contact.
   b. A mother tells her friends that her baby's eyes and nose are just like hers.
   c. A mother picks up and cuddles her baby girl when she begins to cry.
   d. A grandmother gazes into her new grandson's face, which she holds about 8 inches away from her own; she and the baby make eye-to-eye contact.

9. A woman expresses a need to review her labor and birth experience with the nurse who cared for her while in labor. This behavior is most characteristic of which of the following phases of maternal postpartum adjustment?
   a. Taking-hold (dependent-independent phase)
   b. Taking-in (dependent phase)
   c. Letting-go (interdependent)
   d. Postpartum blues (baby blues)

10. Before discharge, a postpartum woman and her partner ask the nurse about the baby blues. "Our friend said she felt so let down after she had her baby, and we have heard that some women actually become very depressed. Is there anything we can do to prevent this from happening to us or at least to cope with the blues if they occur?" The nurse could tell this couple:
    a. "Postpartum blues usually happen in pregnancies that are high risk or unplanned, so there is no need for you to worry."
    b. "Try to become skillful in breastfeeding and caring for your baby as quickly as you can."
    c. "Get as much rest as you can and sleep when the baby sleeps, because fatigue can precipitate the blues or make them worse."
    d. "I will call your doctor before you leave to get you a prescription for an antidepressant to prevent the blues from happening."

III. THINKING CRITICALLY

1. Jane and Andrew are parents of a newborn girl. Describe what you would teach them regarding the communication process as it relates to their newborn.

   a. Techniques they can use to communicate effectively with their newborn.

   b. The manner in which the baby is able to communicate with them.

2. Allison had a difficult labor that resulted in an emergency cesarean birth under general anesthesia. She did not see her baby until 12 hours after her birth. Allison tells the nurse who brings the baby to her room, "I am so disappointed. I had planned to breastfeed my baby and hold her close, skin to skin, right after her birth just like all the books say. I know that this is so important for our relationship." Describe how the nurse should respond to Allison's concern.

3. Angela is the mother of a 1-day-old boy and a 3-year-old girl. As you prepare Angela for discharge, she states, "My little girl just saw her brother. She says she loves him and cannot wait for him to come home. I am so glad that I do not have to worry about any of that sibling rivalry business!" Indicate how you would respond to Angela's comments.

4. Sara and Ben have just experienced the birth of their first baby. They are very happy with their baby boy but appear very unsure of themselves and are obviously anxious about how to tell what their baby needs. Sara is trying very hard to breastfeed and is having some success but not as much as she had hoped. Both parents express self-doubt about their ability to succeed at the "most important role in our lives."

   a. State the nursing diagnosis that is most appropriate for this couple.

   b. Describe what the nurse caring for this family can do to facilitate the attachment process.

5. Mary and Jim are the parents of three sons. They very much wanted to have a girl this time, but after a long and difficult birth they had another son who weighed 10 pounds. His appearance reflects the difficult birth process: occipital molding, caput succedaneum, and forceps marks on each cheek. Mary and Jim express their disappointment not only in the appearance of their son but also in the fact that they had another boy. "This was supposed to be our last child—now we just do not know what we will do." Discuss how you would facilitate Mary and Jim's attachment to their son and reconcile their fantasy ("dream") child with the reality of their actual child.

6. Dawn and Matthew have just given birth to their first baby. This is the first grandchild for both sets of grandparents. The grandmothers approach the nurse to ask how they can help the new family, stating, "We want to help Dawn and Matthew but at the same time not interfere with what they want to do." Discuss the role of the nurse in helping these grandparents to recognize their importance to the new family and to develop a mutually satisfying relationship with Dawn, Matthew, and the new baby.

7. Jane is 2 days postpartum. When the nurse makes a home visit, Jane is found crying. Jane states, "I have such a let-down feeling. I cannot understand why I feel this way when I should be so happy about the healthy outcome for myself and my baby." Jane's husband confirms her behavior and expresses confusion as well, stating, "I wish I knew what to do to help her." Identify the priority nursing diagnosis and one expected outcome for this situation. Describe the recommended nursing management for the nursing diagnosis you have identified.

Nursing diagnosis   Expected outcome   Nursing management

8. Ali has just become a father with the birth of his first child, a baby boy.

   a. Describe the process Ali will follow as he adjusts to fatherhood.

   b. Identify several measures the nurse caring for Ali's wife and baby boy can use to facilitate his adjustment to father-hood and attachment to his baby.

I. LEARNING KEY TERMS

FILL IN THE BLANKS: Insert the term that corresponds to each of the following descriptions of postpartum complications.

1. _____ Loss of 500 mL or more of blood after vaginal birth or 1000 mL or more after cesarean birth. _____ Excessive blood loss that occurs within 24 hours after birth; it is most often caused by marked uterine hypotonia. _____ Blood loss that occurs more than 24 hours after birth but less than 6 weeks after birth.

2. _____ Marked hypotonia of the uterus; the uterus fails to contract well or maintain contraction.

3. _____ Collection of blood in the connective tissue as a result of blood vessel damage. _____ are the most common type. _____ are usually associated with a forceps-assisted birth, an episiotomy, or primigravidity.

4. _____ Unusual placental adherence in which there is slight penetration of the myometrium by placental trophoblast.

5. _____ Unusual placental adherence in which there is deep penetration of the myometrium by the placenta.

6. _____ Unusual placental adherence in which there is penetration of the uterus by the placenta.

7. _____ Turning of the uterus inside out after birth.

8. _____ Delayed return of the enlarged uterus to normal size and function.

9. _____ Emergency situation in which profuse blood loss (hemorrhage) can result in severely compromised perfusion of body organs. Death may occur.

10. _____ Coagulopathy resulting from an autoimmune disorder in which antiplatelet antibodies decrease the life span of the platelets.

11. _____ Type of hemophilia; it is among the most common congenital clotting defects in North American women of childbearing age.

12. _____ Pathologic form of clotting that is diffuse and consumes large amounts of clotting factors; it is also known as consumptive coagulopathy.

13. _____ Formation of a blood clot or clots inside a blood vessel.

14. _____ Inflammation of a vein with clot formation.

15. _____ Clot involves the superficial saphenous venous system. _____ Clot involvement can extend from the foot to the iliofemoral region.

16. _____ Complication occurring when part of a blood clot dislodges and is carried to the pulmonary artery, where it occludes the vessel and obstructs blood flow to the lungs.

17. _____ or _____ Clinical infection of the genital canal that occurs within 28 days after miscarriage, induced abortion, or childbirth. In the United States, it is defined as a temperature of 38° C or more on 2 successive days of the first 10 postpartum days (not counting the first 24 hours after birth).

18. _____ Infection of the lining of the uterus; it is the most common postpartum infection and usually begins as a localized infection at the placental site.

19. _____ Infection of the breast affecting approximately 2% to 10% of women, soon after childbirth, most of whom are first-time breastfeeding mothers; it almost always is unilateral and develops well after lactation has been established.

135

20. _____ Downward displacement of the uterus, with degrees of displacement from mild to complete.

21. _____ Protrusion of the bladder downward into the vagina that develops when supporting structures in the vesicovaginal septum are injured.

22. _____ Herniation of the anterior rectal wall through the relaxed or ruptured vaginal fascia and rectovaginal septum.

23. _____ Leakage of urine that occurs due to sudden increases in intraabdominal pressure.

24. _____ Perforation between genital tract organs.

25. _____ Perforation between the bladder and the genital tract.

26. _____ Perforation between the urethra and the vagina.

27. _____ Perforation between the rectum or sigmoid colon and the vagina.

28. _____ Device that can be inserted into the vagina for the purpose of supporting the uterus and holding it in the correct position.

29. _____ Surgical procedure used to repair large, symptomatic cystoceles.

30. _____ Surgical procedure used to repair large, symptomatic rectoceles.

31. _____ Predominant classification of mental health disorders in the postpartum period.

32. _____ An intense and pervasive sadness with severe and labile mood swings; it is more serious and persistent than postpartum blues. Intense fears, anger, anxiety, and despondency that persist past the baby's first few weeks are not a normal part of postpartum blues.

33. _____ Syndrome most often characterized by depression, delusions, and thoughts by the mother of harming either herself or her infant.

34. _____ Mood disorder defined by the presence of one or more episodes of abnormally elevated energy levels, cognition, and mood and one or more depressive episodes.

35. _____ A cluster of painful responses experienced by individuals coping with the death of someone with whom they had a close relationship, generally a relative or close friend.

36. _____ Grief response that occurs with reminders of the loss; typically happens on birthdays, death days, and anniversaries; at school events; during changes in the seasons; and during the time of year when the loss occurred.

II. REVIEWING KEY CONCEPTS

1. State the twofold focus of medical management of hemorrhagic shock.

2. Identify the priority nursing interventions for postpartum hemorrhage and hypovolemic shock. Include the rationale for each intervention identified.

3. State the standard of care for bleeding emergencies.

4. Identify measures found to be effective in preventing genital tract infections during the postpartum period.

5. Mary, a pregnant woman at 24 weeks of gestation, has been admitted to the labor unit following a prenatal visit at her health care provider's office. Fetal death is suspected and eventually confirmed. Identify the phase of grief response represented by each of the comments made by Mary as she reacts to her loss. Describe each phase in terms of expected duration, behaviors typically exhibited, and emotions experienced.

a. "The doctor says he cannot find my baby's heart-beat or feel my baby move. He thinks my baby has died. I know you will hear my baby's heartbeat since you have a monitor here. My baby is okay—I just know it!"

b. "I know this never would have happened if I had quit my job as a legal secretary. My mom told me that pregnant women should take it easy. If I had listened, I would have my baby in my arms right now!"

c. "Since my baby died I just cannot seem to concentrate on even the simplest things at home and at work. I always seem to feel tired and out of sorts."

d. "Why did this happen to my baby? Why did it happen to me?"

e. "It is going to be hard. I will always remember my little baby boy and the day he was supposed to be born. But I know that my husband and I have to go on with our lives."

6. Describe how you, as a nurse, would help parents and other family members actualize the loss of their newborn.

7. A woman has been diagnosed with severe postpartum depression. The nurse caring for this woman is concerned that she may harm herself, her baby, or both of them.

a. What questions should the nurse ask to determine whether the woman is considering such a harmful action?

b. The woman admits that she has been thinking that her family and even her baby might be better off without her. Identify the four criteria the nurse could use to determine how serious the woman might be.

8. Methylergonovine (Methergine) 0.2 mg is ordered to be administered intramuscularly to a woman who gave birth vaginally 1 hour ago for a profuse lochial flow with clots. Her fundus is boggy and does not respond well to massage. She is still being treated for preeclampsia with intravenous magnesium sulfate at 1 g/hr. Her blood pressure, measured 5 minutes ago, was 155/98. In fulfilling this order, the nurse would do which of the following?
   a. Measure the woman's blood pressure again 5 minutes after administering the medication.
   b. Question the order based on the woman's hypertensive status.
   c. Recognize that Methergine will counteract the uterine relaxation effects of the magnesium sulfate infusion the woman is receiving.
   d. Tell the woman that the medication will lead to uterine cramping.

9. A postpartum woman in the fourth stage of labor received prostaglandin F_{2a} (Hemabate) 0.25 mg intramuscularly. The expected outcome of care for the administration of this medication would be which of the following?
   a. Relief from the pain of uterine cramping
   b. Prevention of intrauterine infection
   c. Reduction in the blood's ability to clot
   d. Limitation of excessive blood loss that is occurring after birth

10. The nurse responsible for the care of postpartum women should recognize that the first sign of puerperal infection would most likely be which of the following?
    a. Fever with body temperature at 38° C or higher after the first 24 hours following birth
    b. Increased white blood cell count
    c. Foul-smelling profuse lochia
    d. Bradycardia

11. A breastfeeding woman's cesarean birth occurred 2 days ago. Investigation of the pain, tenderness, and swelling in her left leg led to a medical diagnosis of deep vein thrombosis (DVT). Care management for this woman during the acute stage of the DVT would involve which of the following actions? (Circle all that apply.)
    a. Explaining that she will need to stop breastfeeding until anticoagulation therapy is completed
    b. Administering heparin via continuous intravenous drip

c. Placing the woman on bed rest with her left leg elevated

d. Encouraging the woman to change her position frequently when on bed rest

e. Teaching the woman and her family how to administer warfarin (Coumadin) subcutaneously after discharge

f. Telling the woman to use acetaminophen (Tylenol) for discomfort

12. Which of the following would be a priority question to ask a woman experiencing postpartum depression?
    a. Have you thought about hurting yourself?
    b. Does it seem like your mind is filled with cobwebs?
    c. Have you been feeling insecure, fragile, or vulnerable?
    d. Does the responsibility of motherhood seem overwhelming?

13. A woman gave birth to twin girls, one of whom was stillborn. Which of the following nursing actions would be least helpful in supporting the woman as she copes with her loss?
    a. Remind her that she should be happy that one daughter survived and is healthy.
    b. Assist the woman in taking pictures of both babies.
    c. Encourage the woman to hold the deceased twin in her arms to say good-bye.
    d. Offer her the opportunity for counseling to help her with her grief and that of her surviving twin as she gets older.

14. During the acute distress phase of the grief response parents are most likely to experience which of the following? (Circle all that apply.)
    a. Fear and anxiety about future pregnancies
    b. Difficulty with making decisions
    c. Search for meaning

d. Sadness and depression
e. Denial and disbelief
f. Guilt and helplessness

15. A 17-year-old woman experiences a miscarriage at 12 weeks of gestation. When she is informed about the miscarriage she begins to cry, stating that she was upset about her pregnancy at first and now she is being punished for not wanting her baby. Which of the following would be the nurse's best response?
    a. "You are still so young, you probably were not ready for a baby right now."
    b. "This must be so hard for you. I am here if you want to talk."
    c. "At least this happened early in your pregnancy before you felt your baby move."
    d. "God must have a good reason for letting this happen."

16. A woman experiencing heavy postpartum bleeding asks her nurse if there are any herbal remedies she can use as part of her treatment regimen. Which of the following would the nurse discuss with the woman? (Circle all that apply.)
    a. Blue cohosh
    b. Shepherd's purse
    c. St. John's wort
    d. Lavender tea
    e. Lady's Mantle
    f. Red raspberry leaves

17. The nurse caring for a women experiencing postpartum depression would question which of the following medication orders if a woman is breastfeeding?
    a. citalopram (Celexa)
    b. venlafaxine (Effexor)
    c. paroxetine (Paxil)
    d. doxepin (Sinequan)

III. THINKING CRITICALLY

1. Andrea is a multiparous woman (6-5-1-0-7) who gave birth to full-term twins vaginally 1 hour ago. Pitocin was used to augment her labor when hypotonic uterine contractions protracted the active stage of her labor. Special forceps were used to assist the birth of the second twin. Currently her vital signs are stable, her fundus is at the umbilicus, midline and firm, and her lochial flow is moderate to heavy without clots.

   a. Early postpartum hemorrhage is a major concern at this time. State the factors that have increased Andrea's risk for hemorrhage at this time.

   b. During the second hour after birth, the nurse notes that Andrea's perineal pad became saturated in 15 minutes and a large amount of blood had accumulated on the bed under her buttocks. Describe the nurse's initial response to this finding. State the rationale for the action you described.

c. The nurse prepares to administer 10 units of Pitocin intravenously as ordered by Andrea's physician. Explain the guidelines the nurse should follow in fulfilling this order.

d. During the assessment of Andrea, the nurse must be alert for signs of developing hypovolemic shock. Cite the signs the nurse would be watching for.

e. Describe the measures that the nurse should use to support Andrea and her family in an effort to reduce their anxiety.

2. Nurses working on a postpartum unit must be constantly alert for signs and symptoms of puerperal infection in their patients.

a. List the factors that can increase a postpartum woman's risk for puerperal infection.

b. State the typical clinical manifestations of endometritis for which the nurse should be alert when assessing post-partum women.

c. Describe the critical nursing measures that are essential in care management related to puerperal infection.

3. Sara, a primiparous breastfeeding mother at 2 weeks postpartum, calls her nurse-midwife to tell her that her right breast is painful and she's not "feeling well."

a. Explain the assessment findings the nurse-midwife would be alert for to indicate whether Sara is experiencing mastitis.

b. A medical diagnosis of mastitis of Sara's right breast is made. State two nursing diagnoses appropriate for this situation.

c. Describe the treatment measures and health teaching that Sara needs regarding her infection and breastfeeding, because she wishes to continue to breastfeed.

d. Identify several behaviors that Sara should learn to prevent recurrence of mastitis.

4. Susan is a 36-year-old obese multiparous woman (5-4-0-1-4) who experienced a cesarean birth 2 days ago. During this pregnancy, she was able to reduce her smoking of 1 pack of cigarettes each day to 1/2 pack per day. Although she has never experienced a deep vein thrombosis (DVT) or thrombophlebitis, she did develop varicose veins in both legs with her third pregnancy. A major complication of the postpartum period is the development of thromboembolic disease.

a. State the risk factors for this complication that Susan presents.

b. When assessing Susan on the afternoon of her second postpartum day, the nurse notes signs indicative of DVT. List the signs the nurse most likely observed.

c. A medical diagnosis of DVT is confirmed. State one nursing diagnosis appropriate for this situation.

d. Outline the expected care management for Susan during the acute phase of the DVT.

e. Upon discharge Susan will be taking warfarin for at least 3 months. Specify the discharge instructions that Susan and her family should receive.

5. Denise (6-5-0-1-5), a 60-year-old postmenopausal woman, has been diagnosed with cystocele and rectocele.

a. Describe the signs and symptoms Denise most likely exhibited that lead to this diagnosis.

b. Identify two priority nursing diagnoses related to the signs and symptoms Denise is most likely experiencing. Write one expected outcome for each of the nursing diagnoses identified.

c. Outline the care management approach recommended for Denise's health problem.

d. Denise will use a pessary during the day until a surgical repair can be accomplished. Specify the instructions the nurse would give to Denise regarding the use and care of a pessary.

6. Mary, a 35-year-old primiparous woman beginning her second week postpartum, is bottle-feeding her baby. She and her husband, Tom, moved from Buffalo, where they lived all their lives, to Los Angeles 2 months ago to take advantage of a career opportunity for Tom. They live in a community with many other young couples who are also starting families. Last month they joined the Catholic church near their home. Tom tries to help Mary with the baby but he has to spend long hours at work to establish his position. Mary's prenatal record reveals that she often exhibited anxiety about her well-being and that of her baby. During a home visit by a nurse, as part of an early discharge program, Mary tells the nurse that she always wants to sleep and just cannot seem to get enough rest. Mary is very concerned that she is not being a good mother and states, "Sometimes I just do not know what to do to care for my baby the right way, and I am not even breastfeeding my baby. It seems that Tom enjoys spending what little time he has at home with the baby and not with me. I even find myself yelling at him for the silliest things." The nurse recognizes that Mary is exhibiting behaviors strongly suggestive of postpartum depression.

   a. Indicate the signs and symptoms that Mary exhibited that led the nurse to suspect postpartum depression.

   b. Specify the risk factors for postpartum depression that are present in Mary's situation.

   c. Write several questions that the nurse could ask Mary to determine the depth of the postpartum depression that she is experiencing.

   d. Describe the measures the nurse could use to help Mary and Tom cope with postpartum depression.

7. Jane (2-1-0-0-1) is a 21-year-old woman admitted with vaginal bleeding at 13 weeks of gestation. She experiences a miscarriage. Jane is accompanied by her husband, Tom. Her 5-year-old daughter is at home with Jane's mother.

   a. Describe the approach you would take to develop a plan of individualized support measures for Jane as she and her family cope with their loss.

   b. Cite questions and observations you would use to gather the information required to create an individualized plan of care.

   c. Identify the therapeutic communication techniques you should use to help Jane and Tom acknowledge and express their feelings and emotions about their loss.

d. At discharge, Jane is crying. She tells you, "I know it must have been something I did wrong this time because my first pregnancy was okay. We wanted to give our daughter a baby brother or sister." Indicate whether the following responses would be therapeutic (T) or nontherapeutic (N). Specify how you would change the responses determined to be nontherapeutic.

(1). _____ "You are still young. As soon as your body heals, you will be able to try to have another baby."

(2). _____ "What can I do that would help you and Tom cope with what happened?"

(3). _____ "Do not worry. I am sure you did everything you could to have a healthy pregnancy."

(4). _____ "It was probably for the best. Fetal loss at this time is usually the result of defective development."

(5). _____ "You sound like you are blaming yourself for what happened. Let's talk about it."

(6). _____ "This must be difficult for you and your family."

(7). _____ "If it had to happen, it is best that it happened this early in the pregnancy before you and your family became attached to the fetus."

(8). _____ "You really should concentrate on your little daughter rather than thinking so much about the baby you lost."

(9). _____ "I feel sad about the loss that you and Tom are experiencing."

(10). _____ "Would you and Tom like to speak to our hospital's chaplain before you are discharged?"

8. Angela gave birth vaginally to a stillborn fetus at 38 weeks of gestation. In addition to emotional support, her physical needs must be recognized and met. Identify these physical needs and how you would meet them.

9. Anita gave birth to a baby boy who died shortly thereafter as a result of multiple congenital anomalies, including anencephaly. She and her husband, Bill, are provided with the opportunity to see their baby.

a. Discuss how the nurse can help Anita and Bill make a decision about seeing their baby that is right for them.

b. Anita and Bill decide to see their baby. Specify the measures the nurse can use to make the time Anita and Bill spend with their baby as easy as possible and to provide them with an experience that will facilitate the grieving process.

22 Physiologic and Behavioral Adaptations of the Newborn

I. LEARNING KEY TERMS

FILL IN THE BLANKS: Insert the term that corresponds to each of the following descriptions related to newborn characteristics and care.

1. _____ Environment that allows the newborn to maintain a stable normal body temperature.

2. _____ Heat production or generation; for the newborn, it occurs as a result of increased muscle activity.

3. _____ Heat production process unique to the newborn accomplished primarily by brown fat and secondarily by increased metabolic activity in the brain, heart, and liver.

4. _____ Flow of heat from the body surface to cooler ambient air. Two measures to reduce heat loss by this method would be to keep the ambient air at 24° C and wrap the infant.

5. _____ Loss of heat from the body surface to a cooler, solid surface not in direct contact but in relative proximity. To prevent this type of heat loss, cribs and examining tables are placed away from outside windows and care is taken to avoid direct air drafts.

6. _____ Loss of heat that occurs when a liquid is converted to vapor; in the newborn heat loss occurs when moisture from the skin is vaporized. This heat loss can be intensified by failure to dry the newborn directly after birth or by drying the newborn too slowly after a bath.

7. _____ Loss of heat from the body surface to cooler surfaces in direct contact. When admitted to the nursery, the newborn is placed in a warmed crib to minimize heat loss. Placing a protective cover on the scale when weighing the newborn will also minimize heat lost by this method.

8. _____ High body temperature that develops more rapidly in the newborn than in the adult. The newborn has a decreased ability to increase evaporative skin water losses because sweat glands do not function sufficiently to allow the newborn to sweat; serious overheating can cause cerebral damage from dehydration or heat stroke and death.

9. _____ Pinkish, easily blanched areas on the upper eyelids, nose, upper lip, back of head, and nape of neck. They are also known as stork bites or salmon patches.

10. _____ Overlapping of cranial bones to facilitate movement of the fetal head through the maternal pelvis during the process of labor and birth.

11. _____ Generalized, easily identifiable edematous area of the scalp usually over the occiput.

12. _____ Collection of blood between a skull bone and its periosteum as a result of pressure during birth.

13. _____ Bluish-black pigmented areas usually found on back and buttocks but can occur anywhere on the exterior surface of the body including the extremities.

14. _____ Bluish discoloration of the hands and feet, especially when chilled as a result of vasomotor instability and capillary stasis; it occurs for the first 7 to 10 days of life.

15. _____ White, cheesy substance that coats and protects the fetus's skin while in utero.

16. _____ White facial pimples caused by distended sebaceous glands.

17. _____ Yellowish skin discoloration caused by increased levels of serum bilirubin.

18. _____ Thick, tarry, dark green-black stool usually passed within 24 hours of birth.

19. _____ Transient newborn rash characterized by erythematous macules, papules, and small vesicles; it may appear suddenly anywhere on the body.

20. _____ Substance present in the urine of newborns that cause a pink-tinged stain or "brick dust" on the diaper; it is a normal finding and not representative of bleeding.

21. _____ Contraction of the anal sphincter in response to touch; it is a sign of good sphincter tone.

22. _____ Accumulation of fluid in the scrotum, around the testes.

23. _____ Bruising.

24. _____ Heart sound heard when fetal shunts (foramen ovale, ductus arteriosus) remain fully or partially open after birth permitting blood to continue to flow through.

25. _____ Soft, downy hair on face, shoulders, and back.

26. _____ Bleeding into a potential space in the brain that contains loosely arranged connective tissue; it is located beneath the tendinous sheath that connects the frontal and occipital muscles and forms the inner surface of the scalp. The injury occurs as a result of forces that compress and then drag the head through the pelvic outlet.

27. _____ Peeling of the skin that occurs in the term infant a few days after birth; if present at birth, it may be an indication of postmaturity.

28. _____ Flat red to purple birthmark composed of a plexus of newly formed capillaries in the papillary layer of the corium; it varies in size, shape, and location but is usually found on the neck and face. It does not blanch under pressure or disappear.

29. _____ Birthmark consisting of dilated, newly formed capillaries occupying the entire dermal and subdermal layers with associated connective tissue hypertrophy; it is typically a raised, sharply demarcated bright or dark red, rough-surfaced swelling that may proliferate and become more vascular as the infant grows; usually is found as a single lesion on the head.

30. _____ Slightly blood-tinged mucoid vaginal discharge associated with an estrogen decrease after birth.

31. _____ Foreskin.

32. _____ Protein that lines the alveoli resulting in a lower surface tension and alveolar stability with inspiration and expiration.

33. _____ Small, white, firm cysts that can be found on the gum margins and at the tip of the foreskin.

34. _____ Extra digits, fingers or toes. _____ Missing digits.

35. _____ Fused fingers or toes.

36. _____ Variations in the state of consciousness of newborn infants.

37. _____ and _____ The two sleep states. The newborn sleeps about 17 hours a day, with periods of wakefulness. _____ gradually.

38. _____, _____, _____, and _____ The four wake states.

39. _____ The optimum state of arousal in which the infant can be observed smiling, responding to voices, watching faces, vocalizing, and moving in synchrony.

40. _____ Ability of the newborn to modulate its state of consciousness, develop predictable sleep and wake states, and react appropriately to stress.

41. _____ Protective mechanism that allows the infant to become accustomed to environmental stimuli. It is a psychologic and physiologic phenomenon in which the response to a constant or repetitive stimulus is decreased.

42. _____ Quality of alert states and ability to attend to visual and auditory stimuli while alert.

43. _____ Ability of the newborn to comfort itself and reduce stress; one behavior a newborn uses is hand-to-mouth movements with or without sucking.

44. _____ Individual variations in a newborn's primary reaction pattern.

45. _____ Child who demonstrates regularity in bodily functions, readily adapts to change, has a predominantly positive mood and moderate sensory threshold, and approaches new situations or objects with a moderate response.

46. _____ Child who has a low activity level, withdraws with first exposure to new stimuli, is slow to adapt and low in intensity of response, and is somewhat negative in mood.

47. _____ Child who is irregular in bodily function, intense in reactions, generally negative in mood, and resistant to change or new stimuli and often cries loudly for long periods.

II. REVIEWING KEY CONCEPTS

1. The most critical adjustment that a newborn must make at birth is the establishment of respirations. List the factors that are responsible for the initiation of breathing after birth.

MATCHING: Match the description with the appropriate newborn reflex.

2. _____ Place infant supine and then partially flex both legs and apply light pressure with fingers to the soles of the feet — legs extend against examiner's pressure.

3. _____ Place infant supine on flat surface and make a loud abrupt noise (e.g., sharp hand clap)—symmetric abduction and extension of arms, fingers fan out, thumb and forefinger form a C; arms are then adducted into an embracing motion and return to relaxed flexion and movement.

4. _____ Place finger in palm of hand or at base of toes—infant's fingers curl around examiner's finger; toes curl downward.

5. _____ Place infant prone on flat surface, run finger down side of back first on one side and then down the other 4 to 5 cm lateral to spine—body flexes and pelvis swings toward stimulated side.

6. _____ Tap over forehead, bridge of nose, or maxilla when eyes are open— blinks for first four to five taps.

7. _____ Use finger to stroke sole of foot beginning at heel, upward along lateral aspect of sole, and then across ball of foot—all toes hyperextend, with dorsiflexion of big toe.

8. _____ Touch infant's lip, cheek, or corner of mouth with nipple or finger— turns head toward stimulus, opens mouth, takes hold, and sucks.

9. _____ Place infant in a supine neutral position, turn head quickly to one side—arm and leg extend on side to which head is turned while opposite arm and leg flex.

10. _____ Hold infant vertically under the arms or around the trunk allowing one foot to touch a flat surface — alternates flexion and extension of its feet; term infants will use soles of feet and preterm infants will use toes.

11. _____ Touch or depress tip of tongue — infant forces tongue outward.

12. _____ Place infant supine and then extend one leg, press knee downward, and stimulate the bottom of the foot — opposite leg flexes, adducts, and then extends as if the infant is attempting to push away the stimulation.

a. Rooting
b. Grasp
c. Extrusion
d. Glabellar (Myerson)
e. Tonic neck
f. Moro
g. Stepping (walking)
h. Babinski
i. Truncal incurvation (Galant)
j. Magnet
k. Crossed extension

13. During the first 6 to 8 hours after birth, newborns experience a transitional period characterized by three phases of instability. Indicate the timing/duration and typical behaviors for each phase of this transitional period.

    First period of reactivity

    Period of decreased responsiveness

    Second period of reactivity

14. A newborn, at 5 hours old, wakes from a sound sleep and becomes very active and begins to cry. Which of the following signs if exhibited by this newborn would indicate expected adaptation to extrauterine life? (Circle all that apply.)
    a. Increased mucus production
    b. Passage of meconium
    c. Heart rate of 160 beats per minute
    d. Respiratory rate of 24 breaths per minute and irregular
    e. Retraction of sternum with inspiration
    f. Expiratory grunting with nasal flaring

15. When assessing a newborn boy at 12 hours of age, the nurse notes a rash on his abdomen and thighs composed of reddish macules, papules, and small vesicles. The nurse would:
    a. document the finding as erythema toxicum.
    b. isolate the newborn and his mother until infection is ruled out.
    c. apply an antiseptic ointment to each lesion.
    d. request nonallergenic linen from the laundry.

16. A breastfed full-term newborn girl is 12 hours old and is being prepared for early discharge. Which of the following assessment findings, if present, could delay discharge?
    a. Dark green–black stool, tarry in consistency
    b. Yellowish tinge in sclera and on face
    c. Swollen breasts with a scant amount of thin discharge
    d. Blood-tinged mucoid vaginal discharge

17. As part of a thorough assessment, the newborn should be checked for hip dislocation and dysplasia. Which of the following techniques would be used?
    a. Check for syndactyly bilaterally
    b. Stepping or walking reflex
    c. Magnet reflex
    d. Ortolani's maneuver

18. When assessing a newborn after birth, the nurse notes flat, irregular, pinkish marks on the bridge of the nose, nape of neck, and over the eyelids. The areas blanch when pressed with a finger. The nurse would document this finding as:
    a. milia.
    b. nevus vasculosus.
    c. telangiectatic nevi.
    d. nevus flammeus.

III. THINKING CRITICALLY

1. When caring for newborns, especially during the transition period following birth, the nurse recognizes that newborns are at increased risk for cold stress.

    a. Explain the basis for this risk.

    b. State the danger that cold stress poses for the newborn.

    c. Identify one nursing diagnosis and one expected outcome related to this danger.

    d. Describe care measures the nurse should implement to prevent cold stress from occurring.

2. After a long and difficult labor, baby boy James was born with a caput succedaneum and significant molding over the occipital area. Low forceps were used for the birth, resulting in ecchymotic areas on both cheeks. James' parents tell the nurse that they are very concerned that James may have experienced brain damage. Describe what the nurse should tell the parents of James about these assessment findings.

3. During the first 24 hours of life, it is essential that the nurse monitor a newborn's breathing pattern for signs of distress. Create a checklist that could be used by a nurse to determine if a newborn is exhibiting eupnea (normal breathing pattern) or dyspnea (respiratory distress).

4. Susan and Allen are first-time parents of a baby girl. They ask the nurse about their baby's ability to see and hear things around her and to interact with them.

    a. Specify what the nurse should tell these parents about the sensory capabilities of their healthy full-term newborn.

    b. Name four stimuli Susan and Allen could provide for their baby that would help foster her development.

5. Tonya and Sam, an African-American couple, express concern that their new baby girl has several bruises on her back and buttocks. They ask if their baby was injured during birth or in the nursery. Describe the appropriate response of the nurse to this couple's concern.

6. Jaundice in the newborn can represent a normal physiologic response or indicate pathology. Compare and contrast each type of jaundice identified below in terms of causation, characteristics, and significance.

a. Physiologic (nonpathologic) jaundice

b. Pathologic (nonphysiologic) jaundice

c. Breastfeeding-associated jaundice

d. Breast-milk jaundice

23 Nursing Care of the Newborn and Family

I. LEARNING KEY TERMS

FILL IN THE BLANKS: Insert the term that corresponds to each of the following descriptions of newborns and their care.

1. _____ Assessment method used to rapidly assess the newborn's transition to extrauterine existence at 1 and 5 minutes after birth; it is based on five signs that indicate his or her physiologic state, namely: _____, _____, _____, _____, and _____.

2. _____ Device used to suction mucus and secretions from the newborn's mouth and nose immediately after birth and when needed.

3. _____ Automatic sensor usually placed on the upper quadrant of the abdomen immediately below the right or left costal margin; it is attached to the radiant warmer and monitors the newborn's skin temperature.

4. _____ Inflammation of the newborn's eyes from gonorrheal or chlamydial infection contracted by the newborn during passage through the mother's birth canal. _____ or _____ ointment is usually instilled into the newborn's eyes within 1 to 2 hours after birth to prevent this infection.

5. _____ Medication administered intramuscularly to the newborn to prevent hemorrhagic disease of the newborn; it is administered in a dose of 0.5 to 1 mg using a 25-gauge, 5/8- to 7/8-inch needle.

6. _____ Scale currently used to assess and estimate a newborn's gestational age at birth; the initial assessment should be performed within the first 48 hours of life to ensure accuracy and assesses physical and neurologic maturity.

7. _____ Term that describes an infant whose birthweight falls between the 10th and 90th percentiles as a result of growing at a normal rate during fetal life regardless of length of gestation.

8. _____ Term that describes an infant whose birthweight falls above the 90th percentile as a result of growing at an accelerated rate during fetal life regardless of length of gestation.

9. _____ Term that describes an infant whose birthweight falls below the 10th percentile as a result of growing at a restricted rate during fetal life regardless of length of gestation.

10. _____ Infant born between 34 0/7 to 36 6/7 weeks of gestation; this infant has risk factors because of his or her physiologic immaturity that require close attention by nurses working with them.

11. _____ Infant born before the completion of 37 weeks of gestation, regardless of birth weight.

12. _____ Infant born between the beginning of week 38 and the end of week 42 of gestation.

13. _____ Infant born after completion of week 42 of gestation.

14. _____ Infant born after completion of week 42 of gestation and showing the effects of progressive placental insufficiency.

15. _____ Infants born from 37 0/7 to 38 6/7 weeks of gestation; a recent increase in the birth of these infants is associated with elective inductions and elective cesarean births that are scheduled before 39 weeks.

16. _____ Pinpoint hemorrhagic areas acquired during birth that may extend over the upper trunk and face; they are benign if they disappear within 2 to 3 days of birth and no new lesions appear.

17. _____ One of the products derived from the hemoglobin released with the breakdown of red blood cells and the myoglobin in muscle cells; its accumulation in the blood results in a yellowish discoloration of the skin, sclera, and oral mucous membranes.

149

18. _____ Yellowish discoloration of the integument and sclera that first appears after the first 24 hours of life and disappears by the end of the seventh day of life.

19. _____ Test performed to distinguish cutaneous jaundice of the skin from normal skin color. It is performed by applying pressure with a finger over a bony area, usually the nose, forehead, or sternum, for several seconds to empty all capillaries in the spot. The area will appear yellow when the finger is removed if jaundice is present.

20. _____ Level of serum bilirubin, which, if left untreated, can result in sensorineural hearing loss, mild cognitive delays, and deposition of bilirubin in the brain; it typically appears during the first 24 hours following birth.

21. _____ Yellow staining of brain cells that may result in bilirubin encephalopathy.

22. _____ Device used for noninvasive monitoring of bilirubin via cutaneous reflectance measurements; it allows for repetitive estimation of bilirubin and works well on both dark- and light-skinned newborns.

23. _____ Common method used to reduce the level of circulating unconjugated bilirubin or to keep it from increasing; it uses light energy to change the shape and structure of unconjugated bilirubin and convert it to molecules that can be excreted.

24. _____ Blood glucose concentration less than adequate to support neurologic, organ, and tissue function during the early newborn period; the precise level at which this occurs in every neonate is not known although intervention is usually required if the blood glucose level falls below 40 to 45 mg/dL.

25. _____ Serum calcium level less than 7.8 to 8 mg/dL in the term infant and less than 7 mg/dL in the preterm infant.

26. _____ Newborn respiratory rate of 30 breaths per minute or lower.

27. _____ Newborn respiratory rate of 60 breaths per minute or higher.

28. _____ The most important single measure in the prevention of neonatal infection.

29. _____ An alternative device for phototherapy in the treatment of hyperbilirubinemia; it involves a fiberoptic panel attached to an illuminator.

30. _____ Surgical procedure that involves removing the prepuce (foreskin) of the glans penis.

II. REVIEWING KEY CONCEPTS

1. Outline the specific measures nurses should use when caring for newborns to ensure a safe and protective environment.

2. Describe the approach you would use to ensure accuracy when performing each of the following measurements on a newborn.

    a. Weight

    b. Length

    c. Head circumference

    d. Chest circumference

3. Preparing parents for the discharge of their newborn requires informing them about the essential aspects of newborn care. Identify three points that you would emphasize when teaching parents about each of the following aspects of newborn characteristics and care:

    a. Vital signs: temperature and respirations

b. Elimination: urinary and bowel

c. Positioning and holding

d. Safety

e. Hygiene: bathing, cord care, and skin care

4. Nurses caring for newborns are often required to collect blood and urine specimens for laboratory testing. Outline the guidelines nurses should use for each of the following specimen collection techniques.

Heel stick

Venipuncture

Collection bag for specimen collection

5. Maintaining a patent airway and supporting respirations to ensure an adequate oxygen supply in the newborn are essential focuses of nursing care management of the newborn, especially in the early postbirth period.

a. State the four conditions that are essential for maintaining an adequate oxygen supply in the newborn.

b. List four signs that the nurse who is assessing a newborn would recognize as indicative of abnormal breathing.

6. A newborn male is estimated to be at 40 weeks of gestation following an assessment using the New Ballard scale. Which of the following would be a Ballard scale finding consistent with this newborn's full-term status? (Circle all that apply.)
   a. Apical pulse rate of 120 beats per minute, regular, and strong
   b. Popliteal angle of 160 degrees
   c. Weight of 3200 g, placing him at the 50th percentile
   d. Thinning of lanugo with some bald areas
   e. Testes descended into the scrotum
   f. Elbow does not pass midline when arm is pulled across the chest

7. The nurse evaluates the laboratory test results of a full term newborn who is 4 hours old. Which of the following results would require notification of the pediatrician? (Circle all that apply.)
   a. Hemoglobin 20 g/dL
   b. Hematocrit 54%
   c. Glucose 34 mg/dL
   d. Total serum bilirubin 3.1 mg/dL
   e. White blood cell count 24,000/mm^3
   f. Calcium 6 mg/dL

8. A newborn male has been designated as large for gestational age. His mother was diagnosed with gestational diabetes late in her pregnancy. The nurse should be alert for signs of hypoglycemia. Which of the following assessment findings would be consistent with a diagnosis of hypoglycemia?
   a. Hyperthermia
   b. Jitteriness
   c. Loose, watery stools
   d. Laryngospasm

9. A radiant warmer will be used to help a newborn girl to stabilize her temperature. The nurse implementing this care measure should do which of the following?
   a. Undress and dry the infant before placing her under the warmer.
   b. Set the control panel between 35° to 38° C.
   c. Place the thermistor probe on her abdomen just below her umbilical cord.
   d. Assess her rectal temperature every hour until her temperature stabilizes.

10. A newborn male has been scheduled for a circumcision. Essential nursing care measures following this surgical procedure would include which one of the following?
    a. Administer oral acetaminophen every 6 hours for a maximum of 4 doses in 24 hours.
    b. Apply petroleum jelly or A&D ointment to the site with every diaper change.
    c. Check the penis for bleeding every 15 minutes for the first 4 hours.
    d. Teach the parents to remove the yellowish exudate that forms over the glans using a diaper wipe.

11. The doctor has ordered that a newborn receive a hepatitis B vaccination prior to discharge. In fulfilling this order, the nurse should do which of the following? (Circle all that apply.)
    a. Confirm that the mother is hepatitis B positive before the injection is given.
    b. Obtain parental consent prior to administering the vaccination.
    c. Inform the parents that the next vaccine in the series would need to be given in 1 to 2 months.
    d. Administer the injection into the vastus lateralis muscle.
    e. Use a 1-inch, 23-gauge needle.
    f. Insert the needle at a 45-degree angle.

12. The nurse is preparing to administer erythromycin ophthalmic ointment 0.5% to a newborn after birth. Which of the following nursing actions would be appropriate? (Circle all that apply.)
    a. Administer the ointment within 30 minutes of the birth.
    b. Wear gloves.
    c. Cleanse eyes if secretions are present.
    d. Squeeze an ointment ribbon of 1 to 2 inches into the lower conjunctival sac.
    e. Wipe away excess ointment after 1 minute.
    f. Apply the ointment from inner to outer canthus.

III. THINKING CRITICALLY

1. Apgar scoring is a method of newborn assessment used in the immediate postbirth period, at 1 and 5 minutes. Indicate the Apgar score for each of the following newborns.

    a. Baby boy Smith at 1 minute after birth:
    Heart rate—160 beats/min
    Respiratory effort—good, crying vigorously
    Muscle tone—active movement, well flexed
    Reflex irritability—cries with stimulus to soles of feet
    Color—body pink, feet and hands cyanotic
       Score:
       Interpretation:

    b. Baby girl Doe at 5 minutes after birth:
    Heart rate—102 beats/min
    Respiratory effort—slow, irregular with weak cry
    Muscle tone—some flexion of extremities
    Reflex irritability—grimace with stimulus to soles of feet
    Color—pale
       Score:
       Interpretation:

2. Baby girl June was just born.

    a. Outline the protocol that the nurse should follow when assessing June's physical status during the first 2 hours after her birth.

    b. State the nurse's legal responsibility regarding identification of June and her mother after birth.

c. Cite the priority nursing care measures that the nurse must implement to ensure June's well-being and safety during the first 2 hours after birth.

d. Describe the emotional and physiologic benefits of early contact between the mother and her newborn.

3. Baby boy Tim is 24 hours old. The nurse is preparing to perform a physical examination of this newborn before his discharge.

   a. List the actions the nurse should take in order to ensure safety and accuracy. Include the rationale for the actions identified.

   b. Identify the major points that should be assessed as part of this physical examination.

   c. Support the premise that Tim's parents should be present during this examination.

4. Baby girl Susan has an accumulation of mucus in her nasal passages and mouth, making breathing difficult.

   a. State the nursing diagnosis represented by the assessment findings.

   b. List the steps that the nurse should follow when clearing Susan's airway using a bulb syringe.

5. Susan and James are taking their newly circumcised (6 hours postprocedure) baby home. This is their first baby and they express anxiety concerning care of both the circumcision and the umbilical cord.

   a. State one nursing diagnosis related to this situation.

   b. State one expected outcome related to the nursing diagnosis identified.

   c. Specify the instructions that the nurse should give to Susan and James regarding assessment of both sites and the care measures required to facilitate healing.

6. Andrew and Marion are parents of a newborn, 30 hours old, who has developed hyperbilirubinemia. They are very concerned about the color of their baby and the need to put the baby under special lights. "A relative was yellow just like our baby and later died of liver cancer!"

   a. Describe how the nurse should respond to Andrew and Marion's concern.

   b. Describe the blanch test as a method of assessment for jaundice.

   c. Identify the expected assessment findings and physiologic effects related to hyperbilirubinemia.

   d. List the precautions and care measures required by the newborn undergoing phototherapy in order to prevent injury to the newborn yet maintain the effectiveness of the treatment. State the rationale for each action identified.

7. A newborn male has just been circumcised. Explain what the CRIES assessment tool entails and why it would be appropriate to use it at this time.

I. LEARNING KEY TERMS

FILL IN THE BLANKS: Insert the term that corresponds to the following descriptions of breast structures and the breastfeeding process.

1. _____ Structures in the breast that are composed of alveoli, milk ductules, and myoepithelial cells.

2. _____ Milk-producing cells.

3. _____ Breast structure that transports milk from the alveoli to the nipple.

4. _____ Sebaceous glands found on the areola that secrete an oily substance to provide protection against the mechanical stress of sucking and the invasion of pathogens; the odor of the secretion can be a means of communication with the infant.

5. _____ Reflex that occurs when the infant cries, suckles, or rubs against the breast.

6. _____ Cells surrounding alveoli; these cells contract in response to oxytocin, resulting in the milk ejection reflex or let-down.

7. _____ Rounded, pigmented section of tissue surrounding the nipple.

8. _____ The process of milk production.

9. _____ The lactogenic hormone secreted by the anterior pituitary gland in response to the infant's suck and emptying of the breast.

10. _____ Posterior pituitary hormone that triggers the let-down reflex.

11. _____ Nipple type that becomes hard, erect, and protrudes upon stimulation, thereby facilitating latch-on. _____ Nipple type that remains flat and soft and does not protrude even when stimulated.

12. _____ Plastic device that can be placed over the nipple and areola to keep clothing off the nipple and put pressure around the base of the nipple to promote protrusion of the nipple.

13. _____ Herbal or pharmaceutical agent reported to increase breast milk production.

14. _____ Very concentrated, clear yellowish fluid that is high in protein and antibodies; it is present in the breasts before the formation of milk.

15. _____ Difficulty in knowing how to latch on to the breast after having taken a bottle or artificial nipple (pacifier).

16. _____ Newborn behaviors that indicate hunger and a desire to eat such as hand to mouth movements, rooting, and mouth and tongue movements.

17. _____ or _____ Reflex triggered by the contraction of myoepithelial cells. Colostrum, and later milk, is ejected toward the nipple.

18. _____ Reflex stimulated when a hungry baby's lower lip is touched. The baby opens its mouth and begins to suck.

19. _____ Placing the baby onto the breast with the mouth open wide and the tongue down. The nipple and some of the areola should be in the baby's mouth, making a seal between the mouth and the breast to create adequate suction for milk removal.

20. _____ Breast response that occurs around the third to fifth day, when the "milk comes in" and blood supply to the breasts increases. The breasts become tender, swollen, hot and hard, and even shiny and red.

21. _____ Breastfeeding position in which the mother holds the baby's head and shoulders in her hand with the baby's back and body tucked under her arm.

22. _____ Breastfeeding position in which the baby's head is positioned in the crook of the mother's arm and the mother and baby are "tummy to tummy."

23. _____ Health care professional who specializes in breastfeeding and may be available to assist a new mother with breast-feeding while in the hospital or after discharge.

24. _____ Infection of the breast manifested by a swollen, tender breast and sudden onset of flu-like symptoms.

25. _____ Oral infection caused by a fungus or yeast.

26. _____ Short frenu-lum, which interferes with extrusion and effective sucking.

27. _____ Process whereby the infant is gradually introduced to drinking from a cup and eating solid food while breastfeeding or bottle-feeding is reduced by gradually decreasing the number of feedings.

28. _____ Milk that is initially released with breastfeeding; it is bluish white, is composed of part skim milk and part whole milk, and provides primarily lactose, protein, and water-soluble vitamins.

29. _____ Milk that is let down 10 to 20 minutes into the feeding; often called the cream, it is denser in calories from fat necessary for optimal growth and contentment between feedings.

30. _____ Jaundice (hyperbilirubinemia) that occurs in breastfeeding infants as a result of insufficient feeding and infre-quent stooling.

31. _____ Jaundice (hyperbilirubinemia) that occurs in breastfed new-borns between 5 and 10 days of age; they are typically thriving, gaining weight, and stooling normally. A brief interruption of breastfeeding for 12 to 24 hours may be recommended.

II. REVIEWING KEY CONCEPTS

1. A nurse has been asked to participate in a women's health seminar for women of childbearing age in the community. Her topic is "Breastfeeding: The Goals for *Healthy People 2020* and Beyond." Outline the points that this nurse should emphasize to help women appreciate the benefits of breastfeeding and seriously consider breastfeeding when they have a baby.

2. It is important that a breastfeeding woman alter the position she uses for breastfeeding as one means of preserving nipple and areolar integrity. Describe four breastfeeding positions the nurse should demonstrate to a woman who is breastfeeding her newborn.

3. Infants exhibit feeding cues as they recognize and express their hunger.

   a. Identify feeding cues of the infant.

   b. State why the new mother should be guided by these cues when determining the timing of feeding sessions.

4. Proper latch (latch-on) is essential for effective breast-feeding and preservation of nipple and areolar tissue integrity.

   a. Indicate the steps the nurse should teach a breast-feeding woman to follow to ensure a proper latch-on.

   b. When observing a woman breastfeeding, it is essen-tial that the nurse determine the effectiveness of the latch-on. State the signs a nurse should look for that would indicate a proper latch-on.

   c. Describe the way a woman should remove her baby from her breast after feeding is completed.

5. During a home visit, the mother of a 1-week-old in-fant son tells the nurse that she is very concerned about whether her baby is getting enough breast milk. The nurse would tell this mother that at 1 week of age a well-nourished newborn should exhibit which of the following?
   a. Weight gain sufficient to reach his birthweight
   b. A minimum of three bowel movements each day
   c. Approximately 10 to 12 wet diapers each day

d. Breastfeeding at a frequency of every 4 hours or about 6 times each day

6. A woman is trying to calm her fussy baby daughter in preparation for feeding. She exhibits a need for further instruction if she does which of the following?
   a. Swaddles the baby
   b. Dims lights in the room and turns off the television
   c. Gently rocks the baby and talks to her in a low voice
   d. Attempts to get the baby to latch on immediately

7. The nurse should teach breastfeeding mothers about breast care measures to preserve the integrity of the nipples and areola. Which of the following should the nurse include in these instructions?
   a. Cleanse nipples and areola twice a day with mild soap and water.
   b. Apply vitamin E cream to nipples and areola at least four times each day before a feeding.
   c. Insert plastic-lined pads into the bra to absorb leakage and protect clothing.
   d. Place a nipple shell into the bra if nipples are sore.

8. A breastfeeding woman asks the nurse about what birth control she should use during the postpartum period. Which is the best recommendation for a safe, yet effective method during the first 6 weeks after birth?
   a. Combination oral contraceptive that she used before she was pregnant
   b. Barrier method using a combination of a condom and spermicide foam
   c. Resume using the diaphragm she used prior to getting pregnant
   d. Complete breastfeeding—baby only receives breast milk for nourishment

9. A woman has determined that bottle-feeding is the best feeding method for her. Instructions the woman should receive regarding this feeding method should include which of the following?
   a. Provide the infant with supplemental vitamins along with the iron-fortified formula.

b. Sterilize water by boiling, then cool and mix with formula powder or concentrate.
c. Expect a 2-week-old newborn to drink approximately 30 to 60 mL of formula at each feeding.
d. Microwave refrigerated formula for about 2 minutes before feeding the newborn.

10. A nurse is evaluating a woman's breastfeeding technique. Which of the following actions would indicate that the woman needs further instruction regarding breastfeeding to ensure success? (Circle all that apply.)
    a. Washes her breasts and nipples thoroughly with soap and water twice a day
    b. Massages a small amount of breast milk into her nipple and areola before and after each feeding
    c. Lines her bra with a thick plastic-lined pad to absorb leakage
    d. Positions baby supporting back and shoulders securely and then brings her breast toward the baby, putting the nipple in the baby's mouth
    e. Feeds her baby every 2 to 3 hours
    f. Inserts her finger into the corner of her baby's mouth between the gums before removing him from the breast

11. A new breastfeeding mother asks the nurse how to prevent nipple soreness. The nurse tells this woman that the key to preventing sore nipples would be which of the following?
    a. Limiting the length of breastfeeding to no more than 10 minutes on each breast until the milk comes in
    b. Applying lanolin to each nipple and areola after each feeding
    c. Using correct breastfeeding technique
    d. Using nipple shells to protect the nipples and areola between feeding

III. THINKING CRITICALLY

1. Elise and her husband, Mark, are experiencing their first pregnancy. During one of their prenatal visits, they tell the nurse that they are as yet unsure about the method they want to use for feeding their baby. "Everyone has an opinion—some say breastfeeding is best, yet others tell us that bottle-feeding is more convenient, especially because the father can help. What should we do?"

   a. Identify one nursing diagnosis and one expected outcome appropriate for this situation.

   b. Discuss why it is important for the pregnant couple to make this decision together.

c. Indicate why is it preferable to make this decision during the prenatal period rather than waiting until the baby is born.

d. Describe how the nurse could use the decision-making process to assist Elise and Mark to choose the method that is best for them.

2. Mary, as a first-time breastfeeding mother, has many questions. Describe how you would respond to the following questions and comments.

a. "I am so afraid that I will not make enough milk for my baby. My breasts are not as large as some of my friends who breastfeed."

b. "Everyone keeps talking about this let-down that is supposed to happen. What is it and how will I know I have it?"

c. "How can I possibly know if breastfeeding is going well and my baby is getting enough if I cannot tell how many ounces he gets with each feeding?"

d. "It is only the first day that I am breastfeeding and my nipples already feel sore. What can I do to relieve this soreness and prevent it from getting worse?"

e. "My friends all told me to watch out for the fourth day and engorgement. What can I do to keep it from being too bad and to take care of myself when it occurs?"

f. "Every time I breastfeed, I get cramps and my flow seems to get heavier. Is there something wrong with me?"

g. "I am so glad I do not have to worry about getting pregnant again as long as I am breastfeeding. I hate using birth control and my friend told me I do not have to as long as I am breastfeeding."

h. "I would like to keep breastfeeding my baby for at least 6 months but I need to return to work in 6 weeks. What should I do when I am ready to stop breastfeeding my baby?"

3. Susan is 2 days old. She last fed 5 hours ago. Her mother tells the nurse that Susan is so sleepy that she just does not have the heart to wake her.

   a. Identify one nursing diagnosis and one expected outcome appropriate for this newborn.

   b. Discuss the approach the nurse should take with regard to this situation.

4. Alice has decided that for personal and professional reasons, bottle-feeding with a commercially prepared formula is the feeding method that is best for her. She tells the nurse that she hopes she made a good decision for her baby. "I hope she will be well nourished and feel that I love her even though I am bottle-feeding."

   a. Describe how the nurse should respond to Alice's concern.

   b. State three guidelines for bottle-feeding technique that the nurse should teach Alice to ensure the safety and health of her baby.

5. Prior to discharge, a nurse is evaluating a woman's ability to breastfeed and her newborn's response to breastfeeding.

   a. Identify the factors that the nurse should assess before and during breastfeeding to ensure that this mother and newborn are ready to breastfeed at home.

   b. After determining that breastfeeding is progressing well, the woman is discharged. One week later the nurse calls the woman to discuss breastfeeding. Write several questions this nurse should ask to determine whether breastfeeding is continuing to progress normally.

25 The High Risk Newborn

I. LEARNING KEY TERMS

MATCHING: Match each term with its definition.

1. _____ Birth injury in which the upper nerve plexus is damaged resulting in an immobilized, limp arm with an intact grasp reflex (often remembered by statement "can hold a cup but cannot carry it").

2. _____ Birth injury in which the lower plexus is damaged resulting in wrist drop and relaxed fingers yet arm movement is not restricted (often remembered by statement "can carry a cup but cannot hold it").

3. _____ Infant whose birthweight is less than 2500 g, regardless of gestational age.

4. _____ Infant whose birthweight is less than 1500 g.

5. _____ Infant whose birthweight is less than 1000 g.

6. _____ Infant born before completion of 37 weeks of gestation, regardless of birthweight. These infants are at risk because their organ systems are immature and they lack adequate physiologic reserves to function in an extrauterine environment.

7. _____ Infants born between 34 and 36 6/7 weeks of gestation regardless of birthweight; by nature of their limited gestation, these infants remain at risk for problems related to thermoregulation, hypoglycemia, hyperbilirubinemia, sepsis, and respiratory function.

8. _____ Infant born between the beginning of 38 weeks and the completion of 42 weeks of gestation, regardless of birthweight.

9. _____ An infant born after 42 weeks of gestational age, regardless of birthweight.

10. _____ Infant whose birthweight falls above the 90th percentile on intrauterine growth curves.

11. _____ Infant whose rate of intrauterine growth was restricted and whose birthweight falls below the 10th percentile on intrauterine growth curves.

12. _____ Respiratory pattern commonly seen in preterm infants; such infants exhibit 5- to 10-second respiratory pauses followed by 10 to 15 seconds of compensatory rapid respirations.

a. Late preterm infant

b. Kangaroo care

c. Surfactant

d. Early-onset sepsis

e. Neutral thermal environment

f. Neonatal death

g. Apnea

h. Periodic breathing

i. Premature or preterm infant

j. Large for gestational age

k. Small for gestational age

l. Full term infant

m. Erb palsy

n. Klumpke palsy

o. Low-birth-weight (LBW)

p. Very-low-birth-weight (VLBW)

q. Extremely-low-birth-weight (ELBW)

r. Postterm infant

s. Macrosomia

t. Phototherapy

u. Jaundice

v. Hypoglycemia

13. _____ Cessation of respirations of 20 seconds or more.

14. _____ Surface-active phospholipid secreted by the alveolar epithelium; it reduces the surface tension of fluids that line the alveoli and respiratory passages, resulting in uniform expansion and maintenance of lung expansion at low intraalveolar pressure.

15. _____ The environmental temperature at which oxygen consumption and metabolic rate are minimal but adequate to maintain the body temperature.

16. _____ Death that occurs in the first 27 days of life; it is described as early if it occurs in the first week of life and late if it occurs at 7 to 27 days.

17. _____ Method that can be used to provide maternal or paternal skin-to-skin contact with their newborn and to reduce stress in the infant.

18. _____ Large for gestational age infant; infant is at increased risk for hypoglycemia, hypocalcemia, hyperviscosity, hyperbilirubinemia, and birth trauma.

19. _____ Presence of a bacterial infection in the newborn with symptoms developing within the first 24 to 48 hours of life; infection is acquired in the perinatal period.

20. _____ Noninvasive method used to treat high levels of circulating bilirubin in newborn infant.

21. _____ A transient yellowish discoloration of the skin and sclera that first appears after 24 hours of life and disappears by the end of the seventh day of life.

22. _____ Common condition that occurs in infants of diabetic mothers (IDM) within minutes to hours after birth; signs and symptoms are variable and infant may be asymptomatic or may have tremors, poor feeding, or respiratory distress.

FILL IN THE BLANKS: Insert the term that corresponds to each of the following descriptions.

23. _____ Acronym used to designate certain maternal infections during early pregnancy that are known to be associated with various congenital malformations and disorders.

24. _____ Neonatal infection with this virus can result in disseminated infection, localized CNS disease, or localized infection of the skin, eye, or mouth.

25. _____ Infection with this virus during pregnancy can result in miscarriage, stillbirth, or congenital illness including microcephaly, hearing loss, and cognitive impairment; it is the most common cause of congenital viral infections in the United States.

26. The single most effective measure to reduce health care-associated infections in high risk infants is _____.

27. _____ Group of disorders caused by fetal exposure to alcohol, which can result in growth restriction, dysmorphic facial features, and CNS involvement.

28. _____ Disorder that occurs when the blood groups of the mother and newborn are different; the most common of these are Rh incompatibility and ABO incompatibility.

29. _____ Condition in which the fetus produces large numbers of immature erythrocytes to replace those hemolyzed as a result of severe Rh incompatibility. _____ The most severe form of this condition; it is characterized by marked anemia with hypoxia, cardiac decompensation, cardiomegaly, hepatosplenomegaly, and generalized edema.

30. _____ Blood test used to determine whether maternal blood contains antibodies to the Rh antigen.

31. _____ Blood test performed on cord blood to determine whether fetal blood contains maternal antibodies to the Rh antigen.

32. _____ The term used to describe the set of behaviors exhibited by infants exposed to narcotics in utero.

33. _____ The most accurate sampling medium used to determine presence of drugs to which the newborn has been exposed in utero.

34. _____ Multisystem disease caused by protozoa found in the feces of infected cats.

35. _____ A group of disorders caused by a metabolic defect that results from the absence of, or a change in, a protein, usually an enzyme and mediated by the action of a certain gene. Examples include phenylketonuria and galactosemia.

36. _____ In this disorder the infant is placed on a low phenylalanine diet and this diet is maintained throughout life to prevent severe cognitive impairment.

37. _____ Disorder in which the affected infant does not properly convert galactose into glucose resulting in cataracts, profoundly stunted growth, *E. Coli* sepsis and eventual death of treatment is not implemented early in infancy.

38. _____ Treatment of this disorder involves the lifelong administration of thyroxine.

39. _____ The bone most often fractured at birth, especially in large for gestational age infants and IDMs.

40. _____ Nerve injury occurring at birth in which the diaphragm does not expand adequately, often resulting in respiratory distress.

41. _____ Cooling of the infant's head or entire body to reduce severity of neurologic injury in hypoxic ischemic encephalopathy.

42. _____ Complex, multicausal disorder that affects the developing blood vessels in the eyes; it is often associated with oxygen tensions that are too high for the level of retinal maturity, initially resulting in vasoconstriction and continuing problems after the oxygen is discontinued. Scar tissue formation and consequent visual impairment may be mild or severe.

43. _____ Acute inflammatory disease of the gastrointestinal mucosa commonly complicated by perforation; intestinal ischemia, colonization by pathogenic bacteria, and formula feeding all play an important role in its development.

44. _____ Occurs when the fetal shunt between the left pulmonary artery and the aorta fails to constrict after birth or reopens after constriction has occurred.

45. _____ Chronic lung disease with a multifactorial etiology that includes pulmonary immaturity, surfactant deficiency, lung injury and stretch, barotrauma, inflammation caused by oxygen exposure, fluid overload, ligation of a PDA, and genetic predisposition; it is primarily seen in infants weighing less than 1000 g who are born at less than 28 weeks of gestation.

46. _____ Lung disorder caused by a lack of pulmonary surfactant, which leads to progressive atelectasis, loss of functional residual capacity, and ventilation-perfusion imbalance with an uneven distribution of ventilation; it usually affects preterm infants and a small percentage of term and near-term infants.

47. _____ Combined findings of pulmonary hypertension, right-to-left shunting, and a structurally normal heart; it is also called *persistent fetal circulation* because the syndrome includes reversion to fetal pathways for blood flow.

II. REVIEWING KEY CONCEPTS

1. The clinical manifestations of perinatal drug exposure may occur in any one or all of the following categories: CNS, gastrointestinal, respiratory, and autonomic nervous system signs. List some common signs of each category:

   Central Nervous System

   Gastrointestinal

   Respiratory

   Autonomic Nervous System

2. Explain the relationship between neonatal hypoglycemia and intrauterine hyperinsulism in the infant of a diabetic mother (IDM).

3. IDMs are at risk for a variety of congenital anomalies and problems at birth. List at least two congenital anomalies or disorders in each category below:

   Metabolic

   Cardiac

   Central Nervous System

   Hematologic

4. What measures should the nurse emphasize when managing the care of pregnant women with gestational diabetes to reduce the risk for fetal congenital anomalies?

5. Explain the pathogenesis of Rh incompatibility and ABO incompatibility.

6. An Rh-negative woman (2-2-0-0-2) just gave birth to a healthy term Rh-positive baby boy. The direct and indirect Coombs' test results are both negative. The nurse should do which of the following?
   a. Prepare to administer Rho(D) immune globulin (RhoGAM) to the newborn within 24 hours of his birth.
   b. Observe the newborn closely for signs of jaundice appearing within 24 hours of birth.
   c. Recognize that RhoGAM is not needed because both Coombs' test results are negative.
   d. Administer Rho(D) immune globulin intramuscularly to the woman within 72 hours of her baby's birth.

7. The nursing care management of a newborn whose mother is HIV positive would most likely include which of the following? (Circle all that apply.)
   a. Isolating the newborn in a special nursery
   b. Implementing standard precautions immediately after birth
   c. Telling the mother that she should not breastfeed
   d. Wearing gloves for routine care measures such as feeding
   e. Initiating treatment with antiviral medication(s) as soon as the newborn is confirmed to be HIV positive
   f. Preparing to administer antibiotics to prevent the newborn from developing opportunistic infections

8. The preterm infant is vulnerable to a number of complications related to immaturity of body systems. Identify the potential problems and their physiologic basis for each of the areas listed below.

   Respiratory function

Cardiovascular function

Thermoregulation

Central nervous system function

Nutritional status

Renal function

Hematologic status

Immune status and infection prevention

9. Preterm infants are at increased risk for developing respiratory distress. The nurse should assess for signs that would indicate that the newborn is having difficulty breathing. Which of the following are signs of respiratory distress? (Circle all that apply.)
   a. Use of abdominal muscles to breathe
   b. Tachypnea
   c. Periodic breathing pattern
   d. Suprasternal retraction
   e. Nasal flaring
   f. Acrocyanosis

10. When caring for a preterm infant born at 30 weeks of gestation, the nurse should recognize which of the following as the newborn's primary nursing diagnosis?
    a. Risk for infection related to decreased immune response
    b. Ineffective breathing pattern related to surfactant deficiency and weak respiratory muscle effort
    c. Ineffective thermoregulation related to immature thermoregulation center
    d. Imbalanced nutrition: less than body requirements related to ineffective suck and swallow

11. The nurse is caring for a newborn whose mother had gestational diabetes. His estimated gestational age is 41 weeks, and his birthweight is 4800 g. When assessing this newborn, the nurse should be alert for which of the following?
    a. Fracture of the femur
    b. Hypercalcemia
    c. Blood glucose level less than 40 mg/dL
    d. Signs of a congenital heart defect

III. THINKING CRITICALLY

1. Anne, a preterm newborn who weighs 3 lbs and 12 oz (1800 g) at 34 weeks of gestation, is admitted to the neonatal intensive care unit (NICU) after her birth for observation and supportive care. Anne's nutritional needs are a critical concern in her care. Oral formula feedings are being considered.

   a. State the assessment data that the nurse should document after each of Anne's feedings to indicate feeding method effectiveness.

   b. The nurse determines that Anne's suck is weak and she becomes too fatigued during oral feedings to obtain sufficient nutrients and fluid. The nurse consults with the practitioner and a decision is made to provide intermittent gavage feedings with occasional oral feedings. Describe the guidelines the nurse should follow when inserting the gavage tube.

   c. State the priority nursing diagnosis for Anne.

d. Discuss the principles the nurse should follow before, during, and after a gavage feeding to ensure safety and maximum effectiveness.

e. Outline the protocol that should be followed when advancing Anne to full oral feeding.

2. The nurse is preparing to insert a gavage tube and feed a preterm newborn. As part of the protocol for this procedure, the nurse should consider the determination of optimal feeding tube placement. Describe current evidence-based guidelines for ensuring safety of feeding tube placement in infants.

3. The NICU is a stressful environment for preterm infants and their families.

a. Identify the common sources of stress facing infants and their families in an intensive care environment.

Infant stressors

Family stressors

b. Nurses working in the NICU and parents must be aware of infant behavioral cues and adjust stimuli accordingly. List infant behavioral cues that indicate readiness for interaction and stimulation and behavioral cues that signal a need for a time-out.

Approach behaviors (readiness)

Avoidance behaviors (need for a time-out)

c. Identify specific measures that can be used to protect infants from overstimulation and yet provide appropriate stimulation to meet the developmental and emotional needs of infants.

d. Specify the guidelines that should be followed regarding infant positioning.

4. Marion is beginning her 43rd week of pregnancy.

    a. Support this statement: Perinatal mortality is significantly higher in the postterm neonate.

    b. State the assessment findings that are typical of a postterm infant.

    c. Discuss the two major complications that can be experienced by a postterm infant.

5. A 26-week neonate who is medically stable is receiving intravenous total parenteral nutrition. Minimal enteral (trophic) feedings with maternal breast milk are being considered. Describe the concept of these trophic feedings in preterm infants and the reported advantages and disadvantages.

6. Anita and Juan are the parents of a 2-day-old preterm newborn boy. Their baby, who is 27 weeks gestation and weighs 1 kg, is in the NICU and will be in the hospital for several weeks. The nurse caring for this baby recognizes that he must also provide supportive care for Anita and Juan.

    a. As parents of a preterm infant, Anita and Juan must accomplish several tasks as they develop a relationship with their baby boy and prepare to care for him. Identify these tasks and a nursing care measure that can be used to help Anita and Juan successfully accomplish the task.

    b. State the behaviors the nurse should assess as he observes Anita and Juan with their baby. Categorize these behaviors in terms of behaviors that indicate effective coping and those that would indicate ineffective coping and maladaptation.

26 21st Century Pediatric Nursing

I. LEARNING KEY TERMS

MATCHING: Match each term with its corresponding definition.

1. _____ Figures describing rates of occurrence for events such as death in children.

2. _____ Collection, interpretation, and integration of valid important, patient-reported, and nurse-observed research-derived information.

3. _____ Interaction with patients in which boundaries are blurred and the nurse's personal needs may be served rather than the patient's.

4. _____ Figures describing the incidence or number of individuals who have died over a specific period of time.

5. _____ Clinical judgment about individual, family, or community responses to actual and potential health problems.

6. _____ The prevalence of a specific illness in the population at a particular time.

7. _____ Therapeutic care that minimizes the psychologic and physical distress experienced by children and their families.

8. _____ The philosophy that recognizes the family as the constant in a child's life that service systems must support and enhance.

9. _____ Meaningful interaction with caring, well-defined boundaries separating the nurse from the patient.

10. _____ Single most common form of common chronic disease of childhood.

11. _____ Body mass index equal to or greater than the 95th percentile for children of the same age and gender.

12. _____ Purposeful, goal-oriented thinking that supports and assists others in making judgments based on evidence.

13. _____ A method of problem identification and solving that describes the thinking process of the nurse.

14. _____ The most common form of early dental disease in childhood.

15. _____ Broadened the health care objectives of the past and highlights prevention as the approach to accomplish health goals.

a. Mortality statistics

b. Morbidity statistics

c. Vital statistics

d. Family-centered care

e. Early childhood caries

f. Evidence-based practice

g. Obesity

h. Atraumatic care

i. Nursing process

j. Therapeutic relationship

k. Nontherapeutic relationships

l. *Healthy People 2020*

m. Critical thinking

n. Low birth weight

o. Injuries

p. Respiratory tract infections

q. Acute illness

r. Suicide

s. Infant mortality rate

t. Asthma

u. Nursing diagnosis

16. _____ Leading cause of death in children over 1 year of age, with the majority being motor vehicle accident related.

17. _____ Occurs 2 to 3 times more often in children than all other illnesses.

18. _____ Major indicator of infant health and a significant predictor of infant mortality.

19. _____ Symptoms severe enough to limit activity or require medical attention.

20. _____ The number of deaths during the first year of life per 1000 live births.

21. _____ The third-leading cause of death among adolescents 10 to 19 years old.

II. REVIEWING KEY CONCEPTS

1. Which of the following objectives would *not* be considered a priority area for *Healthy People 2020?*
   a. Improving nutritional and infant health
   b. Technologic advances to treat neonates
   c. Reducing violent and abusive behavior
   d. Vaccinating 90% of 2-year-olds

2. Mortality rates are calculated from a:
   a. survey of physicians.
   b. sample of hospital records.
   c. registry of all deaths.
   d. sample of death certificates.

3. Infant mortality for infants in the United States less than 1 year of age:
   a. has dramatically increased.
   b. is the same as it is in developing countries.
   c. is the same as the rate in Japan.
   d. has decreased over the past few years.

4. Which of the following statements about injuries in childhood is false?
   a. Male deaths outnumber female deaths.
   b. After 1 year of age, death rates in children are less than for infants.
   c. Children ages 5 to 14 years have the lowest rate of death.
   d. Caucasians have more deaths for all ages than Hispanics.

5. List three factors that contribute to increasing the morbidity of any disorder in children.

6. Two basic concepts in the philosophy of family-centered pediatric nursing care are:
   a. enabling and empowerment.
   b. empowerment and bias.
   c. enabling and curing.
   d. empowerment and self-control.

7. An example of atraumatic care would be to:
   a. eliminate or minimize distress experienced by a child in a health care setting.
   b. restrict visiting hours to adults only.
   c. perform invasive procedures only in the treatment room.
   d. permit only traditional clinical practices.

MATCHING: Match each role of the pediatric nurse with its corresponding description.

8. _____ A mutual exchange of ideas and opinions.

9. _____ Assists children and families in making informed choices and acting in the child's best interest.

10. _____ Plan of care that fosters growth and development.

11. _____ Determining actions for difficult situations by assigning different weight to the competing moral values.

12. _____ Using a unified interdisciplinary approach to provide holistic care; working together as a member of the health team.

13. _____ Attention to emotional needs (listening/physical presence).

14. _____ Transmitting information about health.

15. _____ Patient's right to be self-governing.

16. _____ Obligation to promote patient's well-being.

17. _____ Concept of fairness.

18. _____ Obligation to minimize or prevent harm.

a. Family advocacy/caring

b. Disease prevention/health promotion

c. Health teaching

d. Support

e. Counseling

f. Coordination/collaboration

g. Ethical decision-making

h. Autonomy

i. Nonmaleficence

j. Beneficence

k. Justice

19. Define quality of care.

20. List 5 specific examples of patient-centered outcome measures identified by the National Quality Forum.

III. THINKING CRITICALLY

1. Generate at least one idea that could be implemented by pediatric nurses to meet the three goals for public health as outlined by *Healthy People 2020*.

2. Using examples from a wide variety of practice areas, describe ways that the pediatric nurse currently fulfills the responsibilities of each of the following broad roles of the nurse.

   a. Family advocacy/caring

   b. Disease prevention/health promotion

   c. Health teaching

   d. Support/counseling

   e. Coordination/collaboration

   f. Ethical decision-making

   g. Research

   h. Health care planning

27 Family, Social, Cultural, and Religious Influences on Child Health Promotion

I. LEARNING KEY TERMS

MATCHING: Match each term with its corresponding definition.

1. _____ Establishment of the rules or guidelines from behavior.

2. _____ Laissez-faire approach; exerting little or no control over children's actions.

3. _____ A refinement of the practice of sending the child to his or her room; based on the premise of removing the reinforcer and using the strategy of unrelated consequences.

4. _____ A system of rules governing conduct.

5. _____ Democratic approach; combining child-rearing practices and emphasizing the reason for rules.

6. _____ Resources for dealing with stress, such as community services, social support, and the adoption of a future orientation.

7. _____ Family situation in which each parent is awarded custody of one or more of the children, thereby separating siblings.

8. _____ Family situation in which the children reside with one parent, with both parents acting as legal guardians and both participating in child rearing.

9. _____ A group of people, living together or in close contact, who take care of one another and provide guidance for their dependent members.

10. _____ Dictatorial approach; trying to control behavior and attitudes through unquestioned mandates.

11. _____ The descriptive term that accommodates a variety of family styles, including communal families, single-parent families, and homosexual families.

12. _____ The unit of care ("the patient") when working with children.

13. _____ Marital relationships.

14. _____ Family unit a person is born into.

15. _____ Blood relationships.

16. _____ The term that describes the concept that parents rear their own children in much the same way as they themselves were reared.

17. _____ The term that describes the support of the family from within, such as adaptability and integration.

18. _____ The term used when role behavior expected of children conflicts with the desirable adult behavior.

a. Family

b. Coping strategies

c. Authoritarian

d. Permissive

e. Authoritative

f. Discipline

g. Limit-setting

h. Time-out

i. Divided, or split, custody

j. Joint custody

k. Consanguineous

l. Affinal

m. Family of origin

n. Household

o. The family

p. Role discontinuity

q. Generational continuity

r. Internal family resources

MATCHING: Match each social, cultural, and religious influence term with its corresponding definition.

19. _____ A commitment and active engagement in a lifelong process that individuals enter into for an ongoing basis with patients, communities, colleagues, and themselves (Tervalon and Murray-Garcia, 1998).

20. _____ The affiliation of a set of people who share a unique cultural, social, and linguistic heritage.

21. _____ The process by which children acquire the beliefs, values, and behaviors of a given society in order to function within that group.

22. _____ Those smaller groups within a culture that possess many characteristics of the larger culture while contributing their own particular values.

23. _____ A pattern of assumptions, beliefs, and practices that unconsciously frames or guides the outlook and decisions of a group of people.

24. _____ The orientation to nursing that includes an awareness of the nurse's own culture; the nurse learns about and becomes able to assess from and share the culture of others.

25. _____ A division of mankind possessing traits that are transmissible by descent and are sufficient to characterize it as a distinct human type.

26. _____ Characterized by intimate, continued, face-to-face contact; mutual support of members; and the ability to order or constrain a considerable proportion of individual members' behavior. Family and peer group are examples.

27. _____ Groups that have limited, intermittent contact and in which there is generally less concern for members' behavior; examples are professional associations and church organizations.

28. _____ When people from different cultures interact.

29. _____ An awareness of cultural similarities and differences.

30. _____ An interactive care process that requires a change in the way the nurse understands and interacts within the work environment to address core cultural issues.

a. Culture

b. Ethnicity

c. Socialization

d. Subculture

e. Cultural humility

f. Race

g. Primary group

h. Transcultural nursing

i. Cultural competency

j. Cultural diversity

k. Secondary group

l. Cultural sensitivity

II. REVIEWING KEY CONCEPTS

1. Which of the following descriptions would *not* be correct using the current definition of the term *family?*
   a. The family is what the patient considers it to be.
   b. The family may be related or unrelated.
   c. The family members are always related by legal ties or genetic relationships and live in the same household.
   d. The family members share a sense of belonging to their own family.

2. Parenting practices differ between small and large families. Which one of the following characteristics is *not* found in small families?
   a. Emphasis is placed on the individual development of the child, with constant pressure to measure up to family expectations.
   b. Adolescents identify more strongly with their parents and rely more on their parents for advice.
   c. More emphasis is placed on the group and less on the individual.
   d. Children's development and achievement are measured against children in the neighborhood and social class.

3. One sibling has always been viewed by his parents as being less dependent than his brother or sister. This sibling is described as affectionate, good-natured, and flexible in this thinking. He identifies with his peer group and is very popular with classmates. His parents tend to place fewer demands on him for household help. From this description, the nurse would expect this sibling to have what birth position within the family?
   a. Firstborn child
   b. Middle child

c. Youngest child

d. An adopted child

4. Which of the following is *not* a description of the discipline "time-out"?
   a. Allows the reinforcer to be maintained
   b. Involves no physical punishment
   c. Offers both parents and child "cooling-off" time
   d. Facilitates the parent's ability to consistently apply the punishment

5. Which of the following is a correct interpretation in the use of reasoning as a form of discipline?
   a. Used for older children when moral issues are involved
   b. Used for younger children to "see the other side" of an issue
   c. Used only in combination with scolding and criticism
   d. Used to allow children a greater degree of attention from parents

6. Areas of concern for parents of adoptive children include:
   a. the initial attachment process.
   b. telling the children that they are adopted.
   c. identity formation of the children during adolescence.
   d. appropriate disciplinary tactics.
   e. a, b, c, d.

7. Which of the following is not an important consideration for parents when telling their children about the decision to divorce?
   a. Initial disclosure should include both parents and siblings.
   b. Time should be allowed for discussion with each child individually.
   c. Initial disclosure should be kept simple and reasons for divorce should not be included.
   d. Parents should physically hold or touch their child to provide feelings of warmth and reassurance.

8. When considering the impact of culture on the pediatric patient, the nurse recognizes that culture:
   a. is synonymous with race.
   b. affects the development of health beliefs.
   c. refers to a group of people with similar physical characteristics.
   d. refers to the universal manner and sequence of growth and development.

9. Cultural beliefs and practices are an important part of nursing assessment, because when analyzed and incorporated into the nursing process, these beliefs:
   a. often assist in the plan of care.
   b. can be manipulated more easily if known.
   c. must be in unison with standard health practices.
   d. are very similar from one culture to another.

10. Adopting a multicultural perspective means that the nurse:
    a. explains that biomedical measures are usually more effective.
    b. uses the patient's traditional health and cultural beliefs.
    c. realizes that most folk remedies have a scientific basis.
    d. uses aspects of the cultural beliefs to develop a plan.

11. Generalizations about cultural groups are important for nurses to know, because this information helps the nurse to:
    a. learn the similarities among all cultures.
    b. learn the unique practices of various groups.
    c. stereotype groups' characteristics.
    d. categorize groups according to their similarities.

12. T F It is recommended that children be told they are adopted before entering school.

13. T F Research has shown that children of divorce suffer no lasting psychological and social difficulties.

14. T F One outcome found in children of divorce is a heightened anxiety about forming enduring relationships as young adults.

15. T F Children of divorce cope better with their feelings of abandonment when there is continuing conflict between parents.

16. T F Preschoolers assume themselves to be the cause of the divorce and interpret the separation as punishment.

17. T F School-age children's teachers and school counselors should be informed about divorce because these children will often display altered behaviors.

18. T F Adolescents have concerns and heightened anxiety and may engage in acting-out behaviors.

MATCHING: Single-parenting, stepparenting, and dual-earner family parenting add stress to the parental role. Match each family type with an expected stressor or concern.

19. _____ Managing shortages of money, time, and energy are major concerns.

20. _____ Overload is a common source of stress, and social activities are significantly curtailed with time demands and scheduling seen as major problems.

21. _____ Requires adjustments for all including complexity in forming new interactions.

a. Single-parenting

b. Stepparenting

c. Dual-earner families

III. THINKING CRITICALLY

1. Ester and Roberto Garcia are the proud new parents of twin boys, Timothy and Thomas. Ester and Roberto have been married less than 1 year. Ester is 17 years old and plans to return to finish high school next year. Roberto finished high school and works with his father in a local auto repair shop. He is taking a week off from work to help Ester at home with Timothy and Thomas. Neither of the parents attended child-parenting classes. You are making a home visit to the couple 1 day after they have brought Timothy and Thomas home from the hospital. As you arrive at the house, you see that both Timothy and Thomas are crying. Ester is trying to give Timothy his bath while Roberto is busy trying to get Thomas to take his formula. Both new parents appear tired, and Roberto admits that they have been up all night with the infants and that either Timothy or Thomas seems to be crying "all the time" and "something must be terribly wrong with them."

   a. Identify three possible basic goals of parenting for this family.

   b. Identify the family's immediate needs.

   c. Identify long-term goals for this family.

   d. Discuss nursing interventions that would foster achievement of these long-term goals.

2. Liseth is a 3-month-old Mexican-American child. She comes to the immunization clinic with her 26-year-old mother, Noemi, her 18-month-old brother, and her 3-year-old sister. One of your goals is to promote continuation of the immunization schedule.

    a. List the questions you should ask to determine whether there are social and cultural influences that affect Noemi's intent to have her children immunized.

    b. Describe specific strategies you would use to communicate with Noemi.

    c. Identify the Hispanic beliefs and practices regarding child rearing that may influence Noemi's approach to child rearing in general and immunization in particular.

3. List and briefly describe the five components of cultural competence.

28 Developmental and Genetic Influences on Child Health Promotion

I. LEARNING KEY TERMS

MATCHING: Match each term with its corresponding definition.

1. _____ A set of skills and competencies peculiar to each developmental stage that children must accomplish or master in order to deal effectively with the environment.

2. _____ An increase in competence and adaptability; aging; most often used to describe a qualitative change.

3. _____ Specific ways in which children deal with stresses.

4. _____ The processes by which developing individuals become acquainted with the world and the objects it contains.

5. _____ Processes whereby early embryonal cells and structures are systematically modified and altered (from broad, global patterns) to achieve specific and characteristic physical and chemical properties.

6. _____ A special class of individual reactions to stressors.

7. _____ The most widely accepted theory of personality development, which emphasizes a healthy personality and was advanced by Erikson; uses the biologic concepts of critical periods and epigenesis, describing key conflicts or more problems that the individual strives to master during critical periods in personality development.

8. _____ Term used by Freud to describe any sensual pleasure.

9. _____ Behaviors exhibited by both children who are abused and those who are depressed.

10. _____ According to Chess and Thomas (1999), a term defined as the manner of thinking, behaving, or reacting that is characteristic of an individual; the way in which a person deals with life.

11. _____ The rate of metabolism when the body is at rest.

12. _____ The work of the child.

13. _____ The most accurate measure of general development; the radiologic determination of osseous maturation.

14. _____ A personal, subjective judgment of one's worthiness derived from and influenced by the social groups in the immediate environment and individuals' perceptions of how they are valued by others.

15. _____ Limited times during a process of growth when the organism is more susceptible to positive or negative influences.

a. Maturation

b. Differentiation

c. Developmental task

d. Cephalocaudal

e. Proximodistal

f. Sensitive period

g. Skeletal age

h. Basal metabolic rate

i. Temperament

j. Psychosexual development

k. Psychosocial development

l. Cognition

m. Self-concept

n. Body image

o. Self-esteem

p. Play

q. Signs of stress

r. Coping

s. Coping strategies

t. Coping styles

176

16. _____ A vital component of self-concept, referring to the subjective concepts and attitudes that individuals have toward their own bodies.

17. _____ The directional pattern of growth and development that proceeds from near to far.

18. _____ Relatively unchanging personality characteristics or outcomes of coping.

19. _____ The term that includes all the notions, beliefs, and convictions that constitute an individual's self-knowledge and influence that individual's relationships with others.

20. _____ The directional trend of growth and development that proceeds from head to tail.

II. REVIEWING KEY CONCEPTS

1. Categorizing growth and behavior into approximate age stages:
   a. helps to account for individual differences in children.
   b. can be applied to all children with some degree of precision.
   c. provides a convenient means to describe the majority of children.
   d. determines the speed of each child's growth.

2. Which of the following is an example of a cephalo-caudal directional trend in development?
   a. Head growth precedes limb growth.
   b. Fingers and toes develop after embryonic limb buds.
   c. Infants manipulate fingers after they are able to use the whole hand as a unit.
   d. Infants begin to have fine muscle control after gross random muscle movement is established.

3. An average healthy term infant who weighs 7 pounds at birth can be expected to weigh _____ pounds by 12 months of life.
   a. 14
   b. 18
   c. 21
   d. 24

4. Which of the following is considered fixed and precise in the development of children?
   a. The pace and rate of development
   b. The order of development
   c. Physical growth—in particular, height
   d. Growth during the vulnerable period

5. Sensitive periods in development are those times when the child is:
   a. more likely to respond to both positive and negative influences.
   b. more likely to require specific stimulation for physical growth.
   c. less likely to acquire a specific skill if it is not learned during this time.
   d. less likely to be harmed by external conditions.

6. If the height of a 2-year-old is measured as 88 cm, his height at adulthood would be estimated as:
   a. 132 cm.
   b. 176 cm.
   c. 172 cm.
   d. 190 cm.

7. If a newborn measures 19 inches at birth, the expected height at age 4 years would be approximately:
   a. 28.5 inches.
   b. 38 inches.
   c. 43.5 inches.
   d. 48 inches.

8. The best estimate of skeletal age in children can be made using measurements obtained from:
   a. bone height.
   b. facial bone radiography.
   c. hand and wrist radiography.
   d. mandibular size.

9. The nurse determines that a 7-month-old infant who weighs 10 kg needs about:
   a. 500 kcal per day.
   b. 750 kcal per day.
   c. 1000 kcal per day.
   d. 1500 kcal per day.

10. The basal metabolic rate (BMR) is highest in the:
    a. adolescent.
    b. infant over 6 months of age.
    c. school-age child.
    d. infant under 6 months of age.

11. The energy requirement to build tissue:
    a. fluctuates randomly.
    b. fluctuates based on need.
    c. steadily decreases with age.
    d. steadily increases with age.

12. Body temperature in young children and infants responds to:
    a. changes in the environment.
    b. exercise.
    c. emotional upset.
    d. a, b, and c.

13. A mother asks whether her 13-month-old child's sleep behavior is abnormal because he usually sleeps through the night and takes two short naps a day. The nurse's response should indicate that the infant probably:
    a. has a normal sleep pattern.
    b. has periods of sleeplessness at night.
    c. does not have colic.
    d. is at risk for having sleep problems in later life.

MATCHING: Match each attribute of temperament with its corresponding description.

14. _____ Amount of stimulation required to evoke a response.

15. _____ Nature of initial responses to a new stimulus: positive or negative.

16. _____ Regularity in the timing of physiologic functions such as hunger, sleep, and elimination.

17. _____ Energy level of the child's reactions.

18. _____ Level of physical motion during activity.

19. _____ Ease or difficulty with which the child adapts or adjusts to new situations.

20. _____ Length of time a child pursues a given activity and continues it.

21. _____ Ease with which attention can be diverted.

22. _____ Amount of pleasant behavior compared with the unpleasant.

a. Activity

b. Rhythmicity

c. Approach-withdrawal

d. Adaptability

e. Threshold of responsiveness

f. Intensity of reaction

g. Mood

h. Distractibility

i. Attention span and persistence

23. Personality development as viewed by Freud focuses on:
    a. the significance of sexual instincts.
    b. the suppression of psychosexual instincts.
    c. direct observations of adults.
    d. retrospective studies of children.

24. Erikson's theory provides a framework for:
    a. clearly indicating the experience needed to resolve crises.
    b. emphasizing pathologic development.
    c. coping with extraordinary events.
    d. explaining children's behavior in mastering developmental tasks.

25. Erikson's stage of trust vs. mistrust corresponds to Freud's:
    a. anal stage.
    b. oral stage.
    c. phallic stage.
    d. guilt stage.

26. For adolescents, their struggle to fit the roles they have played and those they hope to play is best outlined by:
    a. Freud's latency period.
    b. Freud's phallic stage.
    c. Erikson's identity vs. role confusion stage.
    d. Erikson's intimacy vs. isolation stage.

27. The best-known theory regarding cognitive development was developed by:
    a. Sullivan.
    b. Kohlberg.
    c. Erikson.
    d. Piaget.

28. An important prerequisite for all other mental activity is the child's awareness that an object exists even though it is no longer visible. According to Piaget, this awareness is called:
    a. object permanence.
    b. logical thinking.
    c. egocentricity.
    d. reversibility.

29. The predominant characteristic of Piaget's preoperational period is egocentricity, which according to him, means:
    a. concrete and tangible reasoning.
    b. selfishness and self-centeredness.
    c. inability to see another's perspective.
    d. ability to make deductions and generalize.

30. The stages of moral development that allow for prediction of behavior but not for individual differences are outlined in the moral development theory according to:
    a. Fowler.
    b. Holstein.
    c. Gilligan.
    d. Kohlberg.

31. The difference between religion and spirituality is that spirituality:
    a. requires an organized set of practices.
    b. affects the whole person: mind, body, and spirit.
    c. ensures the individual's desire to differentiate right from wrong.
    d. extends beyond religion.

MATCHING: Match each type of play with the corresponding example of that type of play.

32. _____ Coloring a picture.

33. _____ Using the telephone.

34. _____ Daydreaming.

35. _____ Playing peek-a-boo/patty-cake.

36. _____ Watching a children's puppet show on television.

37. _____ Preparing a puppet show.

38. _____ Learning to ride a bicycle.

39. _____ Swinging.

40. _____ Following each other with wagons.

41. _____ Toddlers playing with blocks in the same room.

a. Sense pleasure

b. Skill play

c. Unoccupied behavior

d. Dramatic play

e. Games

f. Onlooker play

g. Solitary play

h. Parallel play

i. Associative play

j. Cooperative play

42. Which of the following functions of play may be hindered by increasing the early academic achievements of a child?
    a. Intellectual development
    b. Creative development
    c. Sensorimotor development
    d. Moral development

43. The medium that has the most impact on children in America today is:
    a. television.
    b. movies.
    c. comic books.
    d. newspapers.

MATCHING: Match the following genetic terms with the appropriate definition.

44. _____ Agent that causes a birth defect when present in the prenatal environment.

a. Syndrome

45. _____ Occurs when a single anomaly leads to a cascade of anomalies (e.g., Pierre Robin).

b. Association

c. Sequence

46. _____ A non-random pattern of malformations for which a cause has not been established (e.g., VACTERL).

d. Teratogen

47. _____ A recognized pattern of anomalies resulting from a single specific cause (e.g., trisomy 21).

III. THINKING CRITICALLY

Use the following scenario to respond to questions 1 through 3.

An 8-year-old child arrives at the clinic for a health checkup for school. He has historically been in the 50th percentile for both height and weight and is generally considered healthy. He watches television for about 4 to 5 hours each day. He has a family history of heart disease. His mother is concerned about an increase in her son's physical aggressiveness lately. Today the child's height is noted to be in the 50th percentile, but his weight is in the 95th percentile. His serum cholesterol is elevated.

1. Delineate the factors in this patient's history that need to be addressed.

2. Describe at least three strategies this child's parents can use to deal with the child's aggressiveness.

3. Describe what outcomes the nurse could encourage the child and his parents to aim for.

29 Communication, History, and Physical Assessment

I. LEARNING KEY TERMS

MATCHING: Match each term with its corresponding description.

1. _____ An essential parameter of nutritional status; the measurement of height, weight, head circumference, proportions, skinfold thickness, and arm circumference.

2. _____ The capacity to understand what another person is experiencing from within that person's frame of reference.

3. _____ Refers to the composition of the family.

4. _____ Specific reason for the child's visit to the clinic or hospital.

5. _____ Refers to all those individuals who are considered by the family member to be significant to the nuclear unit.

6. _____ Specific review of each body system.

7. _____ Small, distinct, pinpoint hemorrhages 2 mm or less in size; can denote a type of blood disorder such as leukemia.

8. _____ Appears translucent, light pearly pink, or gray.

9. _____ Lateral curvature of the spine.

10. _____ Redness that may be a result of increased blood flow from climatic conditions, local inflammation, infection, skin irritation, allergy, or other dermatoses or may be caused by increased numbers of red blood cells as a compensatory response to chronic hypoxia.

11. _____ Response of the testes to stimulation by cold, touch, emotional excitement, or exercise.

12. _____ Yellow staining of the skin usually caused by bile pigments.

13. _____ Bowel sounds.

14. _____ The amount of elasticity in the skin; determined by grasping the skin on the abdomen or arm between the thumb and index finger, pulling it taut, and quickly releasing it.

15. _____ Large diffuse area that is usually black and blue; caused by hemorrhage of blood into skin; typically a result of injuries.

16. _____ Placing the hands against the skin to feel for abnormalities and tenderness.

a. Empathy

b. Chief complaint

c. Family

d. Family structure

e. Review of systems

f. Anthropometry

g. Recumbent length

h. Stature

i. Tissue turgor

j. Cyanosis

k. Pallor

l. Erythema

m. Ecchymosis

n. Petechiae

o. Jaundice

p. Tympanic membrane

q. Binocularity

r. Strabismus

s. Auscultation

t. Palpation

u. Peristalsis

v. Cremasteric reflex

w. Scoliosis

17. _____ Pallor that may be a sign of anemia, chronic disease, edema, or shock.

18. _____ Using the stethoscope to evaluate breath sounds.

19. _____ A person's standing height.

20. _____ Occurs when one eye deviates from the point of fixation; sometimes called "cross eye."

21. _____ A patient's length measured while the patient is lying down.

22. _____ The ability to visually fixate on one visual field with both eyes simultaneously.

23. _____ A bluish tone to the skin indicating reduced (deoxygenated) hemoglobin.

II. REVIEWING KEY CONCEPTS

1. Mrs. G. has brought her daughter Karen to the clinic as a new patient. Karen, age 12 years, requires a physical examination so that she can play volleyball. Which of the following techniques used by the nurse to establish effective communication during the interview process is not correct?
   a. The nurse introduces himself or herself and asks the names of all family members present.
   b. After the introduction, the nurse is careful to direct questions about Karen to Mrs. G. because she is the best source of information.
   c. After the introduction and explanation of her role, the nurse begins the interview by saying to Karen, "Tell me about your volleyball team."
   d. The nurse chooses to conduct the interview in a quiet area with few distractions.

2. While conducting an assessment of the child, the nurse communicates with the child's family. Which of the following does the nurse recognize as not productive in obtaining information?
   a. Obtaining input from the child, verbal and nonverbal
   b. Observing the relationship between parents and child
   c. Using broad, open-ended questions
   d. Avoiding the use of guiding statements to direct the focus of the interview

3. Anticipatory guidance should:
   a. view family weakness as a competence builder.
   b. focus on problem resolution.
   c. base interventions on needs identified by the nurse.
   d. empower the family to use information to build parenting ability.

4. T F Children are alert to their surroundings and attach meaning to gestures.

5. T F Active attempts to make friends with children before they have had an opportunity to evaluate an unfamiliar person increases their anxiety.

6. T F When communicating with small children the nurse should assume a position that is at eye level with the child.

MATCHING: Match each development stage with its corresponding description of appropriate communication guidelines to be used.

7. _____ Children focus communication on themselves; experiences of others are of no interest to them.

8. _____ Children primarily use and respond to nonverbal communication.

9. _____ Children require explanations and reasons why procedures are being done to them.

10. _____ Children are often willing to discuss their concern with an adult outside the family and often welcome the opportunity to interact with a nurse.

a. Infancy

b. Early childhood

c. School-age years

d. Adolescence

11. Which of the following best describes the appropriate use of play as a communication technique in children?
    a. Small infants have little response to activities that focus on repetitive actions like patting and stroking.
    b. Few clues about intellectual or social developmental progress are obtained from the observation of children's play behaviors.
    c. Therapeutic play has little value in reduction of trauma from illness or hospitalization.
    d. Play sessions serve as assessment tools for determining children's awareness and perception of illness.

12. List eight components of a complete pediatric health history.

13. In eliciting the chief complaint, it would be inappropriate for the nurse to:
    a. limit the chief complaint to a brief statement restricted to one or two symptoms.
    b. use labeling-type questions such as "How are you? Are you sick?" to facilitate information exchange.
    c. record the chief complaint in the child's or parent's own words.
    d. use open-ended neutral questions to elicit information.

14. Which component of the pediatric health history is illustrated by the following? "Nausea and vomiting for 3 days. Started with abdominal cramping after eating hamburger at home. No pain or cramping at present. Unable to keep any foods down but able to drink clear liquids without vomiting. No temperature elevation; no diarrhea."
    a. Chief complaint
    b. Past history
    c. Present illness
    d. Review of systems

15. Which of the following components is *not* a part of the past history in a pediatric health history?
    a. Symptom analysis
    b. Allergies
    c. Birth history
    d. Current medications

16. The nurse knows that the best description of the sexual history for a pediatric health history:
    a. includes a discussion of plans for future children.
    b. allows the patient to introduce sexual activity history.

    c. includes a discussion of contraception methods only when the patient discloses current sexual activity.
    d. alerts the nurse to the need for sexually transmitted disease screening.

17. Assessment of family interactions and roles, decision making and problem solving, and communication is known as assessment of:
    a. family structure.
    b. family function.
    c. family composition.
    d. home and community environment.

18. The dietary history of a pediatric patient includes:
    a. a 12-hour dietary intake recall.
    b. a more specific, detailed history for the older child.
    c. financial and cultural factors that influence food selection.
    d. criticism of parents' allowance of nonessential foods.

19. To effectively establish a setting for communication, the nurse, upon entering the room with a child and his mother, introduces herself and explains the purpose of the interview. The child is included in the interaction as the nurse asks his name and age and what he is expecting at his visit today. The nurse next tells them both, "The child is 25 pounds overweight, and his diet and exercise plan must be dreadful for him to be in such appalling shape." Which aspect of effective communication has the nurse disregarded that will most significantly impact the exchange of information during this interview?
    a. Assurance of privacy and confidentiality
    b. Preliminary acquaintance
    c. Directing the focus away from the complaint of fatigue to one of obesity
    d. Injecting her own attitudes and feelings into the interview

20. Mrs. J. brings her 11-month-old daughter to the clinic because she is "sleeping poorly and tugging at her ear when she is awake." Based on the information provided, the nurse can correctly record which of the following?
    a. Chief complaint
    b. Present illness
    c. Past medical history
    d. Symptom analysis

21. Which of the following methods to record dietary intake would the nurse suggest as most reliable for providing qualitative information about the child's diet?
    a. 12-hour recall
    b. 24-hour recall
    c. Food diary for 3-day period
    d. Food frequency questionnaire

22. The nurse is measuring a 20-month-old child's length. The most accurate method to obtain this measurement is with the child:
    a. sitting on the mom's lap.
    b. laying on a recumbent measuring board.
    c. laying on the exam table paper.
    d. standing with head and shoulders against a tape measure on the wall.

23. In examining pediatric patients, the normal head-to-toe sequence is often altered to accommodate the patient's developmental needs. With this approach, the nurse will:
    a. increase the stress and anxiety associated with the assessment of body parts.
    b. record the findings according to the normal sequence.
    c. hinder the trusting nurse-child relationship.
    d. decrease the security of the parent-child relationship.

24. A father brings his 12-month-old son in for the child's regular well-infant examination. The nurse knows that the best approach to the physical examination for this patient will be to:
    a. have the infant sit on the parent's lap to complete as much of the examination as possible.
    b. place the infant on the examining table with parent out of view.
    c. perform examination in head-to-toe direction.
    d. completely undress the child and leave him undressed during the examination.

25. Of the following behaviors, the behavior that indicates to the nurse that a child may be reluctant to participate and cooperate during a physical examination is:
    a. talking to the nurse.
    b. making eye contact with the nurse.
    c. allowing physical touching.
    d. sitting on parent's lap, playing with a doll.

26. The National Center for Health Statistics has revised the growth charts available for pediatric patients aged 2 to 19 years. The new charts include _____ (BMI) for age. The revised charts include all infants and children, regardless of their _____ or _____. Specialized growth charts exist to track growth of _____ infants.

27. The assessment method that provides the best information about the physical growth pattern of a preschool-age child is to:
    a. record child's height and weight measurements on the standardized growth reference chart.
    b. keep a flow sheet for height, weight, and head circumference increases.
    c. obtain a history of sibling growth patterns.
    d. measure the height, weight, and head circumference of the child.

28. T F Breastfed infants grow faster than bottle-fed infants during the 6- to 18-month age period.

29. T F Growth is a continuous but uneven process, and the most reliable evaluation lies in comparison of growth measurements over a given time period (e.g., over a year).

30. T F Growth measurements during the physical examination should be age-specific and include length, height, weight, skinfold thickness, and arm and head circumference.

31. Head circumference is:
    a. measured in all children up to the age of 24 months.
    b. equal to chest circumference at about 1 to 2 years of age.
    c. about 8 to 9 cm smaller than chest circumference during childhood.
    d. measured slightly below the eyebrows and pinna of the ears.

32. In infants and small children, the _____ pulse should be taken because it is the most reliable. This pulse should be counted for _____ because of the possibility of irregularities in rhythm.

33. Which of the following observations would not be recorded as part of the child's general appearance?
    a. Impression of child's nutritional status
    b. Behavior, interactions with parents
    c. Hygiene, cleanliness
    d. Vital signs

34. When assessing a 7-year-old child's lymph nodes, the nurse uses the distal portions of the fingers and gently but firmly presses in a circular motion along the occipital and postauricular node areas. The nurse records the findings as "tender, enlarged, warm lymph nodes." The nurse knows that the:
    a. findings are within normal limits for the child's age.
    b. assessment technique was incorrect and should be repeated.
    c. findings suggest infection or inflammation in the scalp area or external ear canal.
    d. recording of the information is complete because it includes temperature and tenderness.

35. The nurse recognizes that an assessment finding of the head and neck that does not need referral is:
    a. head lag before 6 months of age.
    b. hyperextension of the head with pain on flexion.
    c. palpable thyroid gland including isthmus and lobes.
    d. closure of the anterior fontanel at the age of 9 months.

36. Normal findings on examination of the pupils may be recorded as PERRLA, which means: _____

_____

37. Which of the following assessments is an expected finding in the child's eye examination?
    a. Opaque red reflex of the eye
    b. Ophthalmoscopic examination reflecting veins that are darker in color and about one-fourth larger in size than the arteries
    c. Strabismus in the 12-month-old infant
    d. Five-year-old child who reads the Snellen eye chart at the 20/40 level

38. Four-year-old Billy has been brought to the clinic by his parents because they have recently noticed a foul odor in the mouth accompanied by a discharge from the right naris. The nurse knows that this is most likely to suggest:
    a. poor dental hygiene.
    b. a foreign body in the nose.
    c. gingival disease.
    d. thumb-sucking.

39. On auscultation of 8-year-old Tammie's lung fields, the nurse hears inspiratory sounds that are louder, longer, and higher-pitched than on expiration. These sounds are heard over the chest, except for over the scapula and sternum. These sounds are:
    a. bronchovesicular breath sounds.
    b. vesicular breath sounds.
    c. bronchial breath sounds.
    d. adventitious breath sounds.

40. Closure of the pulmonic and aortic valves:
    a. S_1.
    b. S_2.
    c. S_3.
    d. S_4.

41. In performing an examination for scoliosis, the nurse understands that which of the following is an incorrect method?
    a. The child should be examined in only his or her underpants (and bra, if an older girl).
    b. The child should stand erect with the nurse observing from behind.
    c. The child should squat down with hands extended forward so that the nurse can observe for asymmetry of the shoulder blades.
    d. The child should bend forward so that the back is parallel to the floor and the nurse can observe from behind.

42. The most important procedure for examining the heart includes:
    a. inspection.
    b. palpation.
    c. auscultation.
    d. percussion.

43. Which of the following organs is located in the lower right quadrant of the abdomen?
    a. Bladder
    b. Liver
    c. Ovaries
    d. Appendix

III. THINKING CRITICALLY

1. Compare and contrast between adults and children in the following nursing situations:

   a. The guidelines for communicating with and interviewing adults vs. the guidelines for communicating with and interviewing children

   b. Communicating with families vs. communicating with adults

   c. Taking a health history from an adult vs. taking a health history from a child

2. Describe the differences between the ear canal of an infant and the ear canal of a school-age child.

3. Compare and contrast the differences in skin color changes between light-skinned and dark-skinned individuals.

30 Pain Assessment and Management

I. LEARNING KEY TERMS

MATCHING: Match each term with its corresponding definition or description.

1. _____ Vocalization, facial expression, and body movements that have been associated with pain.

2. _____ Distraction, relaxation, and guided imagery to help decrease pain perception.

3. _____ Skin-to-skin holding of an infant.

4. _____ Eutectic mixture of local anesthetics.

5. _____ Pain not relieved with the usual scheduled dose of pain medication.

6. _____ A multidimensional pain instrument to assess patient and parental perceptions of the pain experience in a manner appropriate for the cognitive-developmental level of children and adolescents.

7. _____ A multidimensional pain instrument for children and adolescents that is used to assess three dimensions of pain: location, intensity, and quality.

8. _____ Pain assessment tool that consists of six photographs of Caucasian child's face representing no hurt to biggest hurt possible; also includes vertical scale with numbers from 0 to 100.

9. _____ A pain assessment tool that uses six caricatures of a child's face representing no hurt to biggest hurt child could ever have.

10. _____ Interval scale that includes five categories of behavior: facial expression (F), leg movement (L), activity (A), cry (C), and consolability (C); commonly used in children ages 2 months to 7 years.

11. _____ A Likert-style pain scale used in children 8 years and older that uses numbers 0 to 10 to denote intensity of pain.

12. _____ Pain that persists for 3 months or more beyond the expected period of healing.

13. _____ The use of swaddling, non-nutritive sucking, and concentrated oral sucrose during a newborn heelstick.

a. Kangaroo care

b. Multimodal analgesia

c. Distress behaviors

d. Chronic pain

e. Nonpharmacologic techniques

f. Pediatric Pain Questionnaire (PPQ)

g. Wong-Baker Faces Pain Rating Scale

h. Adolescent Pediatric Pain Tool (APPT)

i. Oucher

j. FLACC Postoperative Pain Tool

k. Numerical rating scale

l. EMLA

m. Breakthrough pain

II. REVIEWING KEY CONCEPTS

1. In regard to pain assessment, nurses tend to:
   a. underestimate the existence of pain in children but not in adults.
   b. underestimate the existence of pain in both children and adults.
   c. overestimate the existence of pain in children but not in adults.
   d. overestimate the existence of pain in both children and adults.

2. When using patient-controlled analgesia (PCA) with children, the:
   a. drug of choice is meperidine.
   b. parent should control the dosing.
   c. nurse should control the dosing.
   d. drug of choice is morphine.

3. The anesthetic cream EMLA is applied:
   a. before invasive procedures.
   b. as preoperative oral sedation.
   c. for chronic cancer pain.
   d. postoperatively.

4. For postoperative or cancer pain control, analgesics should be administered:
   a. as needed.
   b. around the clock.
   c. before the pain escalates.
   d. after the pain peaks.

5. The most common side effect from opioid therapy is:
   a. respiratory depression.
   b. pruritus.
   c. nausea and vomiting.
   d. constipation.

6. T F   Children may not realize how much they are hurting when they are in constant pain.

7. T F   Narcotics are no more dangerous for children than they are for adults.

8. T F   Children cannot tell you where they hurt.

9. T F   A 3-year-old child can use a pain scale.

10. T F   Children tolerate pain better than adults.

11. T F   Children may not admit having pain in order to avoid an injection.

12. T F   Infants do not feel pain.

13. T F   Children may believe that the nurse knows how they feel.

14. A needle-free system containing 1% buffered lidocaine provides a rapid onset of action to reduce pain associated with peripheral IV insertions or blood draws. This is called:
    a. EMLA
    b. J-tip
    c. Refrigerant spray
    d. Transdermal patch

15. T F   Virtual reality has been identified as a potentially effective tool for pain management.

16. By _____ to _____ years of age most children are able to use the 0 to 10 numeric rating scale that is currently used by adolescents and adults.

17. The _____ or _____ is an important source of information during assessment.

18. The Non-communicating Children's Pain Checklist is a pain measurement tool specifically designed for children with _____.

19. Self-report observational scales and interview questionnaires for pain may not be a reliable measure of pain assessment in _____ children.

20. List the five classifications of complementary and alternative medicine (CAM) therapies and give an example of each.

III. THINKING CRITICALLY

1. Which pain assessment method is useful for measuring pain in infants and preverbal children who do not have the language skills to communicate that they are in pain? Why is this the most effective way of measuring pain in infants and preverbal children?

2. Which pain assessment scales are most suitable to use to assess pain in a 6-year-old child?

3. How do infants who spend 1 to 3 hours in kangaroo care benefit from this therapy?

4. Define a ceiling effect. Describe the major difference between opioids and nonopioids regarding a ceiling effect.

31 The Infant and Family

I. LEARNING KEY TERMS

MATCHING: Match each term with its corresponding definition or description.

1. _____ Between ages 4 and 8 months, the infant progresses through the first stage of separation-individuation and begins to have some awareness of self and mother as separate beings.

2. _____ Vaccination; responsible for the decline of infectious diseases over the past 60 years.

3. _____ The unexpected and abrupt death of an infant under 1 year of age that remains unexplained after a complete postmortem examination, including an investigation of the death scene and a review of the case history; the leading cause of death in children between the ages of 1 month and 1 year.

4. _____ A sign of inadequate growth resulting from inability to obtain or use calories required for growth.

5. _____ Cessation of breathing for 20 seconds or more.

6. _____ A major accomplishment of cognitive development that develops at approximately 9 to 10 months of age; the realization that objects continue to exist after they leave one's visual field.

7. _____ The process of giving up one method of feeding for another; usually refers to relinquishing the breast or bottle for a cup.

8. _____ Fusion of two ocular images that begins to develop at 6 weeks and should be well established by age 4 months.

9. _____ Paroxysmal abdominal pain manifested by a duration of more than 3 hours and by drawing up of the legs to the abdomen in an infant under the age of 3 months.

10. _____ Behaviors that demonstrate a preference for the mother and are a result of the 5- to 6-month-old infant developing the ability to distinguish the mother or other primary caregiver from other individuals; results from improving cognitive development and peaks at 8 months of age.

11. _____ An acquired condition that occurs as a result of cranial molding during infancy; incidence has increased dramatically since implementation of the Back to Sleep campaign.

a. Binocularity

b. Object permanence

c. Stranger fear

d. Attachment

e. Weaning

f. Immunization

g. Failure to thrive

h. Separation anxiety

i. Colic

j. Sudden infant death syndrome (SIDS)

k. World Health Organization

l. Positional plagiocephaly

m. Apnea

n. Stereopsis (depth perception)

12. _____ A characteristic behavior of social development that occurs in the second half of the first year of life; depends on the interaction rather than reflex.

13. _____ These standardized reference growth curves are globally representative of infant growth velocity and reflect breastfeeding as the feeding norm for infants.

14. _____ Begins to develop by age 7 to 9 months but may not be fully mature until 2 or 3 years of age, thus increasing the infant's and younger toddler's risk of falling.

II. REVIEWING KEY CONCEPTS

1. A healthy 6-month-old infant is seen in the well-child clinic with a hemoglobin of 9.0. The nurse is aware that this represents:
   a. a critical lab value requiring immediate intervention.
   b. physiologic anemia.
   c. iron deficiency.
   d. chronic hypoxemia.

2. The age at which most infants can roll from back to abdomen is:
   a. 3 months.
   b. 6 months.
   c. 9 months.
   d. 12 months.

3. The child's anterior fontanel usually closes by:
   a. 3 to 6 months.
   b. 7 to 9 months.
   c. 12 to 18 months.
   d. 24 months.

4. Which of the following characteristics of vision begins to develop by 6 weeks of age and should be well established by age 4 months?
   a. Corneal reflex
   b. Stereopsis
   c. Binocularity
   d. Strabismus

5. Which of the following assessment findings would be considered most abnormal?
   a. The infant who displays head lag at 3 months of age
   b. The infant who displays head lag at 6 months of age
   c. The infant who begins to roll from front to back at 4 months
   d. The infant who begins to roll from front to back at 6 months

6. Which one of the following play activities would be least appropriate to suggest to the mother for her 3-month-old infant to promote auditory and tactile stimulation?
   a. Playing music and singing along
   b. Using rattles
   c. Using an infant swing
   d. Placing toys out of infant's reach

7. Reactive attachment disorder stems from:
   a. crying and vocalizing to the mother.
   b. clinging to the mother.
   c. crying when the mother leaves the room.
   d. maladaptive or absent attachment.

8. If a mother is concerned about the fact that her 14-month-old infant is not walking, the nurse would particularly want to evaluate whether the infant:
   a. pulls up to the furniture.
   b. uses a pincer grasp.
   c. transfers objects.
   d. has developed object permanence.

9. Colic is said to be more common in the infant who:
   a. is between 3 and 6 months of age.
   b. has a difficult temperament.
   c. has other congenital abnormalities.
   d. has signs of failure to thrive.

10. The nurse should withhold the vaccine if the child:
    a. has a low-grade fever.
    b. is currently taking antibiotics.
    c. has a moderately acute illness without fever.
    d. was born prematurely.

11. Which of the following techniques has been demonstrated by research to be most successful when two or more immunizations are given at one visit?
    a. Inject the less painful immunization first.
    b. Use an air bubble to clear the needle after the injection.
    c. Inject the immunizations simultaneously.
    d. Apply a topical anesthetic to the site for a minimum of 1 hour.

12. What is the third-leading cause of infant mortality in the United States?
    a. Falls
    b. Motor vehicle accidents
    c. SIDS
    d. Accidental poisoning

13. Honey should be avoided in infants younger than 12 months of age because of its association with the occurrence of:
    a. SIDS.
    b. food allergy.
    c. infant botulism.
    d. pertussis.

14. A mother of a 4-month-old tells the clinic nurse that her infant son sleeps approximately 24 hours per day, combining naps and night time sleep. The nurse recognizes that this pattern of sleep in infancy is:
    a. a normal sleep pattern for this age.
    b. an abnormal sleep pattern for this age.

15. T F The incidence of SIDS is associated with diphtheria, tetanus, and pertussis vaccines.

16. T F Maternal smoking during and after pregnancy has been implicated as a contributor to SIDS.

17. T F Parents should be advised to position an infant on his or her abdomen to prevent SIDS.

18. T F The nurse should encourage the parents to sleep in the same bed as the infant being monitored for apnea of infancy in order to detect subtle clinical changes.

19. T F Failure to thrive (growth failure) occurs almost exclusively in third-world countries where food shortage and poverty are prevalent.

20. T F Placing a healthy term infant who spits up part of his feedings on his side to sleep will reduce the risk for aspiration and further complications.

MATCHING: Match each term with its corresponding definition or description.

21. _____ This vaccine is administered in early fall and is repeated yearly for ongoing protection; may be given to infants as young as 6 months.

22. _____ Vaccine protects against a number of serious infections caused by *haemophilus influenzae* type b, especially bacterial meningitis, epiglottitis, bacterial pneumonia, septic arthritis, and sepsis.

23. _____ Vaccine protects against Streptococcal pneumococci, which are responsible for a number of bacterial infections in children under 2 years; these include generalized infections such as septicemia and meningitis or localized infections such as otitis media, sinusitis, and pneumonia.

24. _____ This vaccine is administered at 2, 4, and 6 months to protect from pertussis, diphtheria, and tetanus.

25. _____ Vaccine is administered to protect against severe diarrhea in infants and young children.

26. _____ Vaccine now given only by intramuscular route in the United States; protects against muscle paralysis.

a. Inactivated poliovirus vaccine (IPV)

b. Hib

c. Prevnar 13

d. DTaP

e. Influenza vaccine

f. Rotavirus vaccine

III. THINKING CRITICALLY

1. Describe the fine motor and gross motor, language, and social developmental milestones to assess in a 7-month-old infant who is coming to the well-child clinic.

2. List two dietary supplements that should be given in infancy and briefly explain the rationale for administration of each in this age-group.

3. List 5 infant risk factors for SIDS.

4. List 3 factors that are considered protective for SIDS.

5. List 4 risk factors for SIDS.

32 The Toddler and Family

I. LEARNING KEY TERMS

MATCHING: Match each term with its corresponding description.

1. _____ The need to maintain sameness and reliability.

2. _____ The destruction of teeth resulting from the process of bathing the teeth in a cariogenic environment for a prolonged period; most often affects the maxillary incisor and the molars.

3. _____ The child's emergence from a symbiotic fusion with the mother.

4. _____ Soft bacterial deposits that adhere to the teeth and cause dental decay and periodontal disease.

5. _____ A necessary assertion of self-control in the toddler.

6. _____ Those achievements that mark children's assumption of their individual characteristics in the environment.

7. _____ The retreat from one's present pattern of functioning to past levels of behavior.

8. _____ Characterized by the child playing alongside, but not with, other children.

9. _____ The developmental stage in which the toddler relinquishes dependence on others.

10. _____ One of the major tasks of toddlerhood.

a. Autonomy

b. Negativism

c. Ritualism

d. Separation

e. Individuation

f. Parallel play

g. Regression

h. Plaque

i. Early childhood caries

j. Toilet training

II. REVIEWING KEY CONCEPTS

1. Which of the following is *not* considered to be a characteristic of the toddler's developing spirituality?
   a. Associates God with something special
   b. Enjoys routines such as praying at mealtime
   c. Thinking is largely based on fantasy rather than reality
   d. Understands the meaning of fear and punishment

2. Which of the following skills is not necessary for the toddler to acquire before separation and individuation can be achieved?
   a. Object permanence
   b. Lack of anxiety during separation from parents
   c. Delayed gratification
   d. Ability to tolerate a moderate amount of frustration

3. The usual number of words acquired by the age of 2 years is about:
   a. 50.
   b. 100.
   c. 300.
   d. 500.

4. Which of the following types of play increases in frequency as the child moves through the toddler period?
   a. Parallel play
   b. Imitative play
   c. Tactile play
   d. Solitary play

5. Which of the following statements is *false* in regard to toilet training?
   a. Bowel training is usually accomplished after bladder training.
   b. Nighttime bladder training is usually accomplished after bowel training.
   c. The toddler who is impatient with soiled diapers is demonstrating readiness for toilet training.
   d. Fewer wet diapers signal that the toddler is physically ready for toilet training.

6. Which of the following strategies is appropriate for parents to use to prepare a toddler for the birth of a sibling?
   a. Explain the upcoming birth as early in the pregnancy as possible.
   b. Move the toddler to his or her own new room.
   c. Provide a doll for the toddler to imitate parenting.
   d. Tell the toddler that a new playmate will come home soon.

7. The best approach for extinguishing a toddler's attention-seeking behavior of a temper tantrum with head banging is to:
   a. ignore the behavior.
   b. provide time-out.
   c. offer a toy to calm the child.
   d. protect the child from injury.

8. Which of the following statements about stress in toddlers is *true*?
   a. Toddlers are rarely exposed to stress or the results of stress.
   b. Any stress is destructive because toddlers have a limited ability to cope.
   c. Most children are exposed to a stress-free environment.
   d. Small amounts of stress help toddlers develop effective coping skills.

9. Regression in toddlers occurs when there is:
   a. stress.
   b. a threat to their autonomy.
   c. a need to revert to dependency.
   d. a, b, and c.

10. Which of the following statements is *true* in regard to nutritional changes from the infant to the toddler years?
    a. Protein and energy requirements remain high to meet demands for muscle growth.
    b. The needs for minerals such as iron and calcium are easy to meet.
    c. Toddlers enjoy being fed by an adult caretaker.
    d. Toddlers like to experience new tastes and foods.

11. Which of the following methods is most effective for plaque removal?
    a. Brushing and flossing
    b. Annual fluoride treatments
    c. Allowing the child to brush his or her own teeth
    d. Using a large stiff toothbrush

12. Which of the following nutritional requirements increases during the toddler years?
    a. Calories
    b. Proteins
    c. Minerals
    d. Fluids

13. Physiologic anorexia in toddlers is characterized by:
    a. strong taste preferences.
    b. extreme changes in appetite from day to day.
    c. heightened awareness of social aspects of meals.
    d. weight loss and thinner appearance.

14. Healthy ways of serving food to toddlers include:
    a. requiring the child to sit at a table for meals.
    b. permitting nutritious grazing between meals.
    c. discouraging between-meal snacking.
    d. providing rewards for foods consumed.

15. Which of the following strategies is *least appropriate* for the parent to use to help the toddler adjust to the initial dental visit?
    a. Explain to the child that a checkup will not hurt.
    b. Have the child observe his or her brother's examination.
    c. Have the child perform a checkup on a doll.
    d. Ask the dentist to reserve a thorough examination for another visit.

16. Studies indicate that toddlers up to 24 months of age are safer riding in _____ _____ _____ in the _____ position.

17. The parents should consider moving the toddler from the crib to a bed after the toddler:
    a. reaches the age of 2 years.
    b. will stay in bed all night.
    c. reaches a height of 35 inches.
    d. is able to sleep through the night.

18. Give an example of an item that could cause aspiration, burns, or suffocation for each of the following categories of items hazardous to the toddler.

    a. Foods

    b. Play objects

    c. Common household objects

    d. Electrical items

III. THINKING CRITICALLY

1. Describe four areas that the nurse should assess to obtain the information necessary to give adequate anticipatory guidance to the parents of a 12-month-old toddler.

2. Describe three gross motor developmental milestones that a 2-year-old toddler should have accomplished.

3. Describe three fine motor developmental milestones that a 2-year-old toddler should have accomplished.

4. Describe three language developmental milestones that a 2-year-old toddler should have accomplished.

5. Describe how negativism contributes to the toddler's acquisition of a sense of autonomy.

The Preschooler and Family

I. LEARNING KEY TERMS

MATCHING: Match each term with its corresponding definition or description.

1. _____ Play activities that reproduce adult behavior; more typically seen at the end of the preschool period.

2. _____ Infectious disease that has declined greatly since the advent of immunizations and the use of antibiotics and antitoxins.

3. _____ Group activities that have no rigid organization or rules; typical of the preschool period.

4. _____ Partial arousal from a deep, nondreaming sleep.

5. _____ The deliberate attempt to destroy or significantly impair a child's self-esteem.

6. _____ The infliction of harm on a child caused by a parent or other person who fabricates or induces illness in the child.

7. _____ Ascribing lifelike qualities to inanimate objects.

8. _____ Scary dreams that are followed by full waking.

9. _____ The result of a preschooler's transductive reasoning; the belief that thoughts are all powerful.

10. _____ Failure to meet the child's need for affection, attention, and emotional nurturance.

11. _____ Articulation problems that occur when children are pressured to produce sounds ahead of their developmental level.

12. _____ The preschooler's way of understanding, adjusting to, and working out life's experiences.

13. _____ A type of speech pattern that occurs normally in children during the preschool period.

14. _____ The use, persuasion, or coercion of any child to engage in sexually explicit conduct.

15. _____ Deliberate infliction of bodily injury on a child, usually by the child's caregiver.

16. _____ Preschool-aged children have difficulty understanding the concept of tomorrow, yesterday, or next week.

17. _____ The deprivation of necessities such as food, clothing, shelter, supervision, medical care, and education.

a. Sense of initiative

b. Conscience

c. Concept of time

d. Play

e. Magical thinking

f. Animism

g. Associative play

h. Imitative play

i. Imaginary playmates

j. Desensitization period

k. Aggression

l. Stuttering (stammering)

m. Dyslalia

n. Nightmares

o. Sleep terrors

p. Communicable disease

q. Prodromal symptoms

r. Child maltreatment

s. Physical neglect

t. Emotional neglect

u. Emotional abuse

v. Physical abuse

w. Munchausen syndrome by proxy

x. Sexual abuse

18. _____ Behavior that attempts to hurt a person or destroys property; differs from anger.

19. _____ The superego; development in this area is a major task for the preschooler.

20. _____ Intentional bodily injury or neglect, emotional abuse or neglect, and/or sexual abuse of children, usually by adults.

21. _____ A type of conditioning that involves gradual introduction to an intimidating experience to help the child overcome apprehension.

22. _____ A feeling of accomplishment in one's activities; a psychosocial developmental task of the preschool period.

23. _____ Occur between early manifestations of a disease and its overt clinical syndrome.

24. _____ An invented companion that serves many purposes in the preschooler's development.

II. REVIEWING KEY CONCEPTS

1. The approximate age range for the preschool period begins at age _____ years and ends at age _____ years.

2. The average annual weight gain during the preschool years is _____ kg or _____ lb.

3. Which of the following statements about the average preschooler's physical proportions is *true*?
   a. Preschoolers have a squat and potbellied frame.
   b. Preschoolers have a slender but sturdy frame.
   c. The muscle and bones of the preschooler have reached full maturity.
   d. Sexual characteristics can be differentiated in the preschooler.

4. During the preschool years, anticipatory guidance shifts to a focus on:
   a. protection rather than education.
   b. education and correcting dysfluency in speech patterns.
   c. education with an emphasis on reasoning.
   d. protection and safeguarding the immediate environment.

5. The moral and spiritual development of the preschooler is characterized by:
   a. concern for why something is wrong.
   b. actions that are directed toward satisfying the needs of others.
   c. thoughts of loyalty and gratitude.
   d. a very concrete sense of justice.

6. T F Sleep terrors can be described as a partial arousal from a very deep nondreaming sleep.

7. T F Television viewing before bedtime may cause bedtime resistance.

8. T F Preschoolers can independently brush and floss their teeth.

9. T F Preschoolers are more prone to falls than toddlers.

10. T F Preschoolers have a concrete concept of a God with physical characteristics, often similar to an imaginary friend.

11. When educating the preschool child about injury prevention, the parents should:
    a. set a good example.
    b. help children establish safety habits.
    c. be aware that pedestrian/motor vehicle injuries increase in this age group.
    d. a, b, and c.

12. Which of the following statements is incorrect?
    a. Most child abuse occurs in lower socioeconomic populations.
    b. One child is usually the victim in an abusive family, and removal of this child often places the other children at risk.
    c. The abusive family environment is one of chronic stress, including problems of divorce, poverty, unemployment, and poor housing.
    d. Child abuse is a problem of all social groups.

13. The nurse is talking with a 13-year-old child who has revealed that she is being sexually abused. Which of the following is the best guideline for the nurse to utilize?
    a. Promise not to tell what the child reveals to you.
    b. Assure the child that she will not need to report the abuse.
    c. Avoid using leading statements that can distort the child's reporting of the problem.
    d. It is acceptable for the nurse to express anger and shock and to criticize the child's family.

14. According to Erikson, the preschooler's primary psychosocial task of this period is acquiring a sense of:
    a. trust.
    b. autonomy.
    c. initiative.
    d. belonging.

15. Preschoolers engage in group play with similar or identical activities but without rigid organization or rules. This type of play is:
    a. parallel.
    b. associative.
    c. dramatic.
    d. solitary.

16. Some evidence suggests that children who participate in family mealtimes in the home (3 or more meals together) have a decreased risk for:
    a. aggressiveness.
    b. child abuse.
    c. sleep problems.
    d. obesity and unhealthy eating practices.

III. THINKING CRITICALLY

Use the following scenario to respond to questions 1 through 4.

Imagine that you are a nurse on the staff of a pediatric group practice. A mother comes in to discuss her son, who is 37 months old. He will attend the preschool program at a local private school this year. He has attended a home day care program since he was a baby, while his mother worked in her own interior decorating business.

An older woman runs the day care that the child has attended until now. The woman and her helper both treat the 12 children in the program as if they were family. The program is very structured in regard to schedule and routines.

The child's mother tells you that she is looking forward to Jacob's new environment. His teacher is very creative and approaches the classroom from the perspective of the child's development. There will be a lot of choices for activities during the day.

1. Based on the information above, analyze the data presented in relation to the child's needs and the concerns for a smooth transition.

2. Develop an expected outcome that is reasonable to establish for this mother and her child.

3. Describe interventions and strategies that are appropriate for you to suggest to this mother and her child.

4. Explain to the mother the characteristics that indicate the child is ready for preschool.

34 The School-Age Child and Family

I. LEARNING KEY TERMS

MATCHING: Match each term with its corresponding definition.

1. _____ The most common cause of severe injury and death in school-age children.

2. _____ Any recurring activity that intends to cause harm, distress, or control towards another in which there is a perceived imbalance of power between the aggressor(s) and the victim.

3. _____ Developmentally inappropriate degrees of inattention and impulsiveness.

4. _____ The principal oral problem in children and adolescents; if untreated can result in total destruction of the involved teeth.

5. _____ Elementary school children who are left to care for themselves before or after school without supervision of an adult.

6. _____ An inflammatory and degenerative condition involving the gums and tissues supporting the teeth.

7. _____ Basic disturbance in this disorder is a lack of contact with reality and the subsequent development of a world of the child's own.

8. _____ The period in which the secondary sex characteristics begin to develop, typically occurring during preadolescence.

9. _____ Development of symptoms after exposure to trauma.

10. _____ The beginning of the development of secondary sex characteristics.

11. _____ Exarticulated; "knocked out."

12. _____ The child's ability to relate a series of events to mental representations that can be expressed both verbally and symbolically.

13. _____ One of the most important socializing agents in the school-age years.

14. _____ A heterogenous group of disorders manifested by significant difficulties in the acquisition and use of listening, speaking, reading, writing, reasoning, or mathematic skills.

a. Childhood schizophrenia

b. Prepubescence

c. Puberty

d. Latchkey children

e. Dental caries

f. Avulsed tooth

g. Concrete operations

h. Attention deficit hyperactivity disorder

i. Motor vehicle accidents

j. Bullying

k. Periodontal disease

l. Peer group

m. Posttraumatic stress disorder

n. Learning disability

II. REVIEWING KEY CONCEPTS

1. The middle childhood is also referred to as "school age" or the "school years." What ages does this period represent?
   a. Ages 5 to 13 years
   b. Ages 4 to 14 years
   c. Ages 6 to 12 years
   d. Ages 6 to 16 years

2. Physiologically, the middle years begin with _____ and end at _____.

3. T   F   In middle childhood there are fewer stomach upsets, better maintenance of blood sugar levels, and an increased stomach capacity.

4. T   F   Caloric needs are higher in relation to stomach size compared with the needs during preschool years.

5. T   F   The heart is smaller in relation to the rest of the body during the middle years.

6. T   F   During the middle years, the immune system develops little immunity to pathogenic microorganisms.

7. T   F   Backpacks are preferred to other book totes during middle years.

8. T   F   Physical maturity correlates well with emotional and social maturity during the middle years.

9. Generally, the earliest age at which puberty begins is age _____ for girls and age _____ for boys, but it can be normal for either sex after the age of _____ years.

10. T   F   In the middle school years children want to spend more time in the company of peers, and they often prefer peer group activities to family activities.

11. Middle childhood is the time when children:
    I. learn the value of doing things with others.
    II. learn the benefits derived from division of labor in accomplishing goals.
    III. achieve a sense of industry and accomplishment.
    IV. expand interests and engage in tasks that can be carried to completion.
    a. I, II, III, and IV
    b. I, III, and IV
    c. I and IV
    d. II and III

12. A 6-year-old boy is starting in a new neighborhood school. On the first day of school he complains of a headache and tearfully tells his mother he does not want to go. His mother takes him to school, and the nurse is consulted. The nurse recognizes that this is a slow-to-warm-up child and suggests which of the following?
    a. Put him in the classroom with the other children and leave him alone.
    b. Insist that he join and lead the class song.
    c. Include him in activities without assigning him tasks until he willingly participates in activities.
    d. Send him home with his mother because he has a headache.

13. During the school-age years, children learn valuable lessons from age-mates. How is this accomplished?
    a. The child learns to appreciate the varied points of view that are within the peer group.
    b. The child becomes sensitive to the social norms and pressures of the group.
    c. The child's interactions among peers lead to the formation of intimate friendships between same-sex peers.
    d. a, b and c.

14. Children's self-concepts are composed of their:
    a. own critical self-assessment.
    b. idea of self in relation to others.
    c. body image awareness.
    d. a, b, and c.

15. The factor that most influences the amount and manner of discipline and limit setting imposed on school-age children is the:
    a. age of the parent.
    b. education of the parent.
    c. response of the child to rewards and punishments.
    d. ability of the parent to communicate with the school system.

16. To assist school-age children in coping with stress in their lives, the nurse should:
    I. be able to recognize signs that indicate the child is undergoing stress.
    II. teach the child how to recognize signs of stress in herself or himself.
    III. help the child plan a means for dealing with any stress through problem solving.
    IV. reassure the child that the stress is only temporary.
    a. I, II, III, and IV
    b. I, II, and III
    c. I, II, and IV
    d. I and III

17. By the end of middle childhood, children should be able to assume personal responsibility for self-care in the areas of _____, _____, _____, _____, _____, and _____.

18. Important education for parents of a child with ADHD includes information regarding:
    a. side effects of medications.
    b. injury prevention.
    c. environmental modifications.
    d. a, b, and c.

19. T F   Evidence shows that bullying is more common in middle school than in high school children.

III. THINKING CRITICALLY

A 9-year-old boy is brought to the clinic by his mother for a school physical examination. His mother is concerned, because the child wants to join the school soccer team this year. On physical examination, the nurse discovers that since last year there has been an increase of 2 inches in height and a 10-pound weight gain. Health history is unchanged from the previous year. The young boy tells the nurse that he rides his bike more now than last year because he has a new best friend to go riding with.

1. Describe the areas of assessment that the nurse should expand upon.

2. Describe an appropriate response to the mother's concern about her son playing soccer.

3. Describe an educational session that would most benefit this child and his mother.

4. Describe how the mother of this 9-year-old boy can foster his development.

35 The Adolescent and Family

I. LEARNING KEY TERMS

MATCHING: Match each term with its corresponding definition.

1. _____ The masculinizing hormones; secreted in small and gradually increasing amounts up to about 7 or 9 years of age, then followed by a rapid increase in both sexes, the level of androgens in males increasing over that in females with the onset of testicular function.

2. _____ Regular use of drugs for other than the accepted medical purposes; use of drugs resulting in physical or psychologic harm to the user and/or detrimental effects to society.

3. _____ The hormone that increases with the onset of testicular function.

4. _____ Behavior associated with drug use that is voluntary and culturally defined.

5. _____ Behaviors associated with drug use that are physiologic and involuntary; not culturally defined.

6. _____ The initial appearance of menstruation; occurs about 2 years after the appearance of the first pubescent changes.

7. _____ The feminizing hormone; found in low quantities during childhood; secreted in slowly increasing amounts until about age 11 years in both males and females, then followed by a distinction in its secretion between the male and the female.

8. _____ Temporary breast enlargement and tenderness; common during mid-puberty in boys.

9. _____ Eating disorder characterized by binge eating and purging followed by self-deprecating thoughts, a depressed mood, and awareness that the eating pattern is abnormal.

10. _____ A period of transition between childhood and adulthood, beginning with the gradual appearance of secondary sex characteristics at about 11 or 12 years of age and ending with cessation of body growth at 18 to 20 years.

11. _____ The first period of puberty; occurs about 2 years immediately before puberty, when the child is developing preliminary physical changes that herald sexual maturity.

12. _____ Eating disorder characterized by a refusal to maintain a minimally normal body weight; severe weight loss in the absence of obvious physical causes.

13. _____ Occurs in males toward the end of the growth spurt of adolescence.

14. _____ The maturational, hormonal, and growth process that occurs when the reproductive organs begin to function and the secondary sex characteristics develop.

a. Puberty

b. Prepubescence

c. Adolescence

d. Estrogen

e. Androgens

f. Testosterone

g. Menarche

h. Gynecomastia

i. Nocturnal emission

j. Religious beliefs

k. Peer group

l. Obesity

m. Anorexia nervosa

n. Bulimia

o. Drug abuse

p. Drug tolerance

q. Addiction

15. _____ Are strongly influenced by inter-personal relationships with peers as well as adults in their environment.

16. _____ Condition said to exist when a child's BMI is greater than the 95th percentile.

17. _____ Serves as a strong support to adolescents and forms the transitional world between dependence and autonomy.

II. REVIEWING KEY CONCEPTS

1. The normal age range for menarche is usually _____ to _____ years, with the average age being _____ years and _____ months for North American girls.

2. The hormone in the female that causes growth and development of the vagina, uterus, and fallopian tubes, as well as breast enlargement is:
   a. estrogen.
   b. progesterone.
   c. follicle-stimulating hormone.
   d. luteinizing hormone.

3. The adolescent growth spurt is characterized as beginning:
   a. sooner in boys.
   b. between the ages of 9½ and 14½ years in boys.
   c. sooner in girls.
   d. between the ages of 10½ and 16 years in girls.

4. Girls may be considered to have _____ if breast development has not occurred by age 13 or if menarche has not occurred within _____ years of the onset of breast development.

5. The first pubescent change in boys is:
   a. appearance of pubic hair.
   b. testicular enlargement with thinning, reddening, and increased looseness of the scrotum.
   c. penile enlargement.
   d. temporary breast enlargement and tenderness.

6. Which one of the following statements about pattern of growth during adolescence is *true*?
   a. Knowing the correct sequence of the growth pattern is useful only when assessing abnormal growth patterns versus normal growth patterns.
   b. Boys start an increase of muscle mass during early puberty that lasts throughout adolescence.
   c. Boys usually begin puberty and reach maturity about 2 years earlier than girls.
   d. Girls and boys have an increase in linear growth that begins for both during midpuberty.

7. On the average, girls gain _____ to _____ inches in height and _____ to _____ pounds during adolescence, whereas boys gain _____ to _____ inches and _____ to _____ pounds.

8. Which of the following best describes the formal operational thinking that occurs between the ages of 11 and 14 years?
   a. Thought process includes thinking in concrete terms.
   b. Thought process includes information obtained from the environment and peers.
   c. Thought process includes thinking in abstract terms, possibilities, and hypotheses.
   d. All of the above.

9. Jimmy, a 13-year-old, is sent to the school nurse because he and some of his peers were observed chewing tobacco while playing baseball. The nurse knows that the best way to influence Jimmy's behavior for health promotion is:
   a. Tell Jimmy that he will be suspended from school if he continues to chew the tobacco.
   b. Show Jimmy pictures of oral cancers caused by chewing tobacco.
   c. Tell Jimmy about the dangers of chewing tobacco and stress the fact that girls do not like boys who chew tobacco.
   d. Arrange for a local baseball hero to talk with Jimmy and his friends to stress that he does not use chewing tobacco, his friends do not chew tobacco, and chewing tobacco causes ugly teeth.

10. According to Erikson, a key to identity achievement in adolescence is best described as:
   a. related to the adolescent's interactions with others, serving as a mirror and reflecting information back to the adolescent.
   b. linked to the role he or she plays within the family.
   c. related to the adolescent's acceptance of parental guidelines.
   d. related to the adolescent's ability to finalize his or her plans for future accomplishments.

11. The formation of sexual identity development during adolescence usually involves which of the following?
   a. Forming close friendships with same-sex peers during early adolescence
   b. Developing intimate relationships with members of the opposite sex during the later part of adolescence
   c. Developing emotional and social identities separate from those of families
   d. All of the above

12. Advances in cognitive development bring which of the following changes for adolescents?
    a. Their beliefs become more concrete and less rooted in general ideologic principles.
    b. They show an increasing emotional understanding and acceptance of parents' beliefs as their own.
    c. They encounter few new situations or opportunities for decisions because of their past experiences.
    d. They develop a personal value system distinct from that of significant adults in their lives.

13. Compared with school-age children, adolescent peer groups are:
    a. more likely to include peers of the opposite sex.
    b. less autonomous.
    c. less likely to influence members' socialization roles.
    d. more likely to require parental supervision.

14. Of the following male reproductive problems, the one most likely to be identified in an adolescent male is:
    a. hypospadias.
    b. cryptorchidism.
    c. testicular tumor.
    d. urethritis.

15. The adolescent with testicular cancer is most likely to present with which of the following signs and symptoms?
    a. Tender, painful swelling of the testes
    b. A mass in the posterior aspect of the scrotum that transilluminates

c. A heavy, hard mass palpable on the anterior or lateral surface of the testicle
d. An asymptomatic scrotal mass that aches, especially after exercise or penile erection

16. It is important to assess adverse effects of exercise on the reproductive cycle in an adolescent with anorexia nervosa. The signs of adverse effects of exercise on an adolescent's reproductive cycle may include:
    a. dysmenorrhea.
    b. weight loss.
    c. decreased appetite.
    d. amenorrhea.

17. T   F   There is evidence that greater levels of religiosity and spirituality in adolescence are associated with fewer high risk behaviors and more health-promoting behaviors.

18. T   F   Evidence suggests that bariatric surgery in adolescents results in sustained weight loss, a decrease in BMI, and a decrease in the incidence of comorbidities such as type II diabetes.

III. THINKING CRITICALLY

1. Explain the principles of physical growth that are important for adolescent girls to understand if they are concerned about their weight.

2. Explain how a peer group contributes to the development of a sense of identity in the adolescent and why peer groups are an important influence during the adolescent years.

3. Describe three guiding principles to offer to parents of adolescents to help them better communicate with their adolescent child.

4. Explain how an adolescent can benefit from participating in sports.

5. Explain why there has been a recent increased incidence of anorexia and bulimia in the United States.

6. Identify the essential aspects of multidisciplinary treatment for anorexia nervosa and bulimia.

7. Describe the characteristics typically seen with adolescent suicide.

36 Chronic Illness, Disability, and End-of-Life Care

I. LEARNING KEY TERMS

MATCHING: Match each term with its corresponding description.

1. _____ A principle in the care of children with special needs that refers to establishing a normal pattern of living.

2. _____ Actions carried out by a person other than the patient to end the life of the patient suffering from a terminal illness.

3. _____ Coping mechanisms that result in movement away from adjustment; maladaptation to the crisis.

4. _____ The active total care of a patient whose disease is not responsive to curative treatment.

5. _____ The concept of providing palliative care for the child with no reasonable expectation of cure so that he or she can live to the fullest without pain, with choices and dignity, and with family support.

6. _____ Coping mechanisms that result in movement toward adjustment and resolution of the crisis.

7. _____ An emotional response that is manifested through the life span of the parent-child interaction; acceptance interspersed with periods of intensified sorrow for losses, especially at certain landmarks of the child's development (e.g., entry into school, the onset of puberty).

8. _____ The behavioral reaction that occurs when death is the expected or possible outcome of a disorder.

9. _____ A process of recognizing, promoting, and enhancing competence.

10. _____ Behaviors aimed at reducing the tension caused by a crisis.

11. _____ A defense mechanism that is a necessary cushion to prevent disintegration and is a normal response to grieving for any type of loss.

a. Coping mechanisms

b. Normalization

c. Approach behaviors

d. Chronic sorrow

e. Avoidance behaviors

f. Anticipatory grief

g. Palliative care

h. Euthanasia

i. Hospice

j. Denial

k. Empowerment

II. REVIEWING KEY CONCEPTS

1. Technologic advancements have inadvertently increased the incidence of:
   a. deaths.
   b. disabilities.
   c. asthma.
   d. cognitive impairment.

2. A goal that is considered inappropriate for family-centered care is for the nurse to:
   a. maintain the integrity of the family.
   b. empower the family members.
   c. support the family during stressful times.
   d. maintain a high level of control.

3. A major goal in working with the family of a child with special needs is to:

4. Identify one strategy to use to help break patterns of unproductive interaction in parents of a child with special needs.

5. Which of the following factors is more characteristic of a father's pattern than a mother's pattern of adjusting to a chronically ill child? The father is more likely to:
   a. feel a threat to his self-esteem.
   b. report a periodic crisis pattern.
   c. forfeit personal goals.
   d. seek immediate professional counseling.

6. Describe the adaptive tasks of parents who have a child with a chronic condition.

7. The sibling of a child with a chronic disabling condition may feel:
   a. responsibility for caregiving.
   b. differential treatment by parents.
   c. limitations in family resources.
   d. a, b, and c.

8. When the parents of a child with special needs experience chronic sorrow, the process:
   a. of grief is pronounced and self-limiting.
   b. involves social reintegration after grieving.
   c. is characterized by realistic expectations.
   d. is interspersed with periods of intensified grief.

9. List the three common phases of families' responses to the diagnosis of a chronic illness or disability.

10. When the parent of a child who is dying tells the nurse the child is in pain even when the child appears comfortable, the nurse should be sure that:
    a. as needed (prn) pain control measures are instituted.
    b. pain control is administered on a preventive schedule.
    c. parents understand that pain is a physical process.
    d. parents understand that the child is probably in less pain than he or she appears to be.

11. Pain control is often a concern of dying children and their parents. Which of the following strategies should the nurse use to help them deal with this fear?
    a. Assure the parents that the pain will be relieved.
    b. Use heavy sedation to help the child cope with this phase.
    c. Adopt a medication schedule that will prevent the pain from escalating.
    d. Give pain medications intravenously only when the child is near death.

12. List at least five physical signs of approaching death.

13. A family's reaction during the terminal stage of illness involves a period of intense anticipatory grieving characterized by:
    a. depression.
    b. loss of hope.
    c. intensification of fears.
    d. a, b, and c.

14. Complicated grief reactions include symptoms of:
    a. denial.
    b. anger.
    c. pangs of severe emotion.
    d. depression.

15. Which of the following symptoms is considered normal acute grief behavior?
    a. Feeling the need to have friends and relatives around
    b. Feeling an emotional closeness to friends and relatives
    c. Hearing the dead person's voice
    d. a, b, and c

16. After a child's death, which of the following evaluation strategies is most likely to support and guide the family members through the resolution of their loss?
    a. A written questionnaire
    b. A telephone call placed 2 days after the death
    c. Meeting with the family at the time of death
    d. A telephone call placed 6 weeks after the death

17. Which of the following techniques is considered an example of the most therapeutic communication to use with the bereaved family?
    a. Cheerfulness
    b. Interpretation
    c. Validating loss
    d. Reassurance

III. THINKING CRITICALLY

1. Describe how the changes that have occurred in the provision of services have improved the care of children with special needs.

2. Describe why it is necessary for the nurse to assess the family's specific perceptions concerning their child's illness or disability.

3. Describe how children between the ages of 3 and 5 years perceive death.

4. Describe how a preschooler who becomes seriously ill is likely to perceive his or her illness.

5. Describe why adolescents, more than any other age group, have more difficulty coping with death, particularly their own.

I. LEARNING KEY TERMS

MATCHING: Match each term with its corresponding description.

1. _____ Also referred to as partially sighted; refers to visual acuity between 20/70 and 20/200; usually allows child to obtain an education in the standard public school system with the use of normal-sized print.

2. _____ Refers to a person whose hearing disability precludes successful processing of linguistic information through audition, with or without a hearing aid.

3. _____ Visual loss that cannot be corrected with regular prescription lenses.

4. _____ Refers to a person who, generally with the use of a hearing aid, has residual hearing sufficient to enable successful processing of linguistic information through audition.

5. _____ A disability that may range in severity from mild to profound and includes the subsets of deaf and hard-of-hearing; one of the most common disabilities in the United States.

6. _____ Inability to express ideas in any form, either written or verbally.

7. _____ A region found in chromosome analysis that fails to condense during mitosis and is characterized by a nonstaining gap or narrowing.

8. _____ The inability to interpret sound correctly.

9. _____ The facial muscle coordination part of speech.

10. _____ Difficulty in processing details or discrimination among sounds.

11. _____ Technique in which the transmission of the audio portion of a television program is translated into subtitles that appear on the screen.

12. _____ The hearing and interpretation skills of speech.

13. _____ A unit of loudness measured at various frequencies; used to express the degree of hearing impairment.

14. _____ Learning through a step-by-step process in which each step of a skill is taught completely before proceeding to the next activity.

a. Cognitive impairment

b. Educable cognitive impairment

c. Trainable cognitive impairment

d. Task analysis

e. Receptive skills

f. Expressive skills

g. Fragile site

h. Hearing impairment

i. Deaf

j. Hard-of-hearing

k. Aphasia

l. Agnosia

m. Dysacusis

n. Decibel

o. Hearing threshold level

p. American sign language (ASL)/British sign language (BSL)

q. Refraction

r. Teletypewriters/telecommunications devices for the deaf (TDD)

s. Closed captioning

t. Visual impairment

u. School vision

v. Legal blindness

15. _____ Equipment used to help deaf people communicate with each other over the telephone.

16. _____ Generally equivalent to children with moderate levels of cognitive impairment; accounts for approximately 10% of the cognitively impaired population.

17. _____ The measurement of an individual's hearing impairment by means of an audiometer.

18. _____ Corresponds to the mildly impaired group, which constitutes approximately 85% of all people with cognitive impairment.

19. _____ A visual-gestural language using hand signals that roughly correspond to specific words and concepts in the English language.

20. _____ Visual acuity of 20/100 or less and/or a visual field of 20 degrees or less in the better eye; not a medical diagnosis; a legal definition that allows special considerations with regard to taxes, entrance into special school, eligibility for aid, and other benefits.

21. _____ A general term for any type of mental difficulty or deficiency; term is used synonymously with intellectual disability.

22. _____ Refers to the bending of light rays as they pass through the lens of the eye.

II. REVIEWING KEY CONCEPTS

MATCHING: Match the level of cognitive impairment/IQ range with the appropriate example of a child's maturation and/or development.

1. _____ A preschool-age child with noticeable delays in motor development and in speech.

2. _____ An adult who may walk but who needs complete custodial care.

3. _____ A school-age child who is able to walk and who can profit from systematic habit training.

4. _____ A preschool-age child who may not be noticed as cognitively impaired but is slow to walk, feed self, and talk.

a. Mild cognitive impairment (IQ of 50–55 to about 70)

b. Moderate cognitive impairment (IQ of 35–40 to 50–55)

c. Severe cognitive impairment (IQ of 20–25 to 35–40)

d. Profound cognitive impairment (IQ below 20–25)

5. The classification system for cognitive impairment allows for:
   a. achieving the same goals for each person.
   b. identification of needs in four care dimensions.
   c. only intelligence and no other criteria.
   d. an age limit of 12 years.

6. Acquiring social skills for the cognitively impaired child includes:
   a. teaching acceptable sexual behavior.
   b. exposing the child to strangers.
   c. greeting visitors without being overly friendly.
   d. a, b, and c.

7. Define task analysis and describe its use when teaching a cognitively impaired child.

8. Trisomy 21 is also known as:
   a. Jacob syndrome.
   b. Turner syndrome.
   c. Down syndrome.
   d. Klinefelter syndrome.

9. Prenatal testing and genetic counseling for Down syndrome should be offered to all women:
   a. regardless of family history.
   b. with a family history of the disorder and who are of advanced maternal age.
   c. with no family history of the disorder and who are of advanced maternal age.
   d. who become pregnant in their adolescent years.

10. Fragile X syndrome is:
    a. the most common inherited cause of cognitive impairment.
    b. caused by a missing gene on the Y chromosome.
    c. caused by an abnormal gene on chromosome 21.
    d. caused by a missing gene on the X chromosome.

11. Parents of a child with fragile X syndrome should optimally receive _____ _____.

12. The correct term to use for a person who is able to process linguistic information only with the use of a hearing aid is:
    a. deaf-mute.
    b. hard-of-hearing.
    c. deaf.
    d. aphasic.

13. Conductive hearing loss in children is most often a result of:
    a. use of aminoglycosides such as tobramycin and gentamicin.
    b. high noise levels in the neonatal environment.
    c. a congenital defect.
    d. recurrent serous otitis media.

14. In the initial screening of an infant with a suspected hearing impairment, the nurse should be alert for:
    a. absent cry.
    b. consistent lack of the startle reflex.
    c. a louder than usual cry.
    d. absence of babble or voice inflections by age 4 months.

15. In the assessment of a child to identify whether a hearing impairment has developed, the nurse would look for:
    a. a loud monotone voice.
    b. consistent lack of the startle reflex.
    c. a high level of social activity.
    d. attentiveness, especially when someone is talking.

16. All of the following are strategies that will enhance communication with a child who is hearing-impaired *except*:
    a. touching the child lightly to signal presence of a speaker.
    b. speaking at eye level or a 45-degree angle.
    c. using facial expressions to convey a message better.
    d. moving and using animated body language to communicate better.

MATCHING: Match each impairment with its corresponding description.

17. _____ Increased intraocular pressure.

18. _____ Squinted or crossed eyes.

19. _____ Different refractive strength in each eye.

20. _____ Unequal curvatures in refractive apparatus.

21. _____ Opacity of crystalline lens.

22. _____ Farsightedness.

23. _____ Lazy eye.

24. _____ Nearsightedness.

a. Myopia

b. Hyperopia

c. Astigmatism

d. Anisometropia

e. Amblyopia

f. Strabismus

g. Cataracts

h. Glaucoma

25. If a child has a penetrating injury to the eye, the nurse should:
    a. apply an eye patch.
    b. attempt to remove the object.
    c. irrigate the eye.
    d. take the child to the emergency department.

26. Which of the following situations would be considered abnormal?
    a. Presence of a red reflex in a 4-year-old
    b. A toddler with strabismus
    c. A 5-year-old who has hyperopia
    d. A healthy term newborn who does not consistently follow a brightly colored object with his eyes

27. Clinical manifestations of retinoblastoma include:
    a. white reflex (leukokoria).
    b. acquired strabismus.
    c. persistent painful erythematous eyes.
    d. a, b, and c.

28. List at least eight of the strategies that the nurse can use during hospitalization with a child who has lost his or her sight.

29. Which of the following statements is correct about eye care and sports?
    a. Glasses may interfere with the child's ability in sports.
    b. Eye protection gear should be worn for softball.
    c. Contact lenses provide less visual acuity than glasses for sports.
    d. It is usually very difficult to convince children to wear their glasses to play sports.

30. Which of the following examples would be most indicative of a language delay?
    a. A 14-month-old child who has not uttered his first word
    b. A 26-month-old who has not formed his first sentence
    c. An 18-month-old who uses short "telegraphic" phrases
    d. A 4-year-old whose speech is not entirely understandable

III. THINKING CRITICALLY

1. Describe the nursing interventions that should be used when caring for a hospitalized child who is cognitively impaired.

2. Describe why the hearing-impaired child is at a great disadvantage for developing social relationships.

3. Explain why it is difficult to teach a deaf child to speak.

4. Describe the measures that parents should use to help their children preserve their sight.

38 Family-Centered Care of the Child During Illness and Hospitalization

I. LEARNING KEY TERMS

MATCHING: Match each term with its corresponding description.

1. _____ An effective, nondirective modality for helping children deal with their concerns and fears; often helpful to the nurse in gaining insights into children's needs and feelings.

2. _____ Spending time being physically close to the child while using a quiet voice, eye contact, and touch.

3. _____ A psychologic technique reserved for use by trained and qualified therapists as an interpretive method with emotionally disturbed children.

4. _____ The major stress from middle infancy throughout the preschool years, especially for children ages 6 to 30 months.

5. _____ One of the most traumatic hospital experiences for the child and parents.

6. _____ Health care professionals with extensive knowledge of child growth and development and of the special psychosocial needs of hospitalized children.

a. Separation anxiety

b. Presence

c. Emergency admission

d. Child life specialists

e. Play therapy

f. Therapeutic play

II. REVIEWING KEY CONCEPTS

1. Major stressors of hospitalization in children include:
   a. loss of control.
   b. separation.
   c. bodily injury.
   d. pain.
   e. a, b, c, and d.

MATCHING: Match each phase of separation anxiety with the behaviors that are typical of that phase.

2. _____ Inactive; withdraws from others; uninterested in environment; uncommunicative; regression behaviors.

3. _____ Becomes more interested in surroundings; interacts with caregivers; resigned to the situation; rarely seen in hospitalized children; occurs in prolonged parental absences.

4. _____ Cries; screams; attacks stranger physically and verbally; attempts to escape; continuous crying.

a. Protest

b. Despair

c. Detachment

5. T F Preschoolers may demonstrate separation anxiety by refusing to eat, experiencing difficulty in sleeping, crying quietly for their parents, continually asking when the parents will visit, or withdrawing from others.

6. T F Parents of a hospitalized child may experience a sense of helplessness and question the skill level of the staff.

7. What age group is more likely to experience increased stress to hospitalization and loss of peer group contact?
   a. preschooler
   b. middle school-age child
   c. adolescent
   d. early school-age child

8. A toddler is most likely to react to short-term hospitalization with feelings of loss of control that result from altered routines; this is often manifested by:
   a. regression.
   b. withdrawal.
   c. formation of new superficial relationships.
   d. self-assertion and anger.

9. Which of the following risk factors make a child more vulnerable to the stressors of hospitalization?
   a. Male gender
   b. Strong support network
   c. Female gender
   d. Passive temperament

10. The pediatric population in the hospital today is different from the pediatric population of 10 years ago in that the usual length of stay has:
    a. decreased and the acuity has increased.
    b. increased and the acuity has decreased.
    c. increased and the acuity has increased.
    d. decreased and the acuity has decreased.

11. Describe at least three posthospital behaviors commonly observed in young children.

12. Siblings who visit their brother or sister in the hospital have an increased tendency to exhibit which of the following behaviors?
    a. Resentment
    b. Anger
    c. Guilt
    d. Acceptance
    e. a, b, and c

13. To help the parents deal with the issues related to separation while their child is hospitalized, the nurse should suggest that parents:
    a. quietly leave while the child is distracted or asleep.
    b. make the surroundings familiar with the child's toys from home.
    c. encourage infrequent parental visits to help decrease the child's frequency of disappointment.
    d. visit over one extended time if rooming-in is impossible.

14. One technique used during hospitalization that can minimize the disruption in the routine of the school-age child who is not critically ill is:
    a. stop school activities.
    b. wear hospital scrubs.
    c. encourage self-care.
    d. watch television.

15. Preparing children for intrusive procedures usually increases their:
    a. feelings of control.
    b. fear.
    c. stress.
    d. misconceptions.

16. Whenever performing a painful procedure on a child, the nurse should attempt to:
    a. perform the procedure in the playroom.
    b. use techniques such as drawing or doll play to help the child understand the procedure.
    c. perform the procedure quickly.
    d. have the parents leave during the procedure.

17. Which of the following reactions to surgery is most typical of an adolescent's reaction to fear of bodily injury?
    a. Concern about the pain
    b. Concern about the procedure itself
    c. Concern about the scar
    d. Understanding explanations literally

18. Identify 3 factors that affect parents' reactions to their child's illness.

19. Describe how toddlers manifest fear of bodily injury.

20. Describe how preschoolers manifest fear of bodily injury.

21. Describe how school-age children manifest fear of bodily injury.

III. THINKING CRITICALLY

1. Describe at least three nursing interventions to use to promote positive family relationships.

2. Considering developmental and safety needs, what types of toys should be recommended for a 4-year-old child who is hospitalized?

3. Describe the strategies a nurse should use to establish a trusting relationship with hospitalized school-age children.

39 Pediatric Variations of Nursing Interventions

I. LEARNING KEY TERMS

MATCHING: Match each term with its corresponding description.

1. _____ Provides for total alimentary needs when feeding by way of the gastrointestinal tract is impossible, inadequate, or hazardous; also known as *hyperalimentation*.

2. _____ Designed for patients documented or suspected to be infected or colonized with highly transmissible or epidemiologically important pathogens.

3. _____ A noninvasive method of providing continual monitoring of partial pressure of oxygen in arterial blood that uses an electrode that is attached to the skin.

4. _____ The primary strategy for successful nosocomial infection control; synthesizes the major features of Standard (blood and body fluid) Precautions, designed to reduce the risk of transmission of blood-borne pathogens, and body substance isolation (BSI), designed to reduce the risk of transmission of pathogens from moist body substances; applies to blood, all body fluids, secretions, and excretions, except sweat, regardless of whether or not blood is visible in the body substance.

5. _____ Designed to reduce the risk of transmission of droplets suspended in the air for long periods of time.

6. _____ Designed to reduce the risk of transmission of infectious agents generated from the source person primarily during coughing, sneezing, or talking and during the performance of certain procedures such as suctioning and bronchoscopy.

7. _____ One who is legally under the age of majority but is recognized as having the legal capacity of an adult under circumstances prescribed by state law, such as pregnancy, marriage, high school graduation, living independently, or military service.

8. _____ A simple, continuous, noninvasive method of determining oxygen saturation; used to guide oxygen therapy.

9. _____ Designed to reduce the risk of transmission of epidemiologically important microorganisms by physical transfer of microorganisms to a susceptible host from an infected or colonized person or from a contaminated intermediate object.

10. _____ A physiologic hazard of oxygen therapy, wherein the respiratory center has adapted to the continuously higher arterial carbon dioxide levels; hypoxia becomes the more powerful stimulus for respiration; occurs when oxygen is administered and the hypoxic drive is removed, resulting in hypoventilation, increased arterial carbon dioxide levels, and unconsciousness.

a. Informed consent

b. Emancipated minor

c. Standard Precautions

d. Transmission-based precautions

e. Airborne precautions

f. Droplet precautions

g. Contact precautions

h. Intermittent infusion device

i. Central venous access device

j. Oxygen-induced carbon dioxide narcosis

k. Pulse oximetry

l. Transcutaneous oxygen monitoring

m. Total parenteral nutrition

11. _____ A device that is an alternative to keeping an intravenous line intact for intermittent use; the device remains in place and is flushed after infusion of medication.

12. _____ Refers to the legal and ethical requirement that the patient clearly, fully, and completely understands the proposed medical treatment to be performed, including significant risks associated with the treatment.

13. _____ Used for frequent total parenteral nutrition (hyperalimentation), blood sampling, or antibiotic therapy and for the management of long-term chemotherapy.

II. REVIEWING KEY CONCEPTS

1. When the parents are divorced, who must consent to medical treatment of the child?
   a. The child
   b. Either parent
   c. Both parents
   d. The legal guardian

2. The nurse is preparing to administer an oral analgesic to a 4-year-old. The nurse's best approach to involve the child's cooperation is reflected in the statement:
   a. Do you want to take this medicine now? It tastes yummy.
   b. It's time for your pain medicine. Would you like water or some Gatorade to drink with it?
   c. Here's your medicine. Do you want me to give it to you or would you rather your mother give it?
   d. Here is your pain medicine. If you don't take it you'll have lots of pain.

3. If a child needs support during an invasive procedure, the nurse should:
   a. inform the parents about how the child did after the procedure.
   b. ask the parents to stay in the room, where they can have eye contact with the child.
   c. decide whether parental presence will be beneficial and try to let the parents choose.
   d. encourage the parents to stay close by to console the child immediately following the procedure.

4. List at least five strategies the nurse can use to support the child during and after a procedure.

5. Describe at least one play activity for each of the following procedures.

   a. Ambulation

   b. Range of motion

   c. Injections

   d. Deep breathing

   e. Extending the environment

   f. Soaks

   g. Fluid intake

6. To prepare a breastfed infant physically for surgery, the nurse would expect to:
   a. permit breastfeeding up to 4 hours before surgery.
   b. withhold breastfeeding as of midnight the night before surgery.
   c. withhold breastfeeding from 4 to 8 hours before surgery.
   d. replace breast milk with formula and permit feeding up to 2 hours before surgery.

7. The most atraumatic choice for a preanesthetic medication in a 5-year-old scheduled for a tonsillectomy would be:
   a. intramuscular morphine sulfate.
   b. intravenous midazolam through an established site.
   c. intramuscular promethazine, chlorpromazine, and meperidine.
   d. oral promethazine, chlorpromazine, and meperidine.

8. Fear of induction of anesthesia by mask can be minimized by applying:
   a. the mask quickly and with assurance.
   b. an opaque mask.
   c. the mask while the child is sitting.
   d. the mask while the child is supine.

9. An increased heart rate, increased respiratory rate, and increased blood pressure in the immediate post-operative period of a young child would most likely indicate:
   a. pain.
   b. infection.
   c. shock.
   d. increased intracranial pressure.

10. The strategies that would be considered an organizational attempt to improve compliance of the family with a young child would be to:
    a. incorporate teaching principles that are known to enhance understanding.
    b. encourage the family to adapt to the hospital medication schedules.
    c. evaluate and reduce the time the family waits for their appointment.
    d. a, b, and c.

11. Which of the following examples of a child's food intake is the best sample of adequate documentation?
    a. Child ate about a cup of cereal with ½ cup of milk.
    b. Child ate an adequate breakfast.
    c. Child ate 80% of the breakfast served.
    d. Parent states that child ate an adequate breakfast.

12. After cleft lip surgery, the nurse should protect the operative site by using:
    a. arm and leg restraints.
    b. elbow restraints.
    c. a jacket restraint.
    d. a mummy restraint.

13. The best positioning technique for a lumbar puncture in a neonate is a:
    a. side-lying position with neck flexion.
    b. sitting position.
    c. side-lying position with modified neck extension.
    d. side-lying position with knees to chest.

14. The most frequently used site for bone marrow aspiration in children is the:
    a. femur.
    b. sternum.
    c. tibia.
    d. iliac crest.

15. To avoid the complication of necrotizing osteochondritis when performing infant heel puncture, the puncture should be:
    a. no deeper than 4.2 mm and on the inner aspect of the heel.
    b. no deeper than 2.4 mm and on the outer aspect of the heel.
    c. no deeper than 2.4 mm and on the inner aspect of the heel.
    d. no deeper than 4.2 mm and on the outer aspect of the heel.

16. To obtain a sputum specimen for tuberculosis testing in an infant, the nurse would optimally:
    a. have the infant cough.
    b. obtain mucus from the throat.
    c. insert a suction catheter into the back of the throat.
    d. perform gastric lavage in the morning before breakfast.

17. Of the following choices for measuring 1 teaspoon of medication at home, the best device for the nurse to instruct the parent to use at home is the:
    a. household soup spoon.
    b. household measuring spoon.
    c. hospital's USP standard dropper.
    d. calibrated hollow-handled medicine spoon.

18. All of the following techniques for medication administration to an infant are acceptable except:
    a. adding the medication to the infant's 8 oz bottle of formula.
    b. allowing the infant to sit in the parent's lap during administration.
    c. allowing the infant to suck the medication from an empty nipple.
    d. inserting the needleless syringe into the side of the mouth while the infant nurses.

19. When determining the needle length for intramuscular injection of medication into a child, the nurse should:
    a. choose a 1-inch needle for a 4-month-old infant.
    b. use a needle length that is too short rather than one that is too long.
    c. choose a half-inch needle for a 4-month-old infant.
    d. grasp the muscle between the thumb and forefinger, choosing a length that is less than half the distance.

20. The preferred site for intramuscular injection in an infant is the:
    a. deltoid muscle.
    b. dorsogluteal.
    c. vastus lateralis.
    d. ventrogluteal.

21. Total parenteral nutrition (TPN) is infused by way of a central intravenous line because:
    a. other medications need to be infused with the TPN.
    b. several attempts to administer it peripherally have probably occurred.
    c. there is less risk of infection.
    d. the glucose in the solution is irritating to the smaller veins.

22. To instill eyedrops in an infant whose eyelids are clenched shut, the nurse should:
    a. apply finger pressure to the lacrimal punctum.
    b. place the drops in the nasal corner where the lids meet and wait until the infant opens the lid.
    c. administer the eyedrops before nap time.
    d. a, b, and c.

23. During intermittent or continuous enteral feedings, the nurse should:
    a. push the formula gradually through the feeding tube.
    b. use a parenteral burette to calibrate the feeding times.
    c. give the infant a pacifier for sucking.
    d. hang the feeding container from an IV pole.

24. A 3-year-old child with cystic fibrosis has a skin-level-feeding device and is being cared for in the home. The mother calls the skin specialist and says the skin around the skin-level device is moist and beefy red but there is no evidence of foul odor, bleeding, or formula leakage. The nurse is aware that this finding is:
    a. a skin infection.
    b. normal granulation tissue.
    c. a reason to change the skin-level device.
    d. a reason to discontinue using this device.

25. One of the major advantages of the recently developed skin-level devices for feeding children is that the button device:
    a. does not clog as easily as other devices.
    b. eliminates the need for frequent bubbling.
    c. is less expensive than the traditional devices.
    d. allows the child more mobility.

26. A 7-year-old child is being prepared for bowel surgery. The best agent for bowel cleansing in this child is:
    a. a pediatric Fleet enema.
    b. a commercially prepared hypertonic enema solution.
    c. an oral polyethylene glycol–electrolyte solution.
    d. plain water enemas.

27. In order to protect the pouch, a young child with an ostomy may need to:
    a. wear a loose-fitting one-piece outfit.
    b. begin toilet training at a later than usual age.
    c. limit activity to avoid skin damage.
    d. use elbow restraints at all times.

28. In an infant with an unpouched colostomy, optimal skin care around the stoma would include:
    a. barrier substance such as zinc oxide.
    b. larger diaper than the one usually worn.
    c. stoma powder mixed with skin barrier.
    d. a, b, and c.

29. A 10-year-old girl diagnosed with leukemia has an implanted port. The advantage(s) of such a device include:
    a. Requires no dressing unless accessed for blood draw or infusion.
    b. Change in body appearance is minimal or negligible.
    c. No limitations on physical activity (except some contact sports).
    d. a, b, and c.

III. THINKING CRITICALLY

1. Discuss the purpose, rationale, and requirements for the use of medical-surgical restraints in children.

2. Discuss the current evidence as well as best practice for verifying NG tube placement in a young (18-month-old) pediatric patient.

3. Describe and briefly discuss the use of end-tidal carbon dioxide monitoring ($ETCO_2$) in a child recovering from moderate procedural sedation.

40 Respiratory Dysfunction

I. LEARNING KEY TERMS

MATCHING: Match each term with its corresponding description.

1. _____ A measurement of the maximum flow of air that can be forcefully exhaled in 1 second; a key measurement of pulmonary function.

2. _____ A worsening of symptoms, either abrupt or progressive.

3. _____ Cessation of breathing for more than 20 seconds or for a shorter period of time when associated with hypoxemia or bradycardia.

4. _____ Exposure to environmental tobacco smoke; a well-established danger to children.

5. _____ Involves stimulating the production of sweat with a special device (stimulation with 3-mA electric current), collecting the sweat on filter paper, and measuring the sweat electrolytes; used in the diagnosis of cystic fibrosis.

6. _____ Inability of the respiratory apparatus to maintain adequate oxygenation of the blood, with or without carbon dioxide retention.

7. _____ A serious obstructive inflammatory process in the upper airway that occurs most often in children 2 to 8 years of age.

8. _____ In general, applies to two conditions: increased work of breathing with near normal gas exchange function or the inability to maintain normal blood gas tensions that develops from carbon dioxide retention with subsequent hypoxemia and acidosis.

9. _____ Characterized by hoarseness and a "barking" cough.

10. _____ The earliest manifestation of cystic fibrosis where the small intestine is blocked with thick, puttylike, tenacious, mucilaginous meconium in the newborn.

11. _____ The child insists on sitting upright and leaning forward with the chin thrust out, mouth open, and tongue protruding.

12. _____ Irritants such as house dust mites, whose prevention (or reduced exposure to) is the goal of nonpharmacologic therapy for asthma.

13. _____ An infection of the mucosa of the upper trachea with features of both croup and epiglottis.

a. Bacterial tracheitis

b. Croup

c. Tripod position

d. Acute epiglottitis

e. Passive smoking

f. Exacerbation

g. Peak expiratory flow rate (PEFR)

h. Allergen

i. Meconium ileus

j. Respiratory insufficiency

k. Respiratory failure

l. Pertussis

m. Sweat chloride test

n. Direct observation therapy (DOT)

o. Airway clearance therapies

p. Apnea

14. _____ Considered to be the cornerstone treatment for children and adolescents with cystic fibrosis.

15. _____ Observation of medication being taken by trained observer; often used with tuberculosis medications to shorten therapy and improve effectiveness.

16. _____ Highly contagious respiratory disease in nonvaccinated children; young infants demonstrate a characteristic expiratory whoop but older children may only have a cough.

II. REVIEWING KEY CONCEPTS

1. Most respiratory infections in children are caused by:
   a. pneumococci.
   b. viruses.
   c. streptococci.
   d. *Haemophilus influenzae.*

2. The most likely reason that the respiratory infection rate increases drastically in the age range from 3 to 6 months is that the:
   a. infant's exposure to pathogens is greatly increased during this time.
   b. viral agents that are mild in older children are extremely severe in infants.
   c. maternal antibodies have decreased and the infant's own antibody production is immature.
   d. diameter of the airways is smaller in the infant than in the older child.

3. The primary concern of the nurse when giving tips for how to increase humidity in the home of a child with a respiratory infection should be to make sure the child has:
   a. continuous contact with the humidification source.
   b. a warm humidification source.
   c. a humidification source that is safe.
   d. a cool humidification source.

4. Which of the following is the best choice for the child with a respiratory disorder who needs rest but is resisting staying in bed?
   a. Be sure the mother takes the advice seriously.
   b. Allow the child to play quietly on the bed or floor.
   c. Insist that the child play quietly in bed.
   d. Allow the child to cry until he or she stays in bed.

5. The best technique to prevent spread of nasopharyngitis is:
   a. prompt immunization.
   b. to avoid contact with infected people.
   c. mist vaporization.
   d. to ensure adequate fluid intake.

6. Group A β-hemolytic streptococcal (GABHS) infection is usually a:
   a. serious infection of the upper airway.
   b. common cause of pharyngitis in children over the age of 15 years.
   c. brief illness that places the child at risk for serious sequelae.
   d. disease of the heart, lungs, joints, and central nervous system.

7. In the postoperative period following a tonsillectomy, the child should be:
   a. placed in the Trendelenburg position.
   b. encouraged to cough and deep breathe.
   c. suctioned vigorously to clear the airway.
   d. placed on bed rest for the day of surgery.

8. The best pain medication administration regimen for a child in the initial postoperative period following a tonsillectomy is:
   a. at regular intervals.
   b. as needed.

9. Of the foods listed, the most appropriate selection to offer first to an alert child who is in the postoperative period following a tonsillectomy is:
   a. strawberry ice cream.
   b. red cherry-flavored gelatin.
   c. an apple-flavored ice pop.
   d. cold diluted orange juice.

10. Which of the following signs is an early indication of hemorrhage in a child who has had a tonsillectomy?
    a. Continuous swallowing
    b. Decreasing blood pressure
    c. Restlessness
    d. a, b, and c

11. During influenza epidemics, it is generally believed the age group that provides a major source of transmission is the:
    a. infant.
    b. school-age child.
    c. adolescent.
    d. preschool-age child.

12. The clinical manifestations of influenza usually include all of the following *except*:
    a. nausea and vomiting.
    b. fever and chills.
    c. sore throat and dry mucous membranes.
    d. photophobia and myalgia.

13. The infant is predisposed to developing otitis media because the eustachian tubes:
    a. are relatively short and open.
    b. have a limited amount of lymphoid tissue.
    c. are relatively long and narrow.
    d. are completely underdeveloped.

14. An abnormal otoscopic examination would reveal:
    a. visible landmarks.
    b. a light reflex.
    c. an opaque immobile tympanic membrane.
    d. a mobile tympanic membrane.

15. Children with croup syndrome and mild mucosal swelling:
    a. require hospitalization.
    b. will need to be intubated.
    c. can be cared for at home.
    d. are over 6 years old.

16. The nurse should prepare for an impending emergency situation to care for the child with suspected:
    a. spasmodic croup.
    b. laryngotracheobronchitis.
    c. acute spasmodic laryngitis.
    d. epiglottitis.

17. The nurse should suspect epiglottitis if the child has:
    a. cough, sore throat, and agitation.
    b. cough, drooling, and retractions.
    c. absence of cough in the presence of drooling and agitation.
    d. absence of cough, hoarseness, and retractions.

18. In the child who is suspected of having epiglottitis, the nurse should.
    a. have intubation equipment available.
    b. visually inspect the child's oropharynx with a tongue blade.
    c. obtain a throat culture.
    d. prepare to immunize the child for *Haemophilus influenzae.*

19. Since the advent of immunization for *Haemophilus influenzae*, there has been a decrease in the incidence of:
    a. laryngotracheobronchitis.
    b. epiglottitis.
    c. influenza (seasonal).
    d. croup.

20. Which one of the following children is most likely to be hospitalized for treatment of croup?
    a. The 2-year-old child whose croupy cough worsens at night
    b. The 5-year-old child whose croupy cough worsens at night
    c. The 2-year-old child using the accessory muscles to breathe
    d. The 2-year-old child with inspiratory stridor when upright and supine

21. The nurse may anticipate intubation as the care management for the young child diagnosed with:
    a. acute spasmodic laryngitis.
    b. bacterial tracheitis.
    c. acute laryngotracheobronchitis.
    d. acute laryngitis.

22. Respiratory syncytial virus (RSV) is:
    a. an uncommon virus that causes severe bronchiolitis.
    b. an uncommon virus that usually does not require hospitalization.
    c. a common virus that usually causes moderate-to-severe bronchiolitis.
    d. a common virus that usually does not require hospitalization.

23. The use of the monoclonal antibody palivizumab for the prevention of RSV is preferred in high-risk children because:
    a. it is administered intravenously.
    b. of its ease of administration, safety, and effectiveness.
    c. it is licensed only for the prevention of RSV disease.
    d. it is an immune globulin that neutralizes antibodies.

24. Nursing care management of the 6-month-old infant with RSV bronchiolitis will include:
    a. monitoring oxygenation with pulse oximetry.
    b. suctioning nasal secretions before nursing.
    c. ensuring adequate oral fluid intake.
    d. a, b, and c.

25. General signs of pneumonia include:
    a. low fever and nausea.
    b. clear breath sounds and brown sputum.
    c. cough, tachypnea, and retractions.
    d. nasal flaring and tympany with percussion.

26. Because of the potential for empyema, closed chest drainage is most likely to be used in the treatment of:
    a. Haemophilus pneumonia.
    b. mycoplasmal pneumonia.
    c. streptococcal pneumonia.
    d. staphylococcal pneumonia.

27. In an 8-month-old infant admitted to the hospital with pertussis, the nurse should inquire about the:
    a. living conditions of the infant and family.
    b. labor and delivery history of the mother.
    c. immunization status of the infant.
    d. alcohol and drug intake of the mother.

28. The best test to screen for tuberculosis infection is the:
    a. chest radiograph.
    b. tuberculin skin test (TST).
    c. sputum culture.
    d. DNA blood test.

29. The child who has active tuberculosis infection is treated with:
    a. isoniazid.
    b. rifampin.
    c. pyrazinamide.
    d. a combination of the above drugs.

30. Severity of a foreign body aspiration is determined by:
    a. location of the object in the airway.
    b. the type of object aspirated.
    c. the extent of obstruction.
    d. a, b, and c.

31. The term latent tuberculosis infection (LTBI) is used to indicate infection in a person with:
    a. positive TST.
    b. absence of physical findings of disease.
    c. a normal chest radiograph.
    d. a, b, and c.

32. Which of the following questions would be most important for the nurse to ask the parents of a child admitted to the hospital with a diagnosis of reactive airway disease?
    a. "What brings you to the hospital?"
    b. "What is your ethnic background?"
    c. "Do you have a history of asthma in your family?"
    d. "Were your pregnancy and delivery uneventful?"

33. The nurse examines a 6-year-old child with asthma and finds that there is hyperresonance on percussion. Breath sounds are coarse and loud with sonorous crackles throughout the lung fields. Expiration is prolonged; rales can be heard. There is generalized inspiratory and expiratory wheezing. The child has these symptoms two times a week, with nighttime episodes a few times per month. He uses a short-acting β-agonist daily and his FEV_1 is 80%. Based on these findings, the nurse suspects that there is:
    a. moderate persistent asthma.
    b. severe persistent asthma.
    c. mild persistent asthma.
    d. mild intermittent asthma.

34. When preparing for discharge, the nurse would include in the home plan of care for the family of an asthmatic child to:
    a. keep the humidity at home above 50%.
    b. use only feather pillows.
    c. limit animal dander by removing cats and/or dogs.
    d. take long-term control medication even in the absence of symptoms.

35. Which of the following principles should be a part of the home self-management program for a child with asthma?
    a. Individuals must learn not to abuse their medications so that they will not become addicted.
    b. It is easy to treat an asthmatic episode as long as the child knows the symptoms.
    c. Although quite uncommon, asthma is very treatable.
    d. Children with asthma are usually able to participate in the same activities as nonasthmatic children.

36. The principal treatment for the insufficiency that occurs in cystic fibrosis is the administration of:
    a. enemas.
    b. corticosteroids.
    c. antibiotics.
    d. pancreatic enzymes.

37. Which of the following strategies would most likely be contraindicated for a child with cystic fibrosis to use?
    a. Forced expiration
    b. Aerobic exercise
    c. Supplemental oxygen as desired
    d. Percussion and postural drainage

38. Supplements are given in cystic fibrosis in the form of:
    a. multivitamins.
    b. a water-miscible form of fat-soluble vitamins.
    c. pancreatic enzymes.
    d. a, b, and c.

39. List the four cardinal signs of impending respiratory failure.

40. Which of the following represent the early subtle signs of hypoxia?
    a. Peripheral cyanosis
    b. Central cyanosis
    c. Hypotension
    d. Mood changes and restlessness

MATCHING: Match each drug used for pediatric emergency care with its appropriate use during resuscitation.

41. _____ β-adrenergic agonist used as an inhaled bronchodilator.

42. _____ Antibiotic of choice in otitis media when causative organism is a highly resistant pneumococcus.

43. _____ A long-acting ß2-agonist (bronchodilator) that is used twice a day (no more frequently than every 12 hours).

44. _____ A potent muscle relaxant that acts to decrease inflammation and improves pulmonary function and peak flow rate among pediatric patients with severe asthma.

45. _____ First-line drug for pulmonary tuberculosis infection.

46. _____ Considered the cornerstone in the pharmacologic management of asthma.

47. _____ Leukotriene modifier used for long-term management of asthma.

48. _____ Anticholinergic that acts as a bronchodilator to relieve asthma symptoms.

49. _____ When nebulized it has been shown to be effective in improving airway hydration and increasing mucus clearance in patients with CF.

50. _____ A monoclonal antibody that blocks the binding of IgE to mast cells; inhibits the inflammation that is associated with asthma and it is used in patients with moderate to persistent asthma who have confirmed perennial aeroallergen sensitivity.

51. _____ Acts to decrease the viscosity of mucus to improve airway clearance.

52. _____ First-line choice antibiotic for the treatment of acute otitis media.

a. Inhaled corticosteroid

b. Ceftriaxone

c. Magnesium sulphate

d. Singulair

e. Salmeterol

f. Amoxicillin

g. Dornase Alpha (Pulmozyme)

h. Albuterol

i. Ipratropium

j. Omalizumab (Xolair)

k. Hypertonic saline

l. Isoniazid

III. THINKING CRITICALLY

1. Describe the parameters that the nurse should assess to recognize status asthmaticus.

2. Explain the rationale for each of the following clinical manifestations of cystic fibrosis.

   a. Respiratory symptoms

   b. Delayed growth and development

   c. Anorexia

3. Describe the instructions the nurse should give to a mother of a child with tuberculosis infection about returning to school.

41 Gastrointestinal Dysfunction

I. LEARNING KEY TERMS

MATCHING: Match each term with its corresponding description.

1. _____ Induction of IgE antibody formation—initial exposure resulting in an immune response and subsequent exposure inducing a much stronger response.

2. _____ Proteins that are capable of inducing IgE antibody formation.

3. _____ Characterized by extremely long intervals between defecation.

4. _____ The infrequent passage of firm or hard stools or of small, hard masses with associated symptoms such as difficulty in expulsion, blood-streaked bowel movements, and abdominal discomfort; frequency not diagnostic.

5. _____ Stool normally passed within 24 to 36 hours after birth. (Newborns with irregularities in the passing of this stool should be evaluated further for possible congenital anomalies.)

6. _____ Dietary patterns that exclude meat.

7. _____ Used to successfully treat infants with isotonic, hypotonic, and hypertonic dehydration; the first line of treatment for diarrhea and dehydration.

8. _____ Trace elements with a daily requirement of less than 100 mg; exact role in nutrition unclear.

9. _____ Constipation with fecal soiling.

10. _____ Fluid compartment, 40% of which is lost when a child is dehydrated.

11. _____ Elements with daily requirements greater than 100 mg (e.g., calcium, phosphorus, magnesium, sodium, potassium, chloride, and sulfur).

12. _____ Fluid compartment that constitutes over half of the total body water at birth.

a. Macrominerals

b. Microminerals

c. Vegetarianism

d. Allergens

e. Sensitization

f. Extracellular fluid

g. Intracellular fluid

h. Oral rehydration solution

i. Meconium

j. Constipation

k. Obstipation

l. Encopresis

II. REVIEWING KEY CONCEPTS

1. In the United States, protein and energy malnutrition (PEM) occurs when:
   a. the food supply is inadequate.
   b. the food supply may be adequate.
   c. the adults eat first, leaving insufficient food for children.
   d. the diet consists mainly of starch grains.

2. Kwashiorkor occurs in populations in which:
   a. the food supply is inadequate.
   b. the food supply is adequate for protein.
   c. the adults eat first, leaving insufficient food for children.
   d. the diet consists mainly of starch grains.

3. Nutritional marasmus usually occurs in populations in which:
   a. the food supply is inadequate.
   b. the food supply is adequate for protein.
   c. the adults eat first, leaving insufficient food for children.
   d. the diet consists mainly of starch grains.

4. Which of the following diagnostic strategies is considered the most definitive for identifying a cow's milk allergy?
   a. Stool analysis for blood
   b. Serum IgE levels
   c. A reintroduction of milk after elimination from diet
   d. Skin prick or scratch testing

5. A child with a diagnosed food allergy (peanuts) in the school cafeteria suddenly complains of being short of breath and is observed wheezing. The most critical nursing intervention is for the school nurse to:
   a. call the child's parents.
   b. call the child's physician of record.
   c. administer intramuscular epinephrine.
   d. take the child to the nurse's office.

6. Treatment of diagnosed cow's milk allergy in infants ideally involves changing the formula to:
   a. soy-based formula.
   b. goat's milk.
   c. casein/whey hydrolysate milk.
   d. whole milk.

7. Infants and young children are at high risk for fluid and electrolyte imbalance. Which of the following factors contributes to this vulnerability?
   a. Decreased body surface area
   b. Lower metabolic rate
   c. Mature kidney function
   d. Increased extracellular fluid volume

8. _____ dehydration occurs when electrolyte and water deficits are present in balanced proportion.

9. _____ dehydration occurs when the electrolyte deficit exceeds the water deficit. There is a greater loss of extracellular fluid, and plasma sodium concentration is usually _____ than 130 mEq/L.

10. _____ dehydration results from water loss in excess of electrolyte loss. This is often caused by a large _____ of water and/or a large _____ of electrolytes. Plasma sodium concentration is _____ than 150 mEq/L.

11. Which of the following choices most accurately describes dehydration or fluid loss in infants and young children?
    a. As a percentage
    b. In milliliters per kilogram of body weight
    c. By the amount of edema present
    d. By the degree of skin elasticity

12. An infant with moderate dehydration may demonstrate:
    a. mottled skin color and decreased pulse and respirations.
    b. decreased urine output, tachycardia and fever.
    c. dry mucous membranes and capillary filling of more than 2 to 3 seconds.
    d. tachycardia, bulging fontanel and decreased blood pressure.

13. List 8 assessment findings that may be used to determine dehydration in a child.

14. A priority goal in the management of acute diarrhea is:
    a. determining the cause of the diarrhea.
    b. preventing the spread of the infection.
    c. rehydrating of the child.
    d. managing the fever associated with the diarrhea.

15. To confirm the diagnosis of Hirschsprung disease, the nurse prepares the child for:
    a. endoscopy.
    b. sonogram.
    c. rectal biopsy.
    d. esophagoscopy.

16. The nurse would expect to see which of the following clinical manifestations in the child diagnosed with Hirschsprung disease?
    a. History of bloody diarrhea, fever, and vomiting
    b. Irritability, severe abdominal cramps, and fecal soiling
    c. Increased serum lipids and positive stool for O&P (ova and parasites)
    d. Constipation, abdominal distention, and foul-smelling stools.

17. The parents of a 2-month-old with gastroesophageal reflux are counseled by the nurse to include which of the following in the infant's care?
    a. After feeding and burping, place the infant prone for two hours.
    b. After feeding and burping, position the infant in an infant seat with the head elevated 30 degrees.
    c. After feeding and burping, position the infant on his or her back with the head turned to the side.
    d. Increase feeding volume right before bedtime.

18. An 8-year-old has been diagnosed with giardiasis. The nurse should expect which of these signs and symptoms?
    a. Diarrhea with blood in the stools
    b. Nausea and vomiting with a mild fever
    c. Abdominal cramps with intermittent loose stools
    d. Weight loss of 5 lb over the last month

19. The nurse is teaching parents how to collect a specimen for enterobiasis using the test tape diagnostic procedure. Which of the following is included in the explanation?
    a. Use a flashlight to inspect the anal area while the child sleeps.
    b. Perform the test 2 days after the child has received the first dose of mebendazole.
    c. Test all members of the family at the same time using frosted tape.
    d. Collect the tape in the morning before the child has a bowel movement or bath.

20. Children with pinworm infections present with the principal symptom of:
    a. perianal itching.
    b. diarrhea with blood.
    c. evidence of small rice-like worms in their stool and urine.
    d. abdominal pain.

21. Reduction of accidental poisonings in children and infants can be accomplished by:
    a. use of child-resistant containers.
    b. educating parents and grandparents to place products out of reach of small children.
    c. educating parents to place plants out of reach of infants, toddlers, and small children.
    d. a, b, and c.

22. The first action parents should be taught to initiate in an accidental poisoning is to:
    a. induce vomiting.
    b. take the child to the family physician's office or emergency center.
    c. call the poison control center.
    d. follow the instructions on the label of the household product.

23. Gastric decontamination is aimed at removing ingested toxic products by _____, _____, or_____.

24. Which of the following would alert the nurse to possible peritonitis in a child suspected of having appendicitis?
    a. Colicky abdominal pain with guarding of the abdomen
    b. Periumbilical pain that progresses to the lower right quadrant of the abdomen with an elevated WBC
    c. Low-grade fever of 100.6° F with the child having difficulty walking and assuming a side-lying position with the knees flexed toward the chest
    d. Temperature of 103° F, absent bowel sounds, and sudden relief from acute abdominal pain

25. The most common clinical manifestations expected with Meckel diverticulum include:
    a. Fever, vomiting, and constipation
    b. Weight loss, hypotension, and obstruction
    c. Painless rectal bleeding, abdominal pain, or intestinal obstruction
    d. Abdominal pain, bloody diarrhea, and foul-smelling stool

26. A common feature of inflammatory bowel disease is:
    a. growth restriction.
    b. chronic constipation.
    c. obstruction.
    d. burning epigastric pain.

27. In the child with peptic ulcer disease, it would be unlikely to find:
    a. *Helicobacter pylori.*
    b. a blood type O.
    c. a diet consisting of spicy foods.
    d. psychologic factors such as stressful life events.

28. The single most effective strategy to prevent and control hepatitis is _____.

29. _____ is the most important cause of serious gastroenteritis among children 3 to 24 months of age and a significant nosocomial (hospital-acquired) pathogen.

MATCHING: Match each viral hepatitis type with its corresponding description.

30. _____ The highest incidence of this type of hepatitis occurs in preschool and school-age children.

31. _____ Immunity by hepatitis B vaccine is available.

32. _____ Non-A, non-B hepatitis with transmission through the fecal-oral route or with contaminated water.

a. Hepatitis A

b. Hepatitis B

c. Hepatitis C

33. _____ Children with chronic hepatitis B should be tested for this type of hepatitis.

34. _____ The major route of infection in children is mother-to-infant transmission.

d. Hepatitis D

e. Hepatitis E

35. The definition of *biliary atresia* is:
    a. persistent jaundice with elevated direct bilirubin levels.
    b. progressive inflammatory process causing bile duct fibrosis.
    c. absence of bile pigment.
    d. hepatomegaly and palpable liver.

36. The most common early symptom of biliary atresia is:
    a. projectile vomiting.
    b. bloody stools.
    c. acholic stools.
    d. jaundice.

37. _____ is often a significant problem in children with biliary atresia that is addressed by drug therapy or comfort measures such as baths in colloidal oatmeal compounds.

38. To assess for the presence of a cleft palate, the nurse should:
    a. assess the infant's ability to swallow.
    b. assess the color of the infant's oral mucosa.
    c. palpate the hard palate with a gloved finger.
    d. flick the infant's foot and make it cry.

39. One of the major problems for infants born with cleft lip and palate is related to:
    a. rejection by the mother.
    b. feeding problems and weight loss.
    c. apnea and bradycardia.
    d. aspiration pneumonia.

40. Postoperative care for the infant with a cleft palate would *not* include the strategy of:
    a. applying bilateral elbow restraints.
    b. removing restraints one at a time at regular intervals.
    c. placing child in the upright infant seat position.
    d. vigorously suctioning the infant's mouth for secretions.

41. Feeding the infant with surgical repair of either a cleft lip or palate postoperatively includes:
    I. If the infant had cleft lip repair, feeding begins with clear liquids.
    II. Feedings are resumed whenever tolerated after a cleft lip repair.
    III. Cleft palate repair feedings include the use of spoons.
    IV. Cleft palate repair feedings include the use of a cup.
       a. I and II
       b. I, II, III, and IV
       c. I and III
       d. I, II and IV

42. An invagination of one portion of the intestine into another is called:
    a. intussusception.
    b. pyloric stenosis.
    c. tracheoesophageal fistula.
    d. Hirschsprung disease.

43. A 5-month-old infant suspected of having intussusception would most likely have what clinical manifestations?
    a. Crying, vomiting, and currant-jelly-appearing stools
    b. Fever, diarrhea, vomiting, and decreased WBC
    c. Weight gain, constipation, and refusal to eat
    d. Abdominal distention, periodic pain, and hypotension

44. A 5-month-old infant's intussusception is treated with hydrostatic reduction. The nurse should expect care after the reduction to include:
    a. administration of antibiotics.
    b. enema administration to remove remaining stool.
    c. close observation of stools.
    d. blood pressure every 4 hours.

45. The nurse observes frothy saliva in the mouth and nose of the neonate who is a few hours old. When fed, the infant swallows normally, but suddenly the fluid returns through the nose and mouth of the infant. The nurse suspects:
    a. Esophageal atresia
    b. Pyloric stenosis
    c. Anorectal malformation
    d. Biliary atresia

46. A 1-month-old infant is brought to the clinic by his mother. The nurse suspects pyloric stenosis because the mother gives a history of:
    a. diarrhea.
    b. projectile vomiting.
    c. fever and dehydration.
    d. abdominal distention.

47. The preoperative nursing plan for an infant with pyloric obstruction should include:
    a. rehydration by intravenous fluids for fluid and electrolyte imbalance.
    b. nasogastric (NG) tube placement to decompress the stomach.
    c. parental support and reassurance.
    d. a, b, and c.

48. The assessment finding that is most likely to indicate an anorectal malformation is:
    a. abdominal distention and vomiting.
    b. a normal-appearing perineum.
    c. passage of meconium stool after 24 hours.
    d. failure to pass meconium through the anal opening.

49. The most important therapeutic management for the child with celiac disease is:
    a. eliminating corn, rice, and millet from the diet.
    b. adding iron, folic acid, and fat-soluble vitamins to the diet.
    c. eliminating wheat, rye, barley, and oats from the diet.
    d. educating the child's parents about the short-term effects of the disease and the necessity of reading all food labels for content until the disease is in remission.

50. The prognosis for children with short bowel syndrome has improved as a result of:
    a. dietary supplemental vitamin B12 additions.
    b. improvement in surgical procedures to correct the deficiency.
    c. improved home care availability.
    d. total parenteral nutrition and enteral feeding.

51. A common long-term complication after surgical repair of esophageal atresia is:
    a. feeding difficulties.
    b. tracheomalacia.
    c. pneumothorax.
    d. short bowel syndrome.

52. T   F   Asymptomatic young children may have lead levels sufficiently elevated to cause neurologic and intellectual damage.

53. T   F   Lead-based paint from older-built houses remains the most frequent source of lead poisoning in children.

54. T   F   Lead-containing pottery or dishes usually do not contribute to lead poisoning.

55. Describe major principles of emergency treatment for accidental poisoning in a child brought to the emergency department.

56. Describe the 3 phases of parenteral rehydration therapy for the child diagnosed with moderate dehydration.

57. Explain the rationale and methodology for oral rehydration management in a child with mild dehydration.

III. THINKING CRITICALLY

1. Describe the assessment parameters to use with a 3-year-old child complaining of constipation.

2. Differentiate between ulcerative colitis and Crohn disease in regard to pathology, rectal bleeding, diarrhea, pain, anorexia, weight loss, and growth restriction.

16. _____ Includes primarily anatomic abnormalities present at birth that result in abnormal cardiac function, the consequences of which are hypoxemia and heart failure.

17. _____ Refers to an arterial oxygen tension (or pressure) that is less than normal and can be identified by a decreased arterial saturation or a decreased PaO_2.

18. _____ Vital organ function is maintained by intrinsic compensatory mechanism; blood flow is usually normal or increased, but generally uneven or maldistributed in the microcirculation.

19. _____ Disease processes or abnormalities that occur after birth and can be seen in the normal heart or in the presence of congenital heart defects; resulting from factors such as infection, autoimmune responses, environmental factors, and familial tendencies.

20. _____ A reduction in tissue oxygenation that results from low oxygen saturation and PaO_2 and results in impaired cellular processes.

21. _____ A blue discoloration in the mucous membranes, skin, and nail beds of the child with reduced oxygen saturation; results from the presence of deoxygenated hemoglobin (hemoglobin not bound to oxygen); determined subjectively.

II. REVIEWING KEY CONCEPTS

1. During fetal life, oxygenated blood travels into the left atrium through a structure known as the:
   a. truncus arteriosus.
   b. foramen ovale.
   c. sinus venosus.
   d. ductus venosus.

2. In fetal circulation only a small amount of blood flows through the nonfunctioning:
   a. pulmonary circulation.
   b. ductus arteriosus.
   c. hepatic circulation.
   d. ductus venosus.

3. When an abnormal connection exists between the heart chambers (e.g., a septal defect), blood will necessarily flow from an area of higher pressure (left side) to one of lower pressure (right side). This is called a:
   a. left-to-right shunt.
   b. right-to-left shunt.

4. When preparing a child for cardiac catheterization the nurse should:
   a. ask about allergies.
   b. assess and mark distal pulses.
   c. ask about a fever above 100° F.
   d. provide information about the procedure to the child and parents.
   e. a, b, c, and d.

5. Coarctation of the aorta should be suspected when the:
   a. blood pressure is higher in the arms than in the legs.
   b. blood pressure in the right arm is different from the blood pressure in the left arm.
   c. apical pulse is greater than the radial pulse.
   d. point of maximum impulse is shifted to the right.

6. The test in which a transducer is placed behind the heart to obtain images of posterior heart structures is the:
   a. electrocardiogram.
   b. echocardiogram.
   c. transthoracic echocardiography.
   d. two-dimensional echocardiogram.

7. Priority nursing responsibilities after cardiac catheterization in children includes:
   I. monitoring oral fluid intake.
   II. checking pulses below the site of catheterization.
   III. assessing the temperature and color of the affected extremity.
   IV. checking vital signs including blood pressure every 15 minutes.
   V. monitoring blood glucose levels in infants.
   VI. checking the dressing for bleeding.
      a. I, II, and VI
      b. I, II, III, IV, V, and VI
      c. II, III, and VI

8. List five of the most significant complications following a cardiac catheterization in an infant or young child.

9. If bleeding occurs at the insertion site after a cardiac catheterization, the nurse should apply:
   a. warmth to the unaffected extremity.
   b. pressure below the insertion site.
   c. warmth to the affected extremity.
   d. pressure above the insertion site.

10. Signs and symptoms of supraventricular tachycardia (SVT) in an infant or young child include:
    a. pallor.
    b. irritability.
    c. poor feeding.
    d. diaphoresis.
    e. a, b, and c.

11. A 12-month-old would be classified as significantly hypertensive with a blood pressure that:
    a. falls above the 99th percentile one time.
    b. persistently falls between the 95th and 99th percentiles.
    c. falls between the 95th and 99th percentiles one time.
    d. falls below the 99th percentile one time.

12. The nurse is teaching a mother how to administer digoxin (Lanoxin) at home to her 3-year-old child. The nurse tells the mother that as a general rule, digoxin should not be administered to the older child whose pulse is:
    a. 108.
    b. 98.
    c. 78.
    d. 68.

13. An infant is receiving Lanoxin elixir 0.028 mg once daily. Lanoxin is available in an elixir concentration of 50 mcg/mL. The correct dose to draw up and administer is:
    a. 0.56 mL.
    b. 0.28 mL.
    c. 0.84 mL.
    d. 1.12 mL.

14. A 12-month-old infant in heart failure is taking enalapril (ACE inhibitor) and spironolactone. The nurse should be especially alert for:
    a. sodium 142 mEq/L.
    b. potassium 5.0 mEq/L.
    c. potassium 3.1 mEq/L.
    d. sodium 132 mEq/L.

15. Fluid and nutritional guidelines for an infant with congestive heart failure rarely include:
    a. sodium restriction.
    b. sodium supplements.
    c. fluid restriction.
    d. decreased caloric intake.

16. The two main angiotensin-converting enzyme (ACE) inhibitors most commonly used for children with congestive heart failure are:
    a. digoxin and captopril.
    b. enalapril and captopril.
    c. enalapril and furosemide.
    d. spironolactone and captopril.

17. The electrolyte most commonly depleted with diuretic therapy is:
    a. sodium.
    b. chloride.
    c. potassium.
    d. magnesium.

18. The nutritional needs of the infant with congestive heart failure are usually:
    a. the same as an adult's.
    b. less than a healthy infant's.
    c. the same as a healthy infant's.
    d. greater than a healthy infant's.

19. The calories are usually modified for an infant with congestive heart failure by:
    a. feeding every 2 hours.
    b. increasing the volume of each feeding.
    c. increasing the caloric density of the formula.
    d. increasing the feeding duration to 1 hour.

20. Which of the following clinical manifestations is a sign of chronic hypoxemia in a child?
    a. Squatting
    b. Polycythemia
    c. Clubbing
    d. a, b, and c

21. Prostaglandin is administered to the newborn with a congenital heart defect to:
    a. keep the ductus arteriosus open.
    b. close the ductus arteriosus.
    c. keep the foramen ovale open.
    d. close the foramen ovale.

22. Dehydration must be prevented in children who are hypoxemic because dehydration places the child at risk for:
    a. infection.
    b. cerebral vascular accident.
    c. fever.
    d. air embolism.

23. The leading cause of death in the first 3 years after heart transplantation (the greatest risk in the first 6 months) in children is:
    a. heart failure.
    b. infection.
    c. rejection.
    d. renal dysfunction.

MATCHING: Match each specific disorder with its corresponding type of defect. (Defects may be used more than once.)

24. _____ Patent ductus arteriosus

25. _____ Coarctation of the aorta

26. _____ Ventricular septal defect

27. _____ Subvalvular aortic stenosis

28. _____ Hypoplastic left heart syndrome

29. _____ Atrioventricular canal defect

30. _____ Pulmonic stenosis

31. _____ Tetralogy of Fallot

32. _____ Aortic stenosis

33. _____ Tricuspid atresia

34. _____ Valvular aortic stenosis

35. _____ Truncus arteriosus

36. _____ Atrial septal defect

37. _____ Transposition of the great vessels

a. Defects with decreased pulmonary blood flow

b. Mixed defects

c. Defects with increased pulmonary blood flow

d. Obstructive defects

38. Which of the following congenital heart defects usually has the best prognosis?
    a. Tetralogy of Fallot
    b. Ventricular septal defect
    c. Atrial septal defect
    d. Hypoplastic left heart syndrome

39. Which of the following sets of assessment findings are the most frequent clinical manifestations of an atrial septal defect in an infant or child?
    a. Decreased cardiac output and low blood pressure
    b. Heart failure and a murmur
    c. Increased blood pressure and pulse
    d. Dyspnea and bradycardia

40. Parents of the child with a congenital heart defect should know the signs of congestive heart failure, which include:
    a. poor feeding.
    b. sudden weight gain.
    c. increased efforts to breathe.
    d. a, b, and c.

41. A parent and child visit to the intensive care unit before open-heart surgery should ideally take place:
    a. several days before the surgery.
    b. at a busy time with a lot to see and hear.
    c. the day before surgery.
    d. several weeks before the surgery.

42. Tetralogy of Fallot consists of these defects:
    I. VSD
    II. ASD
    III. Right ventricular hypertrophy
    IV. Pulmonic stenosis
    V. Overriding aorta
    VI. Patent ductus arteriosus
       a. II, III, IV, and VI
       b. I, III, IV, and V
       c. II, IV, V, and VI

43. Because an incision is made through muscle, most children consider the most painful part of cardiac surgery to be the:
    a. thoracotomy incision site.
    b. graft site on the leg.
    c. sternotomy incision site.
    d. intravenous insertion sites.

44. An infant who weighs 7 kg has just returned to the intensive care unit following cardiac surgery. The chest tube has drained 40 mL in the past hour. In this situation, what is the first action for the nurse to take?
    a. Notify the surgeon.
    b. Identify any other signs of hemorrhage.
    c. Suction the patient.
    d. Identify any other signs of renal failure.

45. An infant who weighs 7 kg has just returned to the intensive care unit following cardiac surgery. The urine output has been 5 mL in the past hour. In this situation, what is the first action the nurse should take?
    a. Notify the surgeon.
    b. Identify any other signs of hypervolemia.
    c. Suction the patient.
    d. Identify any other signs of renal failure.

46. Following cardiac surgery, fluid *intake* calculations for a child would include:
    a. intravenous fluids.
    b. arterial and CVP line flushes.
    c. fluid used to dilute medications.
    d. a, b, and c.

47. Following cardiac surgery, in addition to hourly recordings of urine, fluid *output* calculations in a child should include:
    a. nasogastric secretions.
    b. blood drawn for analysis.
    c. chest tube drainage.
    d. a, b, and c.

48. One of the most important factors in preventing bacterial endocarditis is:
    a. administration of prophylactic antibiotic therapy.
    b. surgical repair of the defect.
    c. administration of prostaglandin to maintain patent ductus arteriosus.
    d. administration of antibiotics after dental work.

49. The test that provides the most reliable evidence of recent streptococcal infection is the:
    a. throat culture.
    b. Mantoux test.
    c. liver enzymes test.
    d. antistreptolysin O test.

50. The peak age for the incidence of Kawasaki disease is in the:
    a. infant age group.
    b. toddler age group.
    c. school-age group.
    d. adolescent age group.

51. Discharge teaching for a child with Kawasaki disease who received IVIG should include:
    a. Peeling of the hands and feet should be reported immediately.
    b. Arthritis, especially in the weight-bearing joints, should be reported immediately.
    c. Defer measles, mumps, and rubella vaccine for 11 months.
    d. All of the above should be included in the instructions.

52. Most cases of hypertension in young children are a result of:
    a. essential hypertension.
    b. secondary hypertension.
    c. primary hypertension.
    d. structural abnormality or an underlying pathologic process.

53. Elevated cholesterol:
    a. can predict the long-term risk of heart disease for the individual.
    b. can predict the risk of hypertension in adulthood.
    c. plays an important role in causing atherosclerosis.
    d. plays an important role in causing congestive heart failure.

54. Recent concerns regarding the incidence of hypertension in children and adolescents has lead to the recommendation that children older than _____ years receive _____ BP screening.

55. Eleven-year-old Juan is in the clinic to receive booster childhood vaccines. The nurse asks Juan's mother if he has ever had cholesterol screening performed. The mother replies that Juan is too young for such screening. The nurse informs Juan's mother that universal cholesterol screening is recommended for:
    a. all children 5 years old and older.
    b. children aged 9 to 11 years.
    c. adolescents 17 to 21 years of age.
    d. a, b, and c.
    e. b and c.

III. THINKING CRITICALLY

1. Identify the clinical manifestations that could indicate the presence of a congenital heart defect in an infant or young child.

2. List the components of the maternal or child's history that could indicate a high risk for congenital heart disease.

3. Explain why a child with congestive heart failure should be placed on a regimen of oral digitalis and diuretics.

4. Describe how to help families decrease their fear and anxiety and increase their coping behaviors when facing their child's surgery to correct a congenital heart defect.

43 Hematologic and Immunologic Dysfunction

I. LEARNING KEY TERMS

MATCHING: Match each term with its corresponding definition or description.

1. _____ Nosebleed.

2. _____ Heterozygous people who have hemoglobin containing HbA as well as abnormal HbS (sickle hemoglobin).

3. _____ The process that stops bleeding when a blood system vessel is injured.

4. _____ Bleeding into the joints.

5. _____ A condition in which the number of red blood cells and/or hemoglobin concentration is reduced below normal; oxygen-carrying capacity of the blood is diminished; less oxygen is available to the tissues.

6. _____ People who are homozygous with predominantly HbS (sickle hemoglobin).

a. Hemostasis

b. Anemia

c. Sickle cell trait

d. Sickle cell anemia

e. Epistaxis

f. Hemarthrosis

II. REVIEWING KEY CONCEPTS

1. A common term used in describing an abnormal CBC is shift to the left, which is usually caused by a(n):
   a. infection.
   b. anemia.
   c. hemolysis
   d. bleeding.

2. The common childhood anemia that occurs more frequently in toddlers between the ages of 12 and 36 months is _____.

3. At birth the healthy full-term newborn has maternal stores of iron sufficient to last:
   a. 5 to 6 months.
   b. 2 to 3 months.
   c. 8 months.
   d. less than 1 month.

4. The best dietary sources of iron for a 7-month-old infant are?
   I. Whole milk
   II. Oral iron supplements
   III. Iron fortified rice cereal
   IV. Iron-fortified commercial formula
   a. I and II
   b. III and IV
   c. I, II, III, and IV

5. List 3 essential guidelines for the effective administration of oral iron supplements to small children.

6. A 5-year-old with sickle cell anemia is admitted because of diminished RBC production triggered by a viral infection. The episode is characterized by distal ischemia and pain. The crisis the child is most likely to be experiencing is:
   a. vasoocclusive crisis.
   b. splenic sequestration crisis.
   c. aplastic crisis.
   d. hyperhemolytic crisis.

7. Therapeutic management of sickle cell crisis generally includes:
   a. long-term oxygen use to enable the oxygen to reach the sickled RBCs.
   b. an increase in activity to promote circulation in the affected area.
   c. a diet high in iron to decrease anemia.
   d. oral or intravenous hydration for hemodilution.

237

8. In controlling severe pain related to vasoocclusive sickle cell crisis, the plan of care will most likely include:
   a. administration of long-term oxygen.
   b. application of cold compresses to the area.
   c. intramuscular meperidine (Demerol).
   d. intravenous or oral opioids.

9. Treatment for the child with aplastic anemia will most likely include:
   a. administration of testosterone.
   b. administration of iron-chelating agents.
   c. irradiation.
   d. bone marrow transplant.

10. Primary prophylaxis in hemophilia patients involves the infusion of factor VIII:
    a. regularly at the emergency room before joint damage occurs.
    b. regularly at home before the onset of joint damage.
    c. whenever bleeding into a joint occurs.
    d. when bleeding begins to impair joint function.

11. A 5-year-old boy previously diagnosed with hemophilia A is being admitted with hemarthrosis. The nurse knows that which of the following would most likely be included in the plan of care?
    I. Ice packs to the affected area
    II. Application of a splint or sling to immobilize the area
    III. Administration of factor VIII concentrate intramuscularly
    IV. Administration of aspirin or aspirin-containing compounds
    V. Administration of factor VIII concentrate intravenously
    VI. Active range-of-motion exercises
    VII. Teaching him how to administer antihemophilic factor to himself
       a. I, III, and VI
       b. II, III, IV, and VI
       c. I, V, and VII
       d. I, II, V, and VI

12. An acquired hemorrhagic disorder characterized by excessive destruction of platelets and a discoloration caused by petechiae beneath the skin with normal bone marrow is _____.

13. The cancer that occurs with the most frequency in children is:
    a. lymphoma.
    b. neuroblastoma.
    c. leukemia.
    d. melanoma.

14. The primary consequences of leukemia in children are:
    I. Infection, from neutropenia
    II. Anemia, from decreased RBCs
    III. Vascular inflammation, from entanglement and enmeshing of RBCs
    IV. Bleeding, from decreased platelets
       a. I, II, and IV
       b. II, III, and IV
       c. I, II, and III

15. Nursing care for a child with leukemia undergoing chemotherapy with resultant nausea and vomiting should focus on:
    a. administration of an antiemetic after the chemotherapeutic drug is administered.
    b. close observation of the child for side effects from the chemotherapeutic drug.
    c. administration of an antiemetic before the chemotherapeutic drug is given.
    d. avoidance of foods in the child's environment that trigger nausea.

16. A 7-year-old with leukemia is receiving an intravenous dose of a chemotherapeutic drug when he tells his mother that the IV site is burning and stinging. The nurse's priority intervention is to:
    a. call the physician who ordered the drug.
    b. slow down the infusion and observe the child for 20 minutes.
    c. immediately stop the infusion.
    d. reassure the child and his mother that this is a common reaction to chemotherapy.

17. A 16-year-old is receiving radiation for Hodgkin Lymphoma. When providing information about the radiation treatments, the nurse informs the adolescent and his mother that the most common effect of radiation is:
    a. moon face.
    b. nausea and vomiting.
    c. fatigue.
    d. alopecia.

18. Children who develop moon face from short-term steroid therapy used to treat cancer may experience symptoms of:
    a. acute toxicities.
    b. decreased appetite.
    c. permanent facial change.
    d. altered body image.

19. Typically the measure used to control the transmission of infection in the immunocompromised child during hospitalization includes:
    a. use of any semiprivate room.
    b. handwashing.
    c. chemotherapy.
    d. prophylactic antibiotics.

20. Hodgkin disease increases in incidence in children:
    a. under the age of 5 years.
    b. between the ages of 5 and 10 years.
    c. between the ages of 11 and 14 years.
    d. between the ages of 15 and 19 years.

21. The Reed-Sternberg cell is a significant finding because it:
    a. is characteristic of Hodgkin disease.
    b. eliminates the need for a lymph node biopsy for staging.
    c. eliminates the need for laparotomy for staging.
    d. is characteristic of leukemia.

22. In children and adolescents, HIV is most likely to be transmitted:
    a. perinatally from the mother.
    b. through contaminated blood or blood products.
    c. to adolescents engaged in IV drug use.
    d. a, b, and c.

23. The American Academy of Pediatrics recommends that all children infected with HIV receive the routine childhood immunizations, but the nurse recognizes that children with HIV who are receiving intravenous immunoglobulin (IVIG) prophylaxis may not respond to the:
    a. varicella vaccine.
    b. poliovirus vaccine.
    c. measles-mumps-rubella vaccine.
    d. pneumococcal vaccine.

24. _____ _____ _____ is the most common opportunistic infection of children infected with HIV; it occurs most frequently between 3 and 6 months of age.

25. Common clinical manifestations of HIV in young children include all of the following *except*:
    a. oral candidiasis.
    b. chronic diarrhea.
    c. failure to thrive.
    d. frequent URIs.

26. Diagnosis of severe combined immunodeficiency disease (SCID) is primarily based on:
    a. failure to thrive.
    b. delayed development.
    c. feeding problems.
    d. susceptibility to infections.

27. In Wiskott-Aldrich syndrome, the most notable effect of the disease at birth is:
    a. bloody diarrhea.
    b. infection.
    c. eczema.
    d. malignancy.

III. THINKING CRITICALLY

1. Describe the best way to manage pain during a sickle cell crisis that will help avoid clock watching and undermedicating.

2. Identify the emergency measures (with rationales) that are used when a child with hemophilia starts to bleed.

3. Describe the interventions (with rationales) that the nurse should use to maintain skin integrity in a child with a diagnosis of leukemia.

44 Genitourinary Dysfunction

I. LEARNING KEY TERMS

MATCHING: Match each term with its corresponding description.

1. _____ Procedure of separating colloids and crystalline substances by circulating a blood filtrate outside the body and exerting hydrostatic pressure across a semipermeable membrane with simultaneous infusion of a replacement solution.

2. _____ Presence of bacteria in the urine.

3. _____ Fluid accumulation in the abdominal cavity.

4. _____ Accumulation of body fluid in the interstitial spaces and body cavities.

5. _____ Accumulation of nitrogenous waste in the blood, resulting in elevated blood urea nitrogen and creatinine levels.

6. _____ A reduction in the serum albumin level.

7. _____ Inflammation of the bladder.

8. _____ Procedure in which colloids and crystalline substances are separated by using the abdominal cavity as a semipermeable membrane through which water and solute of small molecular size move by osmosis and diffusion based on concentrations on either side of the membrane.

9. _____ Shift of fluid from the plasma to the interstitial spaces, resulting in a reduction in the vascular fluid volume.

10. _____ Inflammation of the urethra.

11. _____ Procedure in which colloids and crystalline substance are separated by circulating the blood outside the body through artificial membranes, which permits a similar passage of water and solutes.

12. _____ Dilation of the renal pelvis from distention caused by a backup of urine above an obstruction.

13. _____ Inflammation of the upper urinary tract and kidneys.

14. _____ The most immediate threat to the life of a child with acute renal failure; excess potassium in the blood; treated with an ion-exchange resin such as Kayexalate and dialysis.

15. _____ Condition in which albumin is lost into the urine because of increased glomerular permeability.

16. _____ The retention of nitrogenous products that produces toxic symptoms; a serious condition that often involves body systems other than the renal system.

17. _____ Febrile urinary tract infection coexisting with systemic signs of bacterial illness; blood culture reveals presence of urinary pathogen.

a. Bacteriuria

b. Cystitis

c. Urethritis

d. Pyelonephritis

e. Urosepsis

f. Hydronephrosis

g. Hyperalbuminuria

h. Hypoalbuminemia

i. Edema

j. Ascites

k. Hypovolemia

l. Azotemia

m. Uremia

n. Hyperkalemia

o. Hemodialysis

p. Peritoneal dialysis

q. Hemofiltration

II. REVIEWING KEY CONCEPTS

1. Which of the following does *not* predispose the child to urinary tract infections?
   a. The short urethra in the young female
   b. The presence of urinary stasis
   c. Urinary reflux
   d. Acidic urine pH

2. _____ male infants younger than 3 months of age have been reported to have a higher incidence of urinary tract infection than other males or females.

3. Clinical manifestations of urinary tract infection in infancy include all but which of the following?
   a. Fever
   b. Poor feeding
   c. Frequent urination
   d. Anemia

4. For the child with nephrosis, one aim of the therapy is to reduce:
   a. excretion of urinary protein.
   b. excretion of fluids.
   c. serum albumin levels.
   d. urinary output.

5. Acute glomerulonephritis is most likely to be suspected when the child presents with the clinical manifestations of:
   a. normal blood pressure, generalized edema, and oliguria.
   b. edema, hematuria, and oliguria.
   c. fatigue, elevated serum lipid levels, and elevated serum protein levels.
   d. temperature elevation, circulatory congestion, and normal creatinine serum levels.

6. The nurse caring for the child with acute glomerulonephritis would expect to:
   a. enforce complete bed rest.
   b. weigh the child daily.
   c. perform peritoneal dialysis.
   d. ensure a diet low in protein.

7. The nurse caring for a child with nephrotic syndrome can expect to administer _____ as the first-line drug therapy.

8. Clinical manifestations of nephrotic syndrome include:
   a. hypercholesterolemia, hypoalbuminemia, edema, and proteinuria.
   b. hematuria, hypertension, periorbital edema, and flank pain.
   c. oliguria, hypocholesterolemia, and hyperalbuminemia.
   d. hematuria, generalized edema, hypertension, and proteinuria.

9. When teaching the family of a child with nephrotic syndrome about prednisone therapy, the nurse includes the information that:
   a. corticosteroid therapy begins after BUN and serum creatinine elevation.
   b. prednisone is administered orally in a dosage of 4 mg/kg of body weight.
   c. after proteinuria and edema resolve, the dose is gradually tapered.
   d. the drug is discontinued as soon as the urine is free from protein.

10. Renal injury, acquired hemolytic anemia, central nervous system symptoms, and thrombocytopenia are characteristic clinical manifestations of the disorder known as:
    a. minimal-change nephrotic syndrome.
    b. Wilms tumor.
    c. hemolytic-uremic syndrome.
    d. vesicoureteral reflux.

11. The most frequent cause of transient acute renal failure in infants and children is:
    a. nephrotoxic agents.
    b. obstructive uropathy.
    c. dehydration.
    d. burn shock.

12. The primary manifestation of acute renal failure is:
    a. edema.
    b. oliguria.
    c. metabolic acidosis.
    d. weight gain and proteinuria.

13. The most immediate threat to the life of the child with acute renal failure is:
    a. hyperkalemia.
    b. anemia.
    c. hypertensive crisis.
    d. cardiac failure from hypovolemia.

14. The drug therapy used for the removal of elevated serum potassium is:
    a. furosemide.
    b. vasopressin.
    c. ion exchange resin.
    d. calcium gluconate.

15. In general, during the oliguric phase of acute renal failure, these electrolytes are withheld:
    a. sodium.
    b. potassium.
    c. chloride.
    d. a and b only.
    e. a, b, and c.

16. Complications of acute renal failure include all of the following *except*:
    a. anemia.
    b. hypertension.
    c. hypernatremia.
    d. cardiac failure with pulmonary edema.

17. The manifestation of chronic renal failure that probably has the most detrimental social consequences for the developing child is:
    a. anemia.
    b. growth restriction.
    c. bone demineralization.
    d. septicemia.

18. Which of the following is included in dietary regulation of the child with chronic renal failure?
    a. Restricting protein intake below the recommended daily allowance
    b. Dietary protein intakes allowed only to the dietary reference intake (DRI) for the child's age
    c. Restricting potassium when creatinine clearance falls below 50 mL/min
    d. Giving vitamin A, E, and K supplements

19. Methods of dialysis for management of renal failure are _____, _____, and _____.

20. _____ is the preferred method of dialysis for children with life-threatening hyperkalemia that needs to be rapidly corrected.

21. _____ dialysis is usually recommended for small children.

22. A child, age 12, had a renal transplant 5 months ago. He now presents to the outpatient clinic with fever, tenderness over the graft area, decreased urinary output, and a slightly elevated blood pressure. The nurse's priority at this time is to:
    a. recognize that the child is probably undergoing acute rejection and to notify the physician immediately.
    b. recognize that this is an episode of increased inflammation within the donor kidney because the child has probably been noncompliant with his immunosuppressant drugs.
    c. obtain urine for culture and sensitivity and a blood count to quickly identify the child's infection before alerting the physician.
    d. recognize that the child is in chronic rejection and that no present therapy can halt the progressive process.

23. Clinical manifestations of a Wilms tumor include:
    a. abdominal swelling.
    b. fatigue.
    c. firm abdomen.
    d. hematuria.
    e. a, b, c, and d.

24. Preoperative nursing care of the child with a Wilms tumor includes:
    a. answering parents' questions regarding postoperative care.
    b. palpating the tumor to determine location and size.
    c. discussing the cosmetic effects of abdominal surgery.
    d. a, b, and c.
    e. a and c.

III. THINKING CRITICALLY

1. Describe the nursing interventions to provide proper nutrition for the child who has minimal-change nephrotic syndrome.

2. Explain how the nurse might help provide diversional activities for a school-age child admitted for acute glomerulonephritis.

3. Explain why a child with glomerulonephritis is placed on a low-protein diet while in acute renal failure.

4. Describe the nursing interventions to promote optimum home care for a 15-year-old who will receive home peritoneal dialysis.

45 Cerebral Dysfunction

I. LEARNING KEY TERMS

MATCHING: Match each term with its corresponding definition or description.

1. _____ Occurring within the anterior two thirds of the brain, mainly the cerebrum; location of a small number (less than 40%) of brain tumors in children.

2. _____ A sign of severe dysfunction of the cerebral cortex characterized by adduction of the arm at the shoulders, flexion of the arm on the chest with the wrist flexed and hands fisted, and extension and adduction of the lower extremities.

3. _____ Brief malfunctions of the brain's electrical system resulting from cortical neuronal discharges; most frequently observed neurologic dysfunction in children; clinical manifestations determined by the site of origin and may include unconsciousness or altered consciousness, involuntary movements, and changes in perception, behaviors, sensations, and posture.

4. _____ A sign of dysfunction at the level of the midbrain; characterized by rigid extension and pronation of the arms and legs; may not be evident when the child is quiet, but can usually be elicited by applying painful stimuli such as pressure of a blunt object on the base of the nail.

5. _____ The most common head injury; a transient and reversible neuronal dysfunction, with instantaneous loss of awareness and responsiveness resulting from trauma to the head and persisting for a relatively short time, usually minutes or hours, followed by amnesia; not always marked by loss of consciousness.

6. _____ Determined by observations of the child's responses to the environment; the earliest indicator of improvement or deterioration in neurologic status.

7. _____ Below the tentorium cerebelli; the location of the majority of tumors (about 60%) in children.

8. _____ The ability to process stimuli and produce verbal and motor responses; one of the two components of consciousness.

9. _____ State of unconsciousness from which the patient cannot be aroused even with painful stimuli.

10. _____ An arousal-waking state that includes the ability to respond to stimuli; one of the two components of consciousness.

11. _____ Depressed cerebral function; the inability to respond to sensory stimuli and to have subjective experiences.

12. _____ An acute inflammation of the meninges and CSF.

13. _____ A high-fat, low-carbohydrate, and adequate protein diet that has been shown to be an efficacious and tolerable treatment for medically refractory seizures.

a. Alertness

b. Bacterial meningitis

c. Unconsciousness

d. Coma

e. Level of consciousness

f. Decorticate posturing

g. Decerebrate posturing

h. Ketogenic diet

i. Infratentorial

j. Supratentorial

k. Seizure

l. Cognitive power

m. Concussion

244

II. REVIEWING KEY CONCEPTS

1. The most common solid tumor in children and the second most common childhood cancer is:
   a. Wilms tumor.
   b. brain tumor.
   c. osteosarcoma.
   d. Ewing Sarcoma.

2. The sign that can be used to indicate increased intracranial pressure in the infant but not in the older child is:
   a. projectile vomiting.
   b. headache.
   c. bulging fontanel.
   d. pulsating fontanel.

3. The best indicator to determine the depth of the comatose state is:
   a. motor activity.
   b. level of consciousness.
   c. reflexes.
   d. vital signs.

4. The nurse's priority when caring for a child during a seizure is to:
   a. intervene to halt the seizure.
   b. restrain the child.
   c. protect the child from injury.
   d. place a solid object between the teeth.

5. Which of the following nursing observations would usually indicate pain in a comatose child?
   a. Increased flaccidity
   b. Increased oxygen saturation
   c. Decreased blood pressure
   d. Increased agitation

6. The activity that has been shown to increase intracranial pressure is:
   a. using earplugs to eliminate noise.
   b. range-of-motion exercises.
   c. suctioning.
   d. osmotherapy.

7. Which of the following neurologic conditions occurs more often in children with a head injury than in adults with a head injury?
   a. Cerebral hyperemia
   b. Hypoxic brain damage
   c. Cerebral edema
   d. Subdural hemorrhage

8. The most important nursing observation following head trauma is assessment of the child's:
   a. head for bruises or lacerations.
   b. level of consciousness.
   c. neurologic signs.
   d. vital signs.

9. Epidural hemorrhage is less common in children under 2 years of age than in adults because:
   a. the middle meningeal artery is embedded in the bone surface of the skull until approximately 2 years of age.
   b. fractures are less likely to lacerate the middle meningeal artery in children under 2 years of age.
   c. separation of the dura from bleeding is more likely to occur in children than in adults.
   d. there is an increased tendency for the skull to fracture in children under 2 years of age.

10. After craniocerebral trauma, children usually have a:
    a. lower frequency of psychologic disturbances than adults.
    b. higher mortality rate than adults.
    c. less favorable prognosis than adults.
    d. higher frequency of psychologic disturbances than adults.

11. The epidemiology of bacterial meningitis has changed in recent years because of the:
    a. diphtheria, pertussis, and tetanus vaccine.
    b. rubella vaccine.
    c. *Haemophilus influenzae* type B vaccine.
    d. hepatitis B vaccine.

12. The most common mode of transmission for bacterial meningitis is:
    a. vascular dissemination of an infection elsewhere.
    b. direct implantation from an invasive procedure.
    c. direct extension from an infection in the mastoid sinuses.
    d. direct extension from an infection in the nasal sinuses.

13. _____ _____ occurs in epidemic form and is the only type readily transmitted by droplet infection from nasopharyngeal secretions; it occurs predominantly in school-age children and adolescents.

14. Secondary problems from bacterial meningitis are most likely to occur in the:
    a. school-aged child.
    b. infant under 2 months of age.
    c. infant over 2 months of age.
    d. child with *H. influenzae* meningitis.

15. Which of the following types of meningitis is self-limiting and least serious?
    a. Meningococcal meningitis
    b. Tuberculous meningitis
    c. *H. influenzae* meningitis
    d. Nonbacterial (aseptic) meningitis

16. The type of seizure, also known as a petit mal seizure, that occurs more often in children between the ages of 4 and 12 years is the:
    a. generalized seizure.
    b. absence seizure.
    c. atonic seizure.
    d. jackknife seizure.

17. The risk factors associated with recurrence of epilepsy include:
    a. polytherapy.
    b. abnormal electroencephalogram (EEG).
    c. frequent seizures on antiepileptic medication.
    d. a, b, and c.

18. Fosphenytoin may be given IV to treat childhood seizures instead of phenytoin because the former drug:
    a. is compatible with glucose and saline solutions.
    b. has fewer complications.
    c. may be given IM.
    d. may be administered at a faster rate.
    e. a, b, c, and d.

19. Risk factors for febrile seizures include:
    a. Family history of febrile seizures.
    b. Viral infections.
    c. Family history of epilepsy.
    d. a and b.
    e. a, b, and c.

20. When a child has a febrile seizure, it is important for the parents to know that the child will:
    a. probably not develop epilepsy.
    b. most likely develop epilepsy.
    c. most likely develop neurologic damage.
    d. usually need tepid sponge baths to control fever.

21. A 6-year-old child is seen in the urgent care unit for a history of seizures at home. He begins to have seizures in the urgent care unit that last more than 5 minutes. IV access has not been successful. The nurse caring for this child is knowledgeable that either of these medications may be given to stop the child's seizures:
    a. IM phenytoin
    b. Rectal diazepam
    c. Buccal midazolam
    d. a and c
    e. b and c

22. Clinical manifestations of hydrocephalus in children older than 18 months include:
    a. headache.
    b. irritability.
    c. lethargy.
    d. vomiting.
    e. a, b, and d.
    f. a, b, c, and d.

23. A 12-month-old with a history of hydrocephalus and ventriculoperitoneal shunt (VP) placement is brought to the ED by his mother who states that he refuses to eat, is afebrile but extremely fussy, and does not play with any of his toys. The diagnostic evaluation for this child will most likely include:
    a. urinary catheterization.
    b. upper GI series.
    c. skull radiographs.
    d. head CT.

III. THINKING CRITICALLY

1. Describe the parameters to assess and the interventions to maintain a stable intracranial pressure in an 8-year-old child who has been unconscious for 3 days.

2. Describe the assessment data that would be most helpful to obtain from the family of a 4-year-old child who is admitted for possible seizure disorder.

3. Describe the benefits of the ketogenic diet in the treatment of childhood seizures.

4. Describe indications for inserting an intracranial pressure (ICP) monitor in a child with a head injury.

46 Endocrine Dysfunction

I. LEARNING KEY TERMS

MATCHING: Match each term with its corresponding definition or description.

1. _____ Protruding eyeballs; occurs in hyperthyroidism.

2. _____ Ketone bodies in the urine.

3. _____ Insatiable thirst.

4. _____ Elevation of the blood glucose; usually caused by illness, growth, or emotional upset.

5. _____ Occurs when serum glucose level exceeds the renal threshold (180 mg/dl) and glucose "spills" into the urine.

6. _____ Insulin reaction; usually caused by bursts of physical activity without additional food or delayed, omitted, or incompletely consumed meals.

7. _____ The condition produced by the presence of ketone bodies in the blood; strong acids lower serum pH.

8. _____ Excessive urination.

9. _____ Hyperventilation that is characteristic of metabolic acidosis; occurs as a result of the respiratory system attempting to eliminate excess carbon dioxide by increased depth and rate of respirations.

10. _____ Carpal spasm elicited by pressure applied to nerves of the upper arm.

11. _____ Premature activation of the hypothalamic pituitary-gonadal axis; early maturation of gonads, secretion of sex hormones, and development of secondary sex characteristics.

12. _____ Carpopedal spasm, muscle twitching, cramps, seizures, and sometimes stridor; indicative of disorders of the parathyroid function.

13. _____ Excess growth hormone after epiphyseal closure; characterized by facial features such as overgrowth of the head, lips, nose, tongue, jaw, and paranasal and mastoid sinuses.

14. _____ Facial muscle spasm elicited by tapping the facial nerve in the region of the parotid gland.

a. Acromegaly

b. Precocious puberty

c. Polyuria

d. Polydipsia

e. Exophthalmos

f. Chvostek sign

g. Trousseau sign

h. Tetany

i. Glycosuria

j. Ketonuria

k. Ketoacidosis

l. Kussmaul respirations

m. Hypoglycemia

n. Hyperglycemia

II. REVIEWING KEY CONCEPTS

1. In a child with hypopituitarism, the growth hormone levels are usually:
   a. elevated after 20 minutes of strenuous exercise.
   b. elevated 45 to 90 minutes after the onset of sleep.
   c. below normal after being stimulated pharmacologically.
   d. below normal at birth.

2. The best time to administer a growth hormone replacement injection is:
   a. midmorning.
   b. at the afternoon nap.
   c. at bedtime.
   d. before breakfast.

3. _____ _____ delay refers to individuals (usually boys) with delayed linear growth, generally beginning as a toddler, and skeletal and sexual maturation that is behind that of age-mates; these children usually achieve normal adult height.

4. Explain the difference between acromegaly and pituitary hyperfunction that would not be considered acromegaly.

5. Recent data suggest that precocious puberty evaluation for a pathologic cause should be performed for Caucasian females younger than _____ years of age or for African American girls younger than ____ years of age; manifestations of sexual development before the age of _____ years in boys would suggest precocious puberty.

6. Parents of the child with precocious puberty need to know that:
   a. dress and activities should be aligned with the child's sexual development.
   b. heterosexual interest will usually be advanced.
   c. the child's mental age is congruent with the chronologic age.
   d. overt manifestations of affection represent sexual advances.

7. The most common cause of thyroid disease in children and adolescents is:
   a. Hashimoto disease (lymphocytic thyroiditis).
   b. Graves disease.
   c. goiter.
   d. thyrotoxicosis.

8. A common cause of secondary hyperparathyroidism is:
   a. maternal hyperparathyroidism.
   b. chronic renal disease.
   c. adenoma.
   d. renal rickets.

9. Pheochromocytoma is a tumor characterized by:
   a. secretion of insulin.
   b. secretion of catecholamines.
   c. adrenal crisis.
   d. myxedema.

10. The parents of a child who has Addison disease should be instructed to:
    a. use extra hydrocortisone only for crises.
    b. discontinue the child's cortisone if side effects develop.
    c. decrease the cortisone dose during times of stress.
    d. report signs of adrenal insufficiency to the physician.

11. Which of the following tests, which yields immediate results, is particularly useful in diagnosing congenital adrenogenital hyperplasia?
    a. Chromosome typing
    b. Pelvic ultrasound
    c. Pelvic x-ray
    d. Testosterone level

12. Definitive treatment for pheochromocytoma consists of:
    a. surgical removal of the thyroid.
    b. administration of potassium.
    c. surgical removal of the tumor.
    d. administration of beta blockers.

13. The primary pathologic defect in children with type 1 DM is:
    a. insulin resistance in which the body fails to use insulin properly.
    b. destruction of pancreatic β cells resulting in absolute insulin deficiency.

14. The pathologic defect described in the previous item is the basis for the lifelong need for _____ administration in type 1 DM and the primary reason that _____ ____ _____ are ineffective in the treatment of type 1 DM.

15. The currently accepted etiology of type 1 DM takes into account:
    a. genetic factors.
    b. autoimmune mechanisms.
    c. environment factors.
    d. a, b, and c.

16. Glycosylated hemoglobin is an acceptable method to:
    a. diagnose diabetes mellitus.
    b. assess the control of diabetes.
    c. assess oxygen saturation of the hemoglobin.
    d. determine blood glucose levels most accurately.

17. The most common acute complication of diabetes that a young child encounters is:
    a. retinopathy.
    b. ketoacidosis.
    c. hypoglycemia.
    d. hyperosmolar nonketotic coma.

18. Exercise for the child with diabetes mellitus:
    a. is restricted to noncontact sports.
    b. may require a decreased intake of carbohydrate.
    c. may necessitate an increased insulin dose.
    d. may require an increased intake of carbohydrate.

19. List the three cardinal signs of type 1 DM.

20. A previously healthy 15-year-old boy is brought to the ED early Saturday morning with a chief complaint of frequent urination. He is afebrile with clear breath sounds bilaterally and upon questioning states that he does have a little bit of an upset stomach. Further history reveals weight loss of 10 pounds or more in the last few months, which parents attributed to a growth spurt and involvement in basketball and soccer. A serum glucose is 520 mg/dL and there is evidence of ketonuria and glycosuria. Based on the above information the nurse anticipates which of these lab values?
    I. Serum pH 7. 27
    II. Serum pH 7.48
    III. Serum potassium 3.5
    IV. Serum potassium 5.4
    V. Serum bicarbonate 12 mmol/L
    VI. Serum bicarbonate 23 mmol/L
       a. I, III, and VI
       b. I, IV, and V
       c. II, III, and VI

21. Conventional management of type 1 DM has consisted of a twice-daily insulin regimen of a combination of _____ and _____ insulin drawn up into the same syringe and injected _____ and before _____.

22. The nurse is teaching 15-year-old Mario about the management of type 1 DM. The management of type 1 DM for the prevention of complications is based on:
    I. a daily insulin regimen.
    II. a periodic insulin regimen.
    III. self blood glucose monitoring.
    IV. a regular exercise regimen.
    V. a balanced diet.
    VI. limited physical exercise.
       a. I, III, and IV
       b. II, IV, and V
       c. I, III, IV, and V

23. Problems of adjustment to diabetes are most likely to occur when it is diagnosed in:
    a. infancy.
    b. adolescence.
    c. the toddler years.
    d. the school-age years.

III. THINKING CRITICALLY

1. Describe the clinical manifestations usually seen in a child with hypopituitarism.

2. Describe the following as they relate to a child with diabetes insipidus (DI):

   a. Clinical manifestations of DI

b. Therapeutic management

3. Identify the symptoms of hypoglycemia in a child with type 1 DM.

4. Describe the interventions to treat hypoglycemia in the child with type 1 DM.

47 Integumentary Dysfunction

I. LEARNING KEY TERMS

MATCHING: Match each term with its corresponding definition or description.

1. _____ Flat, circumscribed, nonpalpable lesion; less than l cm in diameter.

2. _____ Elevated, circumscribed, palpable, encapsulated lesion filled with liquid or semisolid material.

3. _____ Pinpoint, tiny, and sharp circumscribed spots in the superficial layers of the epidermis.

4. _____ Elevated, superficial lesion filled with purulent fluid (e.g., impetigo).

5. _____ Bruises; localized red or purple discoloration caused by extravasation of blood into dermis and subcutaneous tissues.

6. _____ Elevated, firm, circumscribed palpable lesion; deeper in dermis than a papule; 1 to 2 cm in diameter.

7. _____ Reddened area caused by increased amounts of oxygenated blood in the dermal vasculature.

8. _____ Vesicle greater than l cm in diameter.

9. _____ Loss of all or part of epidermis; depressed, moist, and glistening; follows rupture of vesicle or bulla.

10. _____ Elevated, circumscribed, superficial lesion filled with serous fluid; less than 2 cm in diameter (e.g., blister, varicella).

11. _____ Elevated, palpable, firm, circumscribed lesion less than l cm in diameter; brown, red, pink, tan, or bluish-red in color (e.g., wart).

12. _____ Heaped-up keratinized cells, flaky exfoliation; irregular; thick or thin; dry or oily; varied size; silver, white, or tan in color (e.g., psoriasis).

13. _____ Loss of epidermis; linear or hollowed-out crusted area; dermis exposed.

14. _____ Elevated, irregular-shaped area of cutaneous edema; solid, transient, and changing; variable in diameter; pale pink with lighter center (e.g., urticaria, insect bite).

15. _____ Fibrous tissue replacing injured dermis; irregular; pink, red, or white; may be atrophic or hypertrophic.

16. _____ Elevated, flat-topped, firm, rough, superficial lesion greater than l cm in diameter.

17. _____ Rough, thickened epidermis; accentuated skin markings caused by rubbing or irritation; often involves flexor aspect of extremity (e.g., chronic dermatitis).

a. Erythema

b. Ecchymoses

c. Petechiae

d. Macule

e. Patch

f. Plaque

g. Wheal

h. Papule

i. Vesicle

j. Bulla

k. Nodule

l. Pustule

m. Cyst

n. Scale

o. Lichenification

p. Scar

q. Keloid

r. Excoriation

s. Erosion

t. Mesh graft

u. Ulcer

v. Hemostasis

w. Angiogenesis

x. Proliferation phase

18. _____ Irregularly shaped, elevated, progressively enlarging scar; grows beyond boundaries of the wound; caused by excessive collagen formation during healing.

19. _____ Flat, nonpalpable lesion; irregular in shape; greater than 1 cm in diameter.

20. _____ Regeneration of capillaries; the process in which angiocytes regenerate the outer layers of capillaries and endothelial cells producing the lining.

21. _____ Skin is removed from the donor site; tiny grid lock slits are cut into the skin that allow the skin to cover a greater area; results in less desirable cosmetic and functional outcome.

22. _____ The stage of wound healing in which platelets act to seal off the damaged blood vessels and begin to form a stable clot; normally occurs within minutes of the initial injury to the skin.

23. _____ Painful procedure to remove devitalized tissue in order to promote healing.

24. _____ Loss of epidermis and dermis; concave; varies in size; exudative; red or reddish blue (e.g., decubiti).

25. _____ The "beefy" pebbled red tissue usually found in the base of healing wounds.

26. _____ Pediculosis capitis eggs.

27. _____ Procedure in which skin is removed from the donor site and placed intact over the recipient site and sutured in place; used in areas where cosmetic results are most visible.

28. _____ Healing that includes granulation and contracture; characterized clinically by the presence of granulation tissue.

29. _____ The oil that is the offending substance in poisonous plants (ivy, oak, and sumac).

30. _____ Procedure in which skin for graft is obtained from a variety of species, most notably pigs.

31. _____ Procedure in which skin for graft is obtained from human cadavers that are screened for communicable diseases.

y. Urushiol

z. Nits

aa. Granulation

bb. Debridement

cc. Allograft (homograft)

dd. Xenograft

ee. Sheet graft

II. REVIEWING KEY CONCEPTS

1. The nurse recognizes that in the care of a wound to promote healing, it would be *unlikely* to use a treatment plan that includes:
   a. nutritional management with sufficient protein, calories, vitamin C, and zinc.
   b. irrigation of wounds with normal saline.
   c. application of povidone-iodine solution daily.
   d. application of an occlusive dressing.

2. Traditional practices of skin cleansing have been shown to have a cytotoxic effect on healthy cells and minimal effect on controlling infections. Two of these agents are:
   I. hydrogen peroxide.
   II. distilled water.
   III. povidone-iodine solutions.
   IV. topical glucocorticoids.
      a. I and III
      b. II and IV
      c. I, II, III, and IV

3. Care of bacterial skin infections in children may include all of the following *except*:
   a. good handwashing.
   b. keeping the child's fingernails short.
   c. puncturing the surface of the pustule.
   d. application of topical antibiotics.

4. A type of fungal infection of the skin is:
   a. tinea corporis.
   b. herpes simplex type 1.
   c. scabies.
   d. warts.

5. Which of the following statements about scabies is *false?*
   a. Clinical manifestations include intense pruritus—especially at night—and papules, burrows, or vesicles on interdigital surfaces.
   b. Treatment is the application of permethrin 5% with 1% lindane cream or 10% crotamiton as alternatives.
   c. There is great variability in the types of lesions that are formed.
   d. The rash and itching will occur only where mites are present.

6. When removing transparent or hydrocolloid dressings, the nurse or parent should raise one edge of the dressing and _____ _____ ___ ___ _____ to loosen the adhesive.

7. When the nurse teaches parents about pediculosis capitis, instructions should include the fact that lice:
   a. infest black girls with curly hair.
   b. infest white girls with straight hair.
   c. jump or fly from one person to another.
   d. are invisible to the naked eye.

8. In addition to the application of a pediculicide, parents are instructed to:
   a. cut the child's hair to a length of 1 inch.
   b. comb the child's hair daily with a metal nit comb to remove nits.
   c. avoid sending the child to daycare or school until nits are no longer visible.
   d. treat all family members with a pediculicide for 7 days.

9. Treatment for a child with Lyme disease who is over the age of 8 usually includes:
   a. doxycycline.
   b. amoxicillin.
   c. cefuroxime.
   d. erythromycin.

10. An important nursing intervention with Lyme disease in children is to:
    a. educate parents about the prevention of tick exposure.
    b. administer the appropriate antiviral medications within 30 days of exposure.
    c. warn parents about the dangers of insect repellents.
    d. remove the tick from the child so the parent is not exposed.

11. The most effective method for tick removal in a child is to:
    a. use a tweezers or forceps and pull straight up with a steady, even pressure.
    b. apply mineral oil to the back of the tick and wait for it to back out.
    c. use the fingers to pull the tick out with a straight, steady, even pressure.
    d. remove the stinger as quickly as possible.

12. Dog bites in children occur most often:
    a. in girls over 4 years of age.
    b. in boys 5 to 9 years of age.
    c. from stray dogs.
    d. in the lower extremities.

13. An 8-year-old has been bitten on the arm by a neighbor's dog. In addition to the rabies vaccine series, the child should be given:
    a. doxycycline.
    b. tetanus toxoid (Tdap).
    c. intravenous immune globulin (IVIG).
    d. amoxicillin.

14. T   F   The incidence of diaper dermatitis is generally reported as being greater in bottle-fed infants than in breastfed infants.

15. The factors that increase the infant's likelihood of developing diaper dermatitis include:
    I. alkaline pH of urine.
    II. continued wetness on skin.
    III. increased skin permeability to bile salts.
    IV. cloth diapers.
    V. irritants such as soap and alcohol.
       a. I, I, and IV
       b. I, II, and III
       c. I, II, III, and V

16. The best strategies for the nurse to recommend to the parents of an infant with diaper dermatitis is to:
    I. apply 1.0% corticosteroid cream sparingly.
    II. avoid cornstarch because it promotes yeast growth.
    III. use a hand-held dryer on the open lesions.
    IV. apply a skin barrier paste such as zinc oxide.
    V. avoid overwashing the skin, especially with commercial wipes.

VI. when soiling occurs, wipe away the stool but leave as much of the skin barrier paste as possible.
   a. I, II, and III
   b. IV, V, and VI
   c. I, II, III, and V

17. The cause of atopic dermatitis appears to be related to:
   a. inadequate parenting.
   b. congenital heat intolerance.
   c. abnormal function of the skin.
   d. ingestion of milk products.

18. Which of these is *not* an appropriate goal in the management of atopy?
   a. Skin hydration
   b. Provide relief from pruritis
   c. Reduce inflammation
   d. Avoid live virus vaccines
   e. Prevent secondary infections

19. A 16-year-old girl presents to the nurse because of acne on her face, shoulders, and neck areas. After talking with her, the nurse makes a nursing diagnosis of deficient knowledge related to proper skin care. The best strategy for the nurse to include in her plan of care is to:
   a. wash the areas vigorously with antibacterial soap.
   b. brush the hair down on the forehead to conceal the acne areas.
   c. avoid the use of all cosmetics.
   d. gently wash the areas with a mild soap once or twice daily.

20. The practitioner has prescribed isotretinoin for acne for a 16-year-old sexually active girl, and the adolescent returns for a follow-up visit after 1 month of treatment. The follow-up assessment should include:
   a. screening for depression.
   b. cholesterol and triglyceride levels.
   c. a discussion about adequate contraception.
   d. screening about suicidal ideation.
   e. a, b, c, and d.

21. Which of these is not believed to influence the development and course of acne?
   a. Heredity
   b. Hormones
   c. Consumption of oily or greasy foods
   d. Cosmetics containing lanolin, petrolatum, and vegetable oils

22. Burns are caused by _____, _____, and _____ agents.

23. _____ burns are the most common cause of burn injuries in toddlers.

24. Burns involving the epidermis and varying degrees of the dermis that are painful, moist, red, and blistered are known as:
   a. superficial first-degree burns.
   b. partial-thickness second-degree burns.
   c. full-thickness third-degree burns.
   d. fourth-degree burns.

25. The severity of burn injury is determined by:
   a. the body area involved.
   b. the causative agent.
   c. the age of the victim.
   d. a, b, and c.

26. Which one of the following pediatric patients is at higher risk of complications from burn injury?
   a. 12-month-old infant
   b. 3-year-old toddler
   c. 10-year-old school-age child
   d. 15-year-old adolescent

27. Initial emergency care of the burned child should include which of the following?
   a. Stop the burning process for burns with ice packs.
   b. Apply ointments to the burned area before transfer of the child.
   c. Remove jewelry and metal.
   d. Apply neutralizing agents to the skin of chemical burn areas.

28. Which instruction should *not* be included in the teaching plan for the parents of a 2-year-old child who has suffered a minor burn injury?
   a. Wash the wound twice daily with mild soap and tepid water.
   b. Soak the dressing in tepid water before removal to reduce discomfort.
   c. Administer acetaminophen immediately after each dressing change.
   d. Watch the wound margins for redness, edema, or purulent drainage.

29. If fluid replacement for a burned child weighing less than 30 kg is adequate, the nurse should expect the child to:
   a. maintain an hourly urinary output of 30 mL per hour.
   b. maintain an hourly urinary output of 1 to 2 mL/kg per hour.
   c. have an increasing hematocrit.
   d. exhibit normal capillary refill.

30. The child with a major burn injury requires which of the following nutrition plans?
   a. High-protein, high-caloric diet
   b. Vitamin A and C supplements
   c. Supplements of zinc
   d. a, b, and c

31. An 8-year-old child suffered partial second-degree burns of his chest, abdomen, and upper legs while on a recent camping trip. He is scheduled for hydrotherapy each morning for 20 minutes followed by debridement of the wounds. The best nursing action to assist the child at this time would be to:
    a. ensure that pain medication is given before hydrotherapy.
    b. hold breakfast until the child returns from treatment.
    c. offer sedation after the procedure to promote rest.
    d. reassure the child that hydrotherapy is not painful.

Use the following scenario to respond to questions 32 through 34.

A 5-year-old child is brought to the emergency center after his clothes caught on fire while he was playing in the family garage with matches. He has partial-thickness second-degree burns and full-thickness third-degree burns of his anterior chest, anterior abdomen, upper right arm, both shoulders, and right hand. There is singed nasal hair apparent on physical examination and some minor burns apparent on his face. A Foley catheter is inserted, and a small amount of clear urine is obtained. Two IV routes are established for fluid replacement.

32. Based on the information given, the nurse should be careful to observe the child for:
    a. inhalation injury.
    b. facial deformities.
    c. sepsis.
    d. renal failure related to formation of myoglobin.

33. The child has normal bowel sounds 24 hours following admission and is placed on a high-caloric, high-protein diet, of which he eats very little. His hydrotherapy sessions are scheduled right after breakfast and before supper. To increase the child's dietary intake, the best action for the nurse to take is to:
    a. show him a feeding tube and explain to him that if he does not eat more, the tube will need to be inserted.

b. maintain the current meal schedule and stay with him until he eats all of his meal.
    c. rearrange his meal and hydrotherapy schedule.
    d. insist that he stop snacking between meals.

34. The child progressed well with skin grafts and healing and is now ready for discharge. The nurse will know that his parents understand discharge instructions if they make which of the following statements?
    a. "He will need to wear this elastic support bandage for only 1 month."
    b. "He will not be able to participate in any sports until the grafts have taken hold firmly."
    c. "We will visit the teacher and his peers before he returns to school to prepare them for his appearance."
    d. "We will need to protect him from normal activities until he requires no further surgery."

35. When advising parents about the use of sunscreen for their children, the nurse should tell them that:
    a. a waterproof sunscreen with a minimum 15 SPF is recommended for children.
    b. the lower the number of SPF, the higher the protection.
    c. sunscreens are not as effective as sun blockers.
    d. the sunscreen should be applied 1 hour before the child is allowed in the sun.

36. In caring for the child with frostbite, the nurse knows that:
    a. slow thawing is associated with less tissue necrosis.
    b. the frostbitten part appears white or blanched, feels solid, and is without sensation.
    c. rewarming produces a small return of sensation with a small amount of pain.
    d. rewarming is accomplished by rubbing the injured tissue.

III. THINKING CRITICALLY

1. Formulate at least three nursing diagnoses for a child who has atopic dermatitis.

2. Describe the interventions to suggest to the mother of a 3-month-old infant to prevent diaper rash and effective treatment if it occurs.

3. Explain why school-age children are highly susceptible to head lice infestations.

4. Explain the rationale for wearing sterile gown, mask, and gloves while in the hospital room of a child who has sustained a thermal injury.

5. Describe how the nurse can provide atraumatic care when implementing burn care procedures.

48 Musculoskeletal or Articular Dysfunction

I. LEARNING KEY TERMS

MATCHING: Match each term with its corresponding definition or description.

1. _____ Produced by compression of porous bone; appears as a raised or bulging projection at the fracture site; occurs in the most porous portion of the bone; more common in young children.

2. _____ The process of separating opposing bone to encourage regeneration of new bone in the created space; may be used when limbs are of unequal length and new bone is needed to elongate the shorter limb.

3. _____ Occurs when the bone is bent but not broken; a child's flexible bone can be bent 45 degrees or more before breaking.

4. _____ Occurs when a bone is angulated beyond the limits of bending, one side bending and the other side breaking.

5. _____ Used when significant pull must be applied to achieve realignment and immobilization; pins or wires may be used to ensure that the stress is placed on the bone rather than on the surrounding tissue.

6. _____ Fractures in which small fragments of bone break off from the fractured shaft and lie in the surrounding tissue.

7. _____ A fracture in which bone fragments cause damage to other organs or tissues such as the lung or bladder.

8. _____ Fracture that divides the bone fragments.

9. _____ Applied when there are minimal displacements and little muscle spasticity; contraindicated when there is skin damage.

10. _____ Fracture with an open wound through which the bone is protruding or has protruded.

11. _____ Used in uncomplicated arm or leg fractures; used to realign bone fragments for immediate cast application.

12. _____ Produced by attaching weight to the distal bone fragment.

13. _____ Black and blue discoloration; the escape of blood into the tissues.

14. _____ Backward force; provided by the body's weight.

15. _____ A fracture that does not produce a break in the skin.

a. Ecchymosis

b. Simple or closed fracture

c. Compound or open fracture

d. Complicated fracture

e. Comminuted fracture

f. Plastic deformation

g. Buckle or torus fracture

h. Greenstick fracture

i. Complete fracture

j. Traction

k. Countertraction

l. Manual traction

m. Skin traction

n. Skeletal traction

o. Distraction

II. REVIEWING KEY CONCEPTS

1. An appropriate nursing intervention for the care of a child with an extremity in a new hip spica plaster cast is:
   a. keeping the cast covered with a sheet.
   b. using the fingertips when handling the cast to prevent pressure areas.
   c. using heated fans or dryers to circulate air and speed the cast-drying process.
   d. turning the child at least every 2 hours to help dry the cast evenly.

2. Bone healing is characteristically more rapid in children because:
   a. children have less constant muscle contraction associated with the fracture.
   b. children's fractures are less severe than adults'.
   c. children have an active growth plate that helps speed repair with deformity less likely to occur.
   d. children have thickened periosteum and more generous blood supply.

3. When caring for a 7-year-old child after application of skeletal traction, the nurse should *not*:
   a. gently massage over pressure areas to stimulate circulation.
   b. release the traction when repositioning the child in bed.
   c. inspect pin sites for bleeding or infection.
   d. assess for alterations in neurovascular status.

MATCHING: Match each type of traction with its corresponding description.

4. _____ A type of running traction in which the pull is only in one direction; it is used to reduce fractures of the femur to realign bone fragments or to fatigue the muscles prior to surgery.

5. _____ Uses a system of wires, rings, and telescoping rods that permits limb lengthening to occur.

6. _____ Device is spring loaded, so making burr holes and shaving hair are not required; used for cervical traction.

7. _____ Uses skin traction on the lower leg and a padded sling under the knee.

8. _____ A type of skin traction with the leg in an extended position; used primarily for short-term immobilization.

9. _____ Skeletal traction in which the lower leg is supported by a boot cast or a calf sling and a pin or wire is placed in the distal fragment of the femur.

10. _____ Used with or without skin or skeletal traction; suspends the leg in a flexed position to relax the hip and hamstring muscles.

11. _____ Consists of a steel halo attached to the head by four screws inserted into the outer skull; several rigid bars connect the halo to a vest that is worn around the chest, thus providing greater mobility of the rest of the body while avoiding cervical spinal motion altogether.

12. _____ May be accomplished by insertion of Gardner-Wells tongs through burr holes in the skull.

a. Gardner-Wells tongs

b. Buck extension

c. Russell traction

d. 90-degree–90-degree traction

e. Balance suspension traction

f. Halo vest or brace

g. Cervical traction

h. Bryant traction

i. Ilizarov external fixator (IEF)

13. Current best practice recommends skeletal pin site cleaning with:
    a. hydrogen peroxide.
    b. chlorhexidine solution.
    c. povidone-iodine solution.
    d. normal saline.

14. An appropriate intervention for a child with phantom limb pain is to:
    a. reassure the child the sensation will go away about 1 month after amputation.
    b. recommend a psychiatric consult with a pediatric specialist.
    c. acknowledge the child's feelings and allow open expression.
    d. encourage the child to ignore the feelings.

15. Stress fractures occur most commonly in the _____ _____ and are more common in _____ and _____ athletes, or _____.

16. Developmental dysplasia of the hip may occur:
    a. in utero.
    b. in infancy.
    c. in early childhood.
    d. a, b, and c.

17. What is the most common management of the newborn with hip dysplasia?
    a. Hip spica cast
    b. Pavlik harness
    c. Buck extension traction
    d. Denise-Brown splint

18. Clubfoot may occur as an isolated deformity or in association with other disorders or syndromes such as:
    a. cerebral palsy.
    b. arthrogryposis.
    c. myelomeningocele.
    d. May occur with any of the above.

19. The priority in teaching parents about a 1-week-old infant being treated for clubfoot is:
    a. skin care.
    b. care of the Pavlik harness.
    c. traction care.
    d. passive range of motion.

20. A 7-year-old boy is diagnosed with Legg-Calvé-Perthes disease. The manifestation that would *not* be consistent with this diagnosis is:
    a. intermittent appearance of a limp on the affected side.
    b. hip soreness, ache, or stiffness that can be constant or intermittent.
    c. pain and limp most evident on arising and at the end of a long day of activities.
    d. specific history of injury to the area.

21. The cause of slipped capital femoral epiphysis is multifactorial and includes:
    I. obesity.
    II. pubertal hormone changes.
    III. physeal architecture.
    IV. overuse injury.
        a. I, II, and IV
        b. I, II, and III

22. Slipped capital femoral epiphysis is suspected when an adolescent or preadolescent:
    a. begins to limp and complains of pain in the hip continuously or intermittently.
    b. has pain without restriction of abduction and internal rotation.
    c. complains of referred pain in the groin.
    d. a and c.

23. An accentuation of the lumbar curvature beyond physiologic limits is termed _____. An abnormally increased convex angulation in the curvature of the thoracic spine is termed _____.

24. Diagnostic evaluation is important for early recognition of scoliosis. The correct procedure for the school nurse conducting this examination would be to view the child:
    a. standing and walking fully clothed to look for uneven hanging of clothing.
    b. from the front to evaluate bone maturity.
    c. from the left and right side while the child is completely undressed.
    d. from behind while the child is bending forward and is wearing only underpants.

25. Nursing implementation directed toward nonsurgical management in an adolescent with scoliosis primarily includes:
    a. promoting self-esteem and positive body image.
    b. promoting immobilization of the legs.
    c. promoting adequate nutrition.
    d. preventing infection.

26. Postoperative priorities of nursing care for the adolescent who has undergone spinal arthrodesis with instrumentation include:
    I. log rolling.
    II. monitoring oxygenation status.
    III. assessment of neurologic status.
    IV. bowel assessment.
    V. monitoring hemodynamic status.
    VI. pain management.
    VII. traction care.
        a. I, II, III, IV, and VII
        b. I, II, III, IV, V, and VI

27. A hospitalized adolescent with scoliosis is 4 days postop and is being prepared for ambulation; when she is helped to a sitting position she suddenly turns pale and complains of shortness of breath and chest pain. The nurse recognizes the symptoms and *immediately*:
    a. calls out for rapid medical assistance.
    b. applies oxygen by nonrebreather face mask.
    c. takes a peripheral blood pressure.
    d. allows the patient to rest before ambulating.

28. The nurse recognizes the adolescent's condition in the previous question as a probable:
    a. orthostatic hypotension.
    b. pulmonary embolism.
    c. fluid volume deficit.
    d. tension pneumothorax.

29. A 3-year-old with suspected osteomyelitis in the lower leg is likely to exhibit:
    a. a history of pain in the affected extremity.
    b. a warm, erythematous lower extremity.
    c. refusal to walk on the affected extremity.
    d. a, b, and c.

30. The nurse can anticipate that the plan of care for the child during the acute phase of osteomyelitis includes:
    I. encouraging the consumption of yogurt.
    II. age-appropriate play activities.
    III. isolation of the child.
    IV. intravenous antibiotics.
    V. weight-bearing exercises for the affected area.
    VI. age-appropriate pain management.
       a. I, II, IV, and VI
       b. II, III, IV, and VI
       c. III and IV

31. Nursing considerations for the patient diagnosed with osteogenesis imperfecta include:
    a. preventing fractures by careful handling.
    b. encouraging the parents to seek genetic counseling.
    c. providing guidelines to the parents to promote optimum development.
    d. a, b, and c.

32. The goal that is most appropriate for the child with juvenile arthritis is for the child to be able to exhibit signs of:
    a. adequate joint function.
    b. improved skin integrity.
    c. weight loss and improved nutritional status.
    d. adequate respiratory function.

33. The majority of children with clinical manifestations of systemic lupus erythematosus present with:
    a. Raynaud phenomenon, especially of the feet and legs.
    b. development of herpes simplex in dry, cracked skin areas.
    c. cutaneous involvement including skin disease as the chief complaint.
    d. patchy areas of alopecia without remission.

34. To promote adequate joint function in the child with juvenile arthritis, the most appropriate nursing intervention would be to:
    a. incorporate therapeutic exercises in play activities.
    b. provide heat to affected joints by use of tub baths.
    c. provide written information for all treatments ordered.
    d. explore and develop activities in which the child can succeed.

35. The nurse formulating the plan of care for a 16-year-old who has undergone a limb salvage procedure for osteosarcoma anticipates that:
    a. pain management will be a priority in the patient's care.
    b. stump care will be required.
    c. body image issues must be discussed.
    d. a and c.
    e. a and b.

III. THINKING CRITICALLY

1. Outline the instructions parents should receive to care for a 2-month-old infant in a Pavlik harness.

2. Describe the six Ps of ischemia from a vascular injury that should always be included in an assessment of the injury.

3. a. Define compartment syndrome and identify the signs and symptoms of this condition.

   b. Identify conditions that predispose to compartment syndrome.

   c. Describe the therapeutic management of compartment syndrome.

49 Neuromuscular or Muscular Dysfunction

I. LEARNING KEY TERMS

MATCHING: Match each term with its corresponding definition or description.

1. _____ A visible defect with an external saclike protrusion that contains meninges, spinal fluid, and nerves.

2. _____ Characterized by wide-based gait; rapid repetitive movements, performed poorly; disintegration of movements of the upper extremities when the child reaches for objects.

3. _____ Visible defect with an external saclike protrusion that encases meninges and spinal fluid but no neural elements.

4. _____ Combination of spastic cerebral palsy and dyskinetic cerebral palsy.

5. _____ Characterized by abnormal involuntary movement such as athetosis, slow, wormlike, writhing movements that usually involve the extremities, trunk, neck, facial muscles, and tongue.

6. _____ May involve one or both sides; hypertonicity with poor control of posture, balance, and coordinated motion; impairment of fine and gross motor skills; abnormal postures and overflow of movement to other parts of the body increased by active attempts at motion.

7. _____ Class of defects involving failure of the osseous spine to close.

a. Spastic cerebral palsy

b. Dyskinetic cerebral palsy

c. Ataxic cerebral palsy

d. Mixed-type cerebral palsy

e. Spina bifida

f. Meningocele

g. Myelomeningocele

II. REVIEWING KEY CONCEPTS

1. The etiology of cerebral palsy (CP) is most commonly related to:
   a. existing prenatal brain abnormalities.
   b. maternal obesity.
   c. postterm birth.
   d. maternal substance abuse.

2. Postnatal factors that may contribute to the development of CP include:
   a. bacterial meningitis.
   b. viral encephalitis.
   c. motor vehicle accidents (MVAs).
   d. child abuse (shaken baby syndrome [traumatic brain injury]).
   e. a, b, c, and d.

3. A child is suspected of having CP because he has clinical manifestations of wide-based gait and rapid repetitive movements of the upper extremities when he reaches for an object. Based on this information,

the clinical classification of CP for this child is most likely:
   a. dyskinetic (nonspastic).
   b. ataxic (nonspastic).
   c. mixed-type (spastic and dyskinetic).
   d. spastic (pyramidal).

4. Disabilities and problems associated with CP usually include:
   a. intelligence testing in the abnormal range.
   b. eye cataracts that will need surgical correction.
   c. seizures with athetosis and diplegia.
   d. coughing and choking while eating.

5. While performing a physical examination on a 6-month-old infant, the nurse suspects possible CP, because the infant:
   a. is able to hold on to the nurse's hands while being pulled to a sitting position.
   b. has no Moro reflex.
   c. has no tonic neck reflex.
   d. has an obligatory tonic neck reflex.

6. The goal of therapeutic management for the child with CP is:
   a. assisting with motor control of voluntary muscle.
   b. maximizing the capabilities of the child.
   c. delaying the development of sensory deprivation.
   d. surgical correction of deformities.

7. The plan of care for a 10-year-old child with CP who is on automatic external defibrillator (AED) and is confined to a wheelchair should include:
   I. transportation safety.
   II. skin care.
   III. dental care.
   IV. seizure precautions.
   V. blood glucose monitoring.
   VI. aspiration precautions.
      a. I, II, IV, and VI
      b. I, II, III, IV, and VI

8. In order to prevent dysfunction in older children with spina bifida, the child and parents are taught:
   a. clean intermittent catheterization.
   b. Foley catheter care.
   c. oral fluid challenge.
   d. bladder irrigations.

9. There is evidence that rates of serious neural tube defects may be decreased with maternal intake of:
   a. ascorbic acid.
   b. folic acid.
   c. muriatic acid.
   d. probiotics

10. Children with spina bifida are at high risk for the development of _____ _____ and should be screened before any surgical procedure for _____ _____.

11. An infant had surgical correction of myelomeningocele and is 5 days postop. The nurse includes in the discharge plan for the parents to:
    I. monitor the operative site for redness or leaking.
    II. breastfeed or feed the infant a commercial formula as tolerated.
    III. perform passive range of motion on the lower extremities twice daily.
    IV. report distended head veins to the practitioner.
    V. place the newborn to sleep on its back.
    VI. pick up or hold the newborn as little as possible.
       a. I, II, III, V, and VI
       b. I, II, III, IV, and V
       c. I, II, III, and V

12. The condition inherited only as an autosomal recessive trait and characterized by progressive weakness and wasting of skeletal muscles caused by degeneration of anterior horn cells is:
    a. Werdnig-Hoffmann disease.
    b. Becker muscular dystrophy.
    c. Kugelberg-Welander disease.
    d. Guillain-Barré syndrome.

13. A major goal in the nursing care of children with muscular dystrophy includes:
    a. promoting strenuous activity and exercise.
    b. promoting high calorie intake.
    c. preventing respiratory tract infection.
    d. preventing cognitive impairment.

14. Because Duchenne Muscular Dystrophy is inherited as an X-linked recessive trait, it is important for the parents of an affected child to:
    a. seek psychological counseling.
    b. screen all female offspring for the condition.
    c. receive genetic counseling.
    d. undergo voluntary sterilization.

15. A priority nursing consideration for the child in the acute phase of Guillain-Barré syndrome is:
    a. careful observation for difficulty in swallowing and respiratory involvement.
    b. prevention of contractures.
    c. prevention of bowel and bladder complications.
    d. prevention of sensory impairment.

16. Nursing interventions for the child hospitalized with tetanus include:
    a. controlling or eliminating stimulation from sound, light, and touch.
    b. observing for location and extent of muscle spasms.
    c. arranging for the child not to be left alone, because these children are mentally alert.
    d. ensuring a patent airway.
    e. a, b, c, and d.

17. A 10-year-old child in the ED has a tetanus-prone wound as a result of an ATV crash. He should therefore receive:
    a. tetanus immune globulin (TIG).
    b. tetanus toxoid (Tdap).
    c. tetanus antitoxin.
    d. a and b.

18. Infant botulism usually presents with symptoms of:
    a. diarrhea and vomiting.
    b. constipation and generalized weakness.
    c. high fever and seizure activity.
    d. failure to thrive.

III. THINKING CRITICALLY

1. Describe how you would intervene to assist a 5-year-old boy with Duchenne Muscular Dystrophy and his parents in regard to avoiding the pitfalls of overprotection.

2. Describe nursing interventions aimed at preventing the complications of Guillain-Barré syndrome.

3. List the primary nursing goals for the initial stabilization in the acute phase of care for an adolescent who arrives at the hospital with paraplegia caused by a spinal cord injury.

4. Describe the phenomenon of autonomic dysreflexia, the signs and symptoms, and management of the condition in an adolescent with spinal cord injury.

Answer Key

CHAPTER 1: 21st CENTURY MATERNITY NURSING

I. Learning Key Terms

1. c   2. g   3. d   4. i   5. f
6. a   7. j   8. b   9. e   10. h
11. Maternity nursing
12. *Healthy People 2020*
13. Millennium Development Goals
14. Integrative health care
15. Telemedicine
16. Doula
17. Health literacy
18. Evidence-based practice
19. Standards of practice
20. Risk management
21. Sentinel event
22. Failure to rescue
23. Standard of care
24. QSEN
25. STEPPS

II. Reviewing Key Concepts

1. See *Infant Mortality in the United States* section that identifies many physical and psychosocial factors; consider access to care, reproductive services for adolescents, incidence of STIs, obesity.
2. See *Increase in High Risk Pregnancies* section for several factors including substance abuse, multiple gestation, cesarean birth rate, and obesity.
3. a, c; conventional Western modalities are included, patient autonomy and decision making is encouraged, and the whole patient and not just the disease process is the primary consideration.
4. c; although the other options are important, inability to pay, which relates to inadequate or no health care insurance, is the most significant barrier.
5. c
6. d; obesity is associated with an increased risk for hypertension and diabetes.

III. Thinking Critically

1. Answer should include the following:
   - Biostatistics and contributing factors
   - Factors associated with high risk pregnancy
   - Benefits of prenatal care; impact of inadequate prenatal care
   - Importance of promoting consumer involvement and self-management; devise ways to encourage participation in prenatal care and overcome barriers
2. Answer should reflect factors associated with IMR, such as the high cost of care management for high risk pregnancies and compromised infants as compared with the cost and effectiveness of early, ongoing, comprehensive prenatal care.
3. See *Social Media* section; explain how you could use social media to improve health care you provide to pregnant women and their families. Identify the precautions you would take to ensure privacy and confidentiality.
4. See *Limited Access to Care* section; address solutions to the identified barriers—be creative and innovative.
5. See *Childbirth Practices* and *Involving Consumers* and *Promoting Self-Management* sections; education and access are critical factors to consider.
6. See *Health Literacy* section; include therapeutic communication techniques, culturally sensitive approaches, and preparation of bilingual written materials in answer.
7. See *Reducing Medical Errors* section and access the *Patient Fact Sheet* identified when formulating your answer.
8. See *International Concerns* section; discuss both female genital mutilation and human trafficking, consider exploring these issues in greater depth, and investigate media reports regarding these issues.

CHAPTER 2: COMMUNITY CARE: THE FAMILY AND CULTURE

I. Learning Key Terms

1. b   2. e   3. d   4. c   5. f   6. g
7. a   8. b   9. e   10. c   11. d   12. a
13. Culture
14. Subculture
15. Cultural relativism
16. Acculturation
17. Assimilation
18. Ethnocentrism
19. Cultural competence
20. Future-oriented
21. Past-oriented
22. Present-oriented
23. Personal space
24. Family
25. Nuclear
26. Extended
27. Single-parent
28. Married-blended
29. Homosexual
30. Multigenerational
31. No-parent
32. Cohabiting-parent
33. Genogram
34. Ecomap

42 Cardiovascular Dysfunction

I. LEARNING KEY TERMS

MATCHING: Match each term with its corresponding description.

1. _____ Abnormally fast heart rate.

2. _____ The consistent elevation of blood pressure beyond values considered to be the upper limits of normal.

3. _____ Abnormally slow heart rate.

4. _____ Refers to abnormalities of the myocardium in which the cardiac muscles' ability to contract is impaired; relatively rare in children.

5. _____ Refers to excessive cholesterol in the blood; believed to play an important role in atherosclerosis development.

6. _____ A general term for excessive lipids (fat) and fatlike substances; believed to play an important role in atherosclerosis development.

7. _____ The first treatment strategy to try for supraventricular tachycardia (SVT); performed by applying ice to the face, massaging one carotid artery, or having the child exhale against a closed glottis.

8. _____ A thickening and flattening of the tips of the fingers and toes; thought to be a result of chronic tissue hypoxemia and polycythemia.

9. _____ Cardiovascular efficiency diminished; microcirculatory perfusion marginal despite compensatory adjustments; tissue hypoxia, metabolic acidosis, and impairment of organ systems function.

10. _____ Procedure in which a radiopaque catheter is inserted through a peripheral blood vessel into the heart; contrast material injected; films taken of the dilution and circulation of the contrast material; used for diagnosis, treatment of valves/vessels, and electrophysiology studies.

11. _____ Slower than normal heart rate.

12. _____ Condition in which actual damage to vital organs occurs and disruption/death occurs even if homeostasis returns to normal with therapy.

13. _____ The inability of the heart to pump an adequate amount of blood to meet the metabolic demands of the body; not a disease; in children, most common in infants; usually secondary to increases in blood volume and pressure from anomalies; result of an excessive workload imposed on normal myocardium.

14. _____ Faster than normal heart rate.

15. _____ An increased number of red blood cells; increases the oxygen carrying capacity of the blood.

a. Congenital heart disease

b. Acquired cardiac disorders

c. Tachycardia

d. Bradycardia

e. Cardiac catheterization

f. Congestive heart failure

g. Hypoxemia

h. Hypoxia

i. Cyanosis

j. Polycythemia

k. Clubbing

l. Hyperlipidemia

m. Hypercholesterolemia

n. Bradydysrhythmias

o. Tachydysrhythmias

p. Cardiomyopathy

q. Vagal maneuvers

r. Hypertension

s. Compensated shock

t. Uncompensated shock

u. Irreversible shock

35. Vulnerable populations
36. Primary prevention
37. Secondary prevention
38. Tertiary prevention

II. Reviewing Key Concepts

1. See *Childbearing Beliefs and Practices* section for a discussion of communication, personal space, time orientation, and family roles including how the nurse should consider each area when communicating with and caring for patients in a culturally sensitive manner.
2. See *Home Care in the Community* and *Guidelines for Nursing Practice* sections to formulate your answer. Consider changes in length of hospital stays, portability of technology, influence of insurance reimbursement, and the need to reduce health care costs in your answer; describe the need for nurses to broaden their scope of practice.
3. See *Community Health Promotion* and *Levels of Preventive Care* sections to formulate your answer.
4. See separate sections for each of the identified vulnerable populations listed to formulate your answer.
5. See *Communication and Technology Applications* section; include warm lines, advice lines, and telephonic nursing assessment, consultation, and education.
6. b; providing explanations, especially when performing tasks that require close contact, can help to avoid misunderstandings; touching the patient, making eye contact, and taking away the right to make decisions can be interpreted by patients in some cultures as invading their personal space.
7. d; choices a, b, and c are incorrect interpretations based on the woman's culture and customs; Native Americans often use cradle boards and avoid handling their newborn often; they should not be fed colostrum.
8. c, e, and f; air movement is considered dangerous; prenatal care should begin late in pregnancy; chamomile tea is thought to ensure effective labor.
9. a, b, d, and e; birthing in an institutional setting is valued and breastfeeding should start as soon as possible after birth.
10. c; the student should be looking at the woman while speaking and asking questions through the interpreter; a normal tone of voice should be used.
11. b, c, and f; a and d are secondary level of prevention and e is tertiary level of prevention.
12. c; it represents primary level of prevention.
13. d; although a and b are appropriate, they are not the most important; gloves are not needed unless the possibility of contacting body substances is present.

III. Thinking Critically

1. Use Table 2-2 to formulate your answer; consider components of communication, personal space, time orientation, and family roles; identify the degree to which each woman/family adheres to their cultures, beliefs, and practices; do not stereotype.

2. a. See questions listed in the *Cultural Competence* box.
   b. See *Childbearing Beliefs and Practices* section; include concepts of communication patterns, space, time, and family roles when formulating your answer.
   c. See Table 2-2 to formulate your answer; remember to determine her individual beliefs and practices to avoid stereotyping.
3. Table 2-2 outlines newborn care guidelines for several ethnic groups, including those Hispanic families are likely to follow.
4. See *Communication—Childbearing Beliefs and Practices* section and Box 2-2 for the content required to answer this question.
5. See *Data Collection and Sources of Community Health Data* section and Box 2-4 for the content required to answer each part of this question.
6. See *Homeless Women* and *Implications for Nursing* sections for the content required to answer each part of this question.
7. See *Migrant Women* section for the content required to answer each part of this question.
8. See *Communication and Technology Applications* section; include questions guided by expected postpartum physical and emotional changes; ask her how she is feeling and managing, condition of her newborn (eating, sleeping, eliminating), response of other family members to newborn, sources of happiness and stress, adequacy of help and support being received, and need for additional support or referrals.
9. See Boxes 2-5 and 2-6 and *Care Management*, the first home care visit section, to answer each component of this exercise, including the approach you would take to prepare, your actions during the visit, safety precautions and infection control measures you would follow, how you would end the visit, and the interventions you would follow after the visit, including documentation of assessments, actions, and responses.
10. See *Home Care in the Community—Perinatal Services and Patient Selection* and *Referral* sections for a and b and *Care Management* for c.
11. See *Home Care in the Community* section; include the following in your answer:
    - Ability to observe firsthand, the home environment and family dynamics; natural; adequacy of resources; safety
    - Teaching can be tailored to the woman, her family, and her home.
    - Services are less expensive than hospital.
    - Can offer measures for prevention, early detection, and treatment.
    - Services may lead to long-term positive effects on parenting and child health.
    - Use research findings and recommendations of professional organizations to validate proposal.
    - Investigate insurance reimbursement for home care.

CHAPTER 3: ASSESSMENT AND HEALTH PROMOTION

I. Learning Key Terms

1. Mons pubis
2. Labia majora
3. Labia minora
4. Prepuce
5. Frenulum
6. Fourchette
7. Clitoris
8. Vaginal vestibule
9. Urethra
10. Perineum
11. Vagina; rugae, Skene's, Bartholin's, hymen
12. Fornices
13. Uterus; cul de sac of Douglas
14. Corpus
15. Isthmus
16. Fundus
17. Endometrium
18. Myometrium
19. Cervix
20. Endocervical; internal os, external os
21. Squamocolumnar junction; transformation
22. Uterine (fallopian) tubes
23. Ovaries; ovulation, estrogen, progesterone, androgen
24. Bony pelvis
25. Breasts
26. Tail of Spence
27. Nipple
28. Areola
29. Montgomery's glands (tubercles)
30. Menarche
31. Puberty
32. Climacteric
33. Menopause
34. Perimenopause
35. Menstruation; endometrial, hypothalamic-pituitary, ovarian, 28 days, the first day of bleeding, 5 days, 3 to 6 days
36. Endometrial; menstrual, proliferative, secretory, ischemic
37. Hypothalamic-pituitary
38. Ovarian; follicular (preovulatory), luteal (postovulatory)
39. Gonadotropin-releasing hormone (GnRH); follicle-stimulating hormone (FSH), luteinizing hormone (LH)
40. Follicle-stimulating hormone
41. Luteinizing hormone (LH)
42. Estrogen; spinnbarkeit
43. Progesterone; basal body
44. Mittelschmerz
45. Prostaglandins
46. Preconception counseling and care
47. Obesity
48. Anorexia nervosa
49. Bulimia nervosa
50. Female genital mutilation (female circumcision, female genital cutting)
51. Intimate partner violence (IPV), wife battering, spouse abuse, domestic, family
52. Increasing tension, battery, calm and remorse, honeymoon

II. Reviewing Key Concepts

1. Guidelines for each component of the procedure are outlined in Box 3-15, *Procedure: Papanicolaou Test.*
2. See *Barriers to Entering Health Care System* section for a full description of each category of issues listed.
3. See *Risky Sexual Practices* section and Box 3-9.
4. See *Violence Against Women* section and Fig. 3-10.
5. See *Nutrition* section and Box 3-7 to formulate your answer.
6. See separate section for each of the substances listed in *Substance Use and Abuse* section.
7. a, d; the woman should perform BSE every month at the end of menstruation when breasts are the least tender; she should use the finger pads of her three middle fingers for palpation.
8. c; self-examination should not be used for self-diagnosis but rather to detect early changes and seek guidance of a health care provider if changes are noted.
9. b; do not ask questions during the examination because it may distract the patient, interfering with relaxation measures she may be using; only offer explanations as needed during the examination.
10. c; women should not use vaginal medications or douche for 24 to 48 hours before the test; OCPs can continue; the best time for the test is midcycle.
11. a; all women should be screened because abuse can happen to any woman; abuse often escalates during pregnancy; the most commonly injured sites are head, neck, chest, abdomen, breasts, and upper extremities. If abuse is suspected the nurse needs to assess further to encourage disclosure and then assist the woman to take action and formulate a plan.
12. b, d, and f; endometrial biopsies are not recommended on a routine basis for most women but women at risk for endometrial cancer should have one done at menopause; mammograms should be done annually for women over 50 years of age and bone mineral density beginning at age 65 (see Table 3-3).
13. a; all women, not just specific groups, should participate in preconception care 1 year before planning to get pregnant.
14. c and e; smoking is associated with preterm birth, not postterm pregnancies; smoking can reduce the age for menopause.
15. c; it is essential to first determine what she drinks and how much; once that is established, then intervention regarding alcohol use that is individualized for her can occur.
16. a, c, and d; cocaine reduces fetal growth and increases the risk for preterm labor and birth; babies

exposed to methamphetamines can have smaller heads; the major concern with using phencyclidine is polydrug abuse and neurobehavioral effects on the neonate.

17. a, b, d, and e; asking "why" questions re-victimizes and blames the victim; the nurse should not talk negatively about the abuser nor talk directly to him about suspicions of abuse.

18. b, e, and f; IPV can occur in any family; battering frequently begins or escalates during pregnancy; women may stay even if the battering is bad because of fear and financial dependence, and shelters often have long waiting lists.

III. Thinking Critically

1. See specific sections for each factor and Boxes 3-10 and 3-11.

2. a. See *Female Reproductive System—External Structures* section; the hymen can be perforated with strenuous exercise, insertion of tampons, masturbation and during GYN examination, as well as during vaginal intercourse.
   b. See Box 3-15; explain what will occur and each guideline to follow for preparation and why each is important for the accuracy of the test; tell her to avoid douching, vaginal medications, and intercourse for 24 hours before the examination; she should not be menstruating.
   c. See *Ovarian Cycle* section; midcycle spotting and pain (mittelschmerz), breast swelling and tenderness, elevated basal body temperature, cervical mucus changes (spinnbarkeit), and other changes in behavior and emotions individual to each woman (premenstrual signs).
   d. See *Internal Structures* section; vaginal secretions are usually acidic and protect the reproductive tract from infection; a douche may alter this acidity and injure the mucosa, thereby increasing the risk for infection; gentle and regular front-to-back washing with mild soap and water is all that is necessary to be clean.

3. See Box 5-1 and *Pelvic Examination* section to formulate answer; consider explanations, education, therapeutic communication, relaxation techniques, and privacy in your answer.

4. a. See *History* section and Box 3-13 for a list and description of components.
   b. Use components of health history as a guide; write questions that are open ended, clear, concise, address only one issue, and progress from general to specific.
   c. See *History* section.

5. Each technique involves cognitive, psychomotor, and affective learning; use a variety of methodologies including discussion (when, how often, why, expected and reportable findings, who to call, what will be done if abnormal findings are experienced); explore feelings regarding self-examination; provide literature with illustrations; demonstrate and have patient redemonstrate using practice models and then self as appropriate.
   a. See Guidelines box, *BSE.*
   b. See *Vulvar Self-Examination* section.

6. See *Cultural Considerations and Communication Variations* section and Cultural Competence box: Communication Variations.
   • Approach the woman in a respectful and calm manner.
   • Consider modifications in the examination to maintain her modesty.
   • Incorporate communication variations such as conversational style, pacing, spacing, eye contact, touch, time orientation.
   • Take time to learn about the woman's cultural beliefs and practices regarding well woman assessment and care.

7. See *Violence Against Women* section including Legal Tip, Boxes 3-10 and 3-11, and Fig. 3-10 for content required to answer all parts of the question.

8. See Box 3-14, *Procedure: Assisting with Pelvic Examination,* and *Pelvic Examination* section for the content required to answer each part of this question.

9. See *Preconception Counseling and Care* section and Box 3-3; this nurse should:
   • Define preconception counseling and care and what it entails and stress the importance of both partners participating.
   • Identify the impact of a woman's health status and lifestyle habits on the developing fetus during the first trimester.
   • Describe how preconception counseling can help a couple choose the best time to begin a pregnancy.

10. See *Nutritional Problems and Eating Disorders* and *Lack of Exercise* sections:
    • Start with 24-hour to 3-day nutritional recall; based on analysis of woman's current nutritional habits, suggest use of My Plate, emphasize complex carbohydrates and foods high in iron and calcium, reduce fat intake, and ensure adequate fluid intake, avoiding those high in sugar, alcohol, or caffeine; use weight changes and activity patterns to determine adequacy of caloric intake.
    • Aerobic exercise: discuss weight bearing versus non–weight-bearing exercises as well as frequency and duration of exercise sessions for maximum benefit.

11. See *Pregnancy* section and Box 3-4.

12. See *Stress* section and Box 3-8 for a listing of typical manifestations of stress, both physical and emotional and how to manage stress; see *Cigarette Smoking* section and Box 3-5 to address the woman's smoking concern.

13. See *Cigarette Smoking* section and Box 3-5.
    • Discuss the impact of smoking on pregnancy using statistics, illustrations, research, and case studies to convince her that smoking does have harmful effects on her, her pregnancy, and on the baby before and after it is born.

- Help her change her behavior by referring her to smoking cessation programs; use motivation of pregnancy to at least limit smoking, if she cannot stop completely.
14. See *Violence Against Women* including *Legal Tip* and *Battering During Pregnancy* sections and Boxes 3-10 and 3-11 for content to answer all parts of this question.

CHAPTER 4: REPRODUCTIVE SYSTEM CONCERNS

I. Learning Key Terms

1. Amenorrhea
2. Hypogonadotropic amenorrhea
3. Female athlete triad
4. Dysmenorrhea
5. Primary dysmenorrhea
6. Secondary dysmenorrhea
7. Premenstrual syndrome (PMS)
8. Premenstrual dysphoric disorder (PMDD)
9. Endometriosis
10. Oligomenorrhea
11. Hypomenorrhea
12. Menorrhagia
13. Metrorrhagia
14. Abnormal uterine bleeding (AUB)
15. Dysfunctional uterine bleeding (DUB)
16. Sexually transmitted infections (STIs)
17. Condom (male, female)
18. Chlamydia
19. Gonorrhea
20. Syphilis; chancre; symmetric maculopapular rash; lymphadenopathy; condylomata lata
21. Pelvic inflammatory disease (PID)
22. Human papillomavirus (HPV)
23. Herpes simplex virus (HSV)
24. Hepatitis A virus (HAV)
25. Hepatitis B virus (HBV)
26. Hepatitis C virus (HCV)
27. Human immunodeficiency virus (HIV); acquired immunodeficiency syndrome (AIDS)
28. Bacterial vaginosis
29. Vulvovaginal candidiasis
30. Trichomoniasis
31. Group B streptococcus (GBS)

II. Reviewing Key Concepts

1. b   2. d   3. a   4. f   5. e   6. c
7. Box 4-3 cites many common risk behaviors according to sexual, drug use–related, and blood-related risks.
8. See Box 4-4 for a full description of Standard Precautions.
9. See *HIV—Screening and Diagnosis* section and Box 4-3 for a description of risky behaviors and clinical manifestations during seroconversion.
10. See *Cancer of the Breast* section and Box 4-5 for the content required to answer each part of this question.
11. See appropriate sections in *Screening and Diagnosis* and *Care Management* sections for a description of each approach.

12. b; the 13-year-old reflects several of the risk factors associated with this menstrual disorder, namely: presently in a growth period, participating in a sport that is stressful, subjectively scored, requires contour revealing clothing, and success is favored by a prepubertal body shape.
13. c; choices a, b, and d all interfere with prostaglandin synthesis, whereas acetaminophen has no antiprostaglandin properties; prostaglandins are a recognized factor in the etiology of dysmenorrhea.
14. b; caffeine should be avoided; other substances listed can be helpful in relieving discomforts of PMS.
15. b, d, e, and f; exercise increases endorphins, dilates blood vessels, and helps to reduce ischemia; peaches and watermelon have a natural diuretic effect.
16. c, d, and f; women taking danazol often experience masculinizing changes; amenorrhea is an outcome of taking this medication; ovulation may not be fully suppressed; therefore birth control is essential because this medication is teratogenic; danazol is taken orally.
17. a; dysmenorrhea is painful menstruation; dysuria is painful urination; dyspnea is difficulty breathing.
18. a; because these infections are often asymptomatic, they can go undetected and untreated causing more damage including ascent of the pathogen into the uterus and pelvis, resulting in PID and infertility; many effective treatment measures are available, including for chlamydia.
19. b; choice a is indicative of candidiasis; choice c is indicative of HSV-2; choice d is indicative of trichomoniasis.
20. b; Flagyl is used to treat bacterial vaginosis and trichomoniasis; ampicillin is effective in the treatment of chlamydia or gonorrhea; acyclovir is used to treat herpes.
21. b; choices a, c, and d are not used to treat GBS infection; acyclovir is used orally to treat herpes; there are no lesions with GBS.
22. d; recurrent infections commonly involve only local symptoms that are less severe; stress reduction, healthy lifestyle practices, and acyclovir can reduce recurrence rate; non-antiviral ointments, especially those containing cortisone, should be avoided—use lidocaine ointment or an antiseptic spray instead.
23. c, e, and f; breast cancer is more common among Caucasian women; the majority of women do not exhibit the identified risk factors; one in eight women could develop breast cancer in her lifetime.
24. b; the right arm should be used as much as possible to maintain mobility and prevent lymphedema; loose nonrestrictive clothing should be worn; tingling and numbness are expected findings for as long as a few months after surgery.
25. a; pain is a common finding; it usually begins a week before the onset of menses; leakage from nipples is not associated with this disorder; surgery is unlikely and is only attempted in a few selected cases; overall cancer risk is 5%.

26. d; fibroadenomas are generally small, unilateral, firm, nontender, moveable lumps located in the upper outer quadrant; borders are discrete and well defined; discharge is not associated with this disorder.

27. c; tamoxifen is an antiestrogenic drug; the woman may experience hot flashes because estrogen activity is blocked; nonhormonal or barrier form of contraception should be used because tamoxifen may be teratogenic.

28. b; ginger and black haw are helpful for menstrual cramping; black cohosh root is effective for some of the symptoms of PMS. See Table 4-2.

III. Thinking Critically

1. See *Hypogonadotropic Amenorrhea* section for the content required to answer each part of this question; Nursing Diagnosis: Disturbed body image related to delayed onset of menstruation and development of secondary sexual characteristics.

2. See *Primary Dysmenorrhea* section and Table 4-2 for the content required to answer each part of this question.

3. See *PMS* and *PMDD* sections for the content required to answer each part of this question; Nursing diagnoses could include acute pain, activity intolerance, disturbed sleep pattern, diarrhea, constipation, ineffective role performance; use assessment findings to determine those that would apply to a particular patient including those that are priority; obtain a detailed history and encourage woman to keep a diary of physical and emotional manifestations (what occurs, when, contributing circumstances) from one cycle to another.

4. See *Endometriosis* section for the content required to answer each part of this question.

5. See *Infections* section, Box 4-3, and Patient Teaching box—*Prevention of Genital Tract Infections* for the content required to answer each part of this question.

6. See *HIV-counseling for HIV Testing* and *Pregnancy and HIV* sections to formulate your answer; include antiviral therapy recommended, use of elective cesarean birth, and not breastfeeding.

7. See *Pelvic Inflammatory Disease* section and Patient Teaching box—*Prevention of Genital Tract Infections in Women* for the content required to answer each part of this question.

8. See *Gonorrhea* section, Patient Teaching box—*Prevention of Genital Tract Infections in Women,* and Table 4-3 for the content required to answer each part of this question; Nursing Diagnosis: Anxiety related to potential effect of STI on future sexual function or risk for ineffective sexuality pattern related to recent diagnosis of STI.

9. See *HPV Management* section for several suggested comfort measures.

10. See *HSV* section for content required to answer each part of this question.

11. See *HIV* section for content required to answer each part of this question; use Sonya's risky behaviors as a basis for discussing prevention measures, including safer sex practices; discuss impact HIV could have on her health and that of her fetus when pregnant.

12. See *Fibrocystic Changes* section and Table 4-6 for content required to answer each part of this question.

13. See *Cancer of Breast* section, Nursing Care Plan—*Woman with Breast Cancer*, Box 4-8, and Patient Teaching Box—*After a Mastectomy* for content required to answer each part of this question.

14. See *Cancer of the Breast—Screening and Diagnosis* section to formulate your answer.

CHAPTER 5: INFERTILITY, CONTRACEPTION, AND ABORTION

I. Learning Key Terms

1. Infertility
2. Fecundity
3. Assisted Reproductive Technology (ART)
4. In vitro fertilization (IVF) and embryo transfer (ET)
5. Intracytoplasmic sperm injection
6. Gamete intrafallopian transfer (GIFT)
7. Zygote intrafallopian transfer (ZIFT)
8. Therapeutic donor insemination
9. Gestational carrier (embryo host)
10. Surrogate motherhood
11. Assisted hatching
12. Donor oocyte
13. Donor embryo (embryo adoption)
14. Therapeutic insemination
15. Cryopreservation
16. Preimplantation genetic diagnosis
17. Semen analysis
18. Hysterosalpingogram
19. Urinary Ovulation Predictor Kit
20. Hysterosalpingo-contrast sonography
21. Contraception
22. Birth control
23. Family planning
24. Contraceptive failure
25. Long Acting Reversible Contraception (LARC)
26. Coitus interruptus
27. Fertility awareness methods
28. Natural family planning
29. Calendar (rhythm) method
30. Standard days method
31. Basal body temperature (BBT)
32. Cervical mucus method
33. Spinnbarkeit
34. Symptothermal
35. Two-day Method of Family Planning
36. Lactation amenorrhea method (LAM)
37. Spermicide
38. Condom
39. Diaphragm
40. Cervical cap
41. Contraceptive sponge

42. Combined Oral Contraceptive (COC)
43. Transdermal contraceptive system (patch)
44. Vaginal contraceptive ring
45. Implanon; Jadelle
46. Plan B One-Step; Next Step
47. Intrauterine device (IUD)
48. Sterilization; bilateral tubal ligation; vasectomy
49. Induced abortion; elective abortion; therapeutic abortion

II. Reviewing Key Concepts

1. See *Cervical Mucus Ovulation-Detection Method* section and Guidelines box, *Cervical Mucus Characteristics.*
   - Alert couple about reestablishment of ovulation after breastfeeding or discontinuing oral contraceptives.
   - Determine whether cycles are ovulatory at any time including menopause, when planning pregnancy, or for timing infertility treatments and diagnostic procedures.
2. See *Abortion* section; preserve life and health of the woman, genetic disorder of the fetus, rape/incest, pregnant woman's request.
3. a, c, d, and e; spermicide should be applied to the surface of the diaphragm and the rim; diaphragm should not be removed for at least 6 hours; it should be washed with warm water and mild soap, and then cornstarch should be applied; it should not be used during menstruation to prevent TSS.
4. b; spinnbarkeit refers to stretchiness of cervical mucus at ovulation to facilitate passage of sperm; there is an LH surge before ovulation; BBT rises in response to increased progesterone after ovulation; cervical mucus becomes thinner and more abundant with ovulation.
5. a; oral contraception provides no protection from STIs; therefore, a condom and spermicide are still recommended to prevent transmission; choices b, c, and d reflect appropriate actions and recognition of side effects.
6. a; although choices b, c, and d are all temporary side effects, the most common is the irregular pattern of vaginal bleeding that occurs; women report that this bleeding is also the most distressing side effect.
7. c; the longer a woman uses DMPA, the more significant the loss of bone mineral density; weight gain not loss can occur.
8. a, d, and e; the string should be checked after menses, before intercourse, at the time of ovulation, and if expulsion is suspected; a missing string or one that becomes longer or shorter should be checked by a health care professional; ParaGard is a copper IUD—it contains no hormone; NSAIDs are safe to use for discomfort.
9. d; Clomid is taken orally; therefore, there is no need to teach the patient's husband how to give an IM injection; b refers to nafarelin and c is used as part of treatment with menotropins.

III. Thinking Critically

1. See *Care Management, Assessment,* and *Psychosocial Implications* sections and Box 5-6 for content required to answer each part of this question.
2. See *Assisted Reproductive Therapies* section and Table 5-2 for the content required to answer each part of this question; answer should discuss such issues as
   - Who should pay? insurance coverage; wealthy versus poor couples
   - Children: Who are their biologic parents? What is their medical history?
   - Availability to married couples only
   - Ownership of ovum, sperm, embryos
   - Attempt to create the "perfect" child
3. See *Contraceptive* section including Care Management and Box 5-8 for content required to answer each part of this question; Nursing Diagnosis: Anxiety related to lack of knowledge regarding contraception.
4. See *Combined Oral Contraceptives* section, Box 5-10, and Table 5-3 for content required to answer each part of this question.
5. See Box 5-11, *Signs of Potential Complications with Intrauterine Devices*, which uses the acronym of PAINS to identify signs of problems; be sure to include in your answer:
   - Teach how and when to check string.
   - Stress importance of appropriate genital hygiene and sexual practices.
   - Inform when IUD needs to be replaced.
6. See *Sterilization* section for content required to answer each part of this question.
7. See *Symptothermal Method* section and Guideline Boxes for content required to answer each part of this question.
8. See *Abortion* section and Box 5-12 for content required to answer each part of this question.
9. See *Medical Abortion* section for a description of the drugs used.
10. See *Emergency Contraception* section for content required to answer each part of this question; be sure to include each of the following in your answer:
    - Explore possibility of pregnancy and options related to continuing pregnancy if it occurs.
    - Explore options for emergency contraception to prevent pregnancy: methods available, how each works, timing, side effects, how administered.
    - Emphasize importance of follow-up to check for effectiveness of method used and occurrence of infection.
    - Discuss methods of contraception and infection prevention measures to prevent recurrence of this situation.

CHAPTER 6: GENETICS, CONCEPTION, AND FETAL DEVELOPMENT

I. Learning Key Terms

1. Conception
2. Gametes; sperm, ovum (egg)

3. Gametogenesis; spermatogenesis, oogenesis
4. Fertilization; ampulla (outer third), zona reaction, diploid (46)
5. Zygote; morula, blastocyst, trophoblast
6. Implantation; chorionic villi, decidua, decidua basalis, decidua capsularis
7. Embryo
8. Fetus
9. Amniotic membranes; chorion, amnion
10. Amniotic fluid
11. Umbilical cord; arteries, vein, Wharton's jelly
12. Placenta; hormones, oxygen, nutrients, wastes, carbon dioxide
13. Viability
14. Pulmonary surfactants; lecithin-sphingomyelin
15. Ductus arteriosus
16. Ductus venosus
17. Foramen ovale
18. Hematopoiesis
19. Quickening
20. Meconium
21. Dizygotic, fraternal
22. Monozygotic, identical

23. j	24. b	25. m	26. h	27. k	28. c
29. l	30. i	31. q	32. a	33. r	34. f
35. o	36. g	37. s	38. d	39. n	40. p
41. t	42. e				

43. Genetic testing
44. Direct or molecular testing
45. Linkage analysis
46. Biochemical testing
47. Cytogenetic testing
48. Predictive testing; presymptomatic; predispositional
49. Carrier screening
50. Pharmacogenomics
51. Gene therapy (transfer)
52. Homologous
53. Homozygous; heterozygous
54. Genotype
55. Phenotype
56. Karyotype
57. Multifactorial
58. Unifactorial
59. Autosomal dominance
60. Autosomal recessive
61. Inborn error of metabolism

II. Reviewing Key Concepts

1. See individual sections for each of these structures in the embryo and fetus.
2. See *Primary Germ Layers* section of the *Embryo and Fetus* and Fig. 6-7, *B,* for identification of tissues and organs that develop from the ectoderm, mesoderm, and endoderm.
3. See Fig. 6-3, a risk factors questionnaire: ask questions that would elicit information regarding health status of family members, abnormal reproductive outcomes, history of maternal disorders, drug exposures, and illnesses, advanced maternal and paternal age, and ethnic origin.
4. See *Genetics—Estimation of Risk* section.
5. See *Human Genome Project* and *Ethical, Legal, Social Implications* sections: consider impact of being able to determine vulnerability to certain disorders and the impact this can have on an individual physically, socially, economically, and emotionally.
6. a; autosomal dominant inheritance is unrelated to exposure to teratogens; each pregnancy has the same potential for expression of the disorder; there is no reduction if one child is already affected; if the gene is inherited, the disorder is always expressed.
7. b; there is a 25% chance females will be carriers; if males inherit the X-chromosome with the defective gene, the disorder will be expressed and they can transmit the gene to female offspring; females are affected if they receive the defective gene from both parents.
8. d; cystic fibrosis, as an inborn error of metabolism, follows an autosomal recessive pattern of inheritance; two defective genes (one from each parent) are required for the disorder to be expressed; she does not have the disorder and the father does not have the defective gene; therefore, none of their children will have the disorder, but there will be a 50% chance they will be carriers of the defective gene.
9. c, e, and f; the sex of a baby is determined at conception; the heart begins to pump blood by the third week, and a beat can be heard with ultrasound by the eighth week of gestation.

III. Thinking Critically

1. a. See Table 6-1 to formulate your answer; use of illustrations and life-size models would facilitate learning.
   b. See *Pulmonary Surfactant* section; discuss how the respiratory system develops including the critical factor, surfactant production; describe how surfactant helps the newborn breathe.
   c. See *Movement of Baby* section; explain that quickening is the woman's perception of fetal movement that occurs at about 16 to 20 weeks of gestation; it will not hurt but can be uncomfortable and interfere with sleep toward the end of pregnancy; fetus will develop its own sleep-wake cycle.
   d. Discuss sensory capability of the fetus using *Sensory Awareness* section; fetus can hear sounds such as parents' voices, respond to light and touch, and perceive temperature and taste.
   e. See *Reproductive System* section; discuss function of X and Y chromosomes; sex of her fetus will become recognizable around 12 weeks of gestation.
   f. See *Multifetal Pregnancy—Twins* section; discuss monozygotic (identical) and dizygotic (fraternal) twinning and how each occurs; emphasize that fraternal twinning tends to occur in some families.
2. See *Genetic Counseling, Genetic Testing,* and *Autosomal Recessive Inheritance* sections.
   a. Tay-Sachs is an autosomal recessive disorder that follows a unifactorial pattern of inheritance;

Mr. G. needs to be tested because he must also be a carrier to produce a child with the disorder; emphasize the nurse's role in terms of emotional support, facilitation of the decision making process, and interpretation of diagnostic test results and how they can influence future childbearing decisions.

b. See *Estimation of Risk* section: There is a 25% chance the child will be unaffected, a 25% chance that the child will express the disorder, and a 50% chance that the child will be a carrier; this pattern is the same for every pregnancy; there is no reduction in risk from one pregnancy to another. See Fig. 6-2.

c. Discuss the nature of this disorder, extent of risk, and consequences if the child inherits the disorder; options available include amniocentesis, continuing or not continuing the pregnancy if the child is affected, and use of reproductive technology or adoption; be sensitive to cultural and religious beliefs; encourage expression of feelings; refer for further counseling or support groups as appropriate.

CHAPTER 7: ANATOMY AND PHYSIOLOGY OF PREGNANCY

I. Learning Key Terms

1. Gravidity
2. Parity
3. Gravida
4. Nulligravida
5. Nullipara
6. Primigravida
7. Primipara
8. Multigravida
9. Multipara
10. Viability
11. Preterm
12. Term
13. Postdate; postterm
14. Human chorionic gonadotropin (hCG)
15. Presumptive changes
16. Probable changes
17. Positive changes
18. Braxton-Hicks contractions
19. Uterine souffle
20. Funic souffle
21. Quickening
22. Supine hypotensive syndrome
23. Pruritus gravidarum
24. Pica

25. c	26. p	27. k	28. t	29. s	30. u
31. j	32. n	33. v	34. b	35. g	36. a
37. o	38. i	39. q	40. e	41. m	42. w
43. f	44. h	45. d	46. r	47. l	48. x

II. Reviewing Key Concepts

1. Nancy (3-1-1-0-1); Marsha (4-2-0-1-2); Linda (4-1-1-1-3).

2. See designated sections in *General Body Systems* section as well as tables cited.
   a. and b. See Table 7-4 for expected changes.
   c. See Table 7-5 for changes in breathing.
   d. See *BMR* section; baseline temperature increases as a result of the increase in BMR and the progesterone effect; women may complain of heat intolerance, and sweating is increased to compensate by dissipating heat.

3. Use the following formula to calculate MAP (see Box 7-2):
$$\frac{Systolic + 2\ (diastolic)}{3} = MAP$$
Answers: 91, 81, 90, 110.

4. a. See Tables 7-3 and 7-4.
   b. See *Circulation and Coagulation Times* section of *Cardiopulmonary System* and Table 7-3.
   c. See *Acid-Base Balance* section and Table 7-3.
   d. See *Fluid and Electrolyte Balance* section.

5. a. See *Renal System* section; slowed passage of more alkaline urine and dilation of the ureters as a result of progesterone increases the risk for UTIs; bladder irritability, nocturia, urinary frequency, and urgency (first and third trimesters after lightening).
   b. See *Gastrointestinal* section; constipation and hemorrhoids; effect of increased progesterone, which decreases peristalsis and intestinal displacement by enlarging uterus.

6. a, c, and e; hCG indicates a positive pregnancy test and is a probable sign of pregnancy along with other changes that can be observed by the examiner; breast tenderness and amenorrhea are presumptive signs; fetal heart sounds are a positive sign of pregnancy.

7. d; gravida (total number of pregnancies including the present one is 5); para (term birth of daughter at 39 weeks = 1; preterm stillbirth at 32 weeks and triplets at 30 weeks = 2; spontaneous abortion at 8 weeks = 1; total number of living children = 4).

8. c; although little change occurs in respiratory rate, breathing becomes more thoracic in nature with the upward displacement of the diaphragm; women normally experience a greater awareness of breathing and may even complain of dyspnea at rest as pregnancy progresses; supine hypotension syndrome with a decrease in systolic pressure as much as 30 mm Hg occurs as a result of vena cava and aorta compression by the uterus when the woman is in a supine position; baseline pulse rate increases by 10 to 15 beats per minute; systolic and diastolic pressure decreases by approximately 5 to 10 mm Hg beginning in the second trimester, returning to first trimester levels in the third trimester.

9. b; friability refers to cervical fragility resulting in slight bleeding when scraped or touched; Chadwick's sign refers to a deep bluish color of cervix and vagina as a result of increased circulation; Hegar's sign refers to softening and compressibility of the lower uterine segment.

III. Thinking Critically

1. a. See *Cervical Changes* section; discuss cervical and vaginal friability and increased vascularity; makes the vagina and cervix softer and more delicate so spotting after intercourse is expected; caution that any bleeding should be reported so it can be evaluated.

   b. *See Pregnancy Tests* section: emphasize the importance of following directions because each brand of test is slightly different; use first-voided morning specimen for the most concentrated urine and notify health care provider regardless of the test result.

   c. See *Vagina and Vulva* and *Renal System* sections: discuss impact of increased vaginal secretions and impact of stasis of urine that contains nutrients and has a high pH; review prevention measures at this time.

   d. See *Breasts* section; discuss changes in breasts such as enlargement of Montgomery's glands and development of lactation structures resulting in larger breasts that are tender during the first trimester; changes in consistency and presence of lumpiness during BSE; changes are bilateral.

   e. See *Uteroplacental Blood Flow, BP,* and *Renal System* sections; discuss supine hypotensive syndrome and importance of the lateral position when at rest; also emphasize safety when changing position from supine to upright and to do so slowly as pregnancy progresses to reduce effects of orthostatic hypotension and dizziness.

   f. See *Respiratory System* section; discuss impact of estrogen-stimulated increase in upper airway vascularity, which increases edema, congestion, and hyperemia of the tissue making nosebleeds more common.

   g. See *Renal System* section; explain that the swelling of her ankles is a result of the pressure of the enlarging uterus and the dependent position of her legs; elevating her legs and exercising them helps decrease edema; caution her to never take someone else's medications or to self-medicate.

   h. See *Musculoskeletal* section; lordosis occurs as a result of the enlargement of the uterus, which decreases abdominal muscle tone and increases mobility of the pelvic joints, tilting the pelvis forward and resulting in lower back pain, a change in posture, and a shifting forward of the center of gravity.

   i. See *Uterine Changes–Contractility* section; the woman is describing false labor contractions because they diminish with activity; these contractions facilitate blood flow and promote oxygen delivery to the fetus; compare these contractions with true labor contractions.

2. See Box 7-1 and *Blood Pressure* section for content required to answer each part of this question.

CHAPTER 8: NURSING CARE OF THE FAMILY DURING PREGNANCY

I. Learning Key Terms

1. Nägele's rule; 3, 7, last menstrual period (LMP), 7, last menstrual period, 9

2. Trimesters
3. Fundal height
4. Developmental Tasks; accepting pregnancy, identifying with role of parent, reordering personal relationships, establishing relationship with fetus, preparing for childbirth
5. Emotional lability
6. Ambivalence
7. Biologic fact of pregnancy, "I am pregnant"; growing fetus as distinct from herself, person to nurture; "I am going to have a baby"; birth, parenting of the child; "I am going to be a mother."
8. Supine hypotensive syndrome; vena cava; abdominal aorta
9. Orthostatic (postural) hypotension
10. Fetal heart rate, fundal height
11. Couvade
12. Couvade syndrome
13. Prescriptions; proscriptions; taboos
14. Doulas
15. Birth plan

II. Reviewing Key Concepts

1. Use Nägele's rule: subtract 3 months and add 7 days and 1 year to the first day of the last menstrual period.
   a. February 12, 2014
   b. October 26, 2013
   c. April 11, 2014

2. See *Cultural Influences* and *Variations in Prenatal Care* sections.
   a. Consider the following factors: beliefs that conflict with typical Western prenatal practices, lack of money and transportation, communication difficulties, concern regarding modesty and gender of health care provider, fear of invasive procedures, view of pregnancy as a healthy state whereas health care providers imply illness, view pregnancy problems as a normal part of pregnancy.
   b. See separate sections for each area.

3. See *Initial Visit* and *Follow-up Visits* in the *Care Management Assessment* section.

4. a. See *Recognizing Potential Complications* section and Box 8-2, *Signs of Potential Complications*, which lists signs according to the first, second, and third trimesters.
   b. • Discuss the signs, possible causes, when and to whom to report.
      • Present the signs verbally and in written form.
      • Provide time to answer questions and discuss concerns; make follow-up phone calls.
      • Gather full information of signs that are reported; use information as a basis for action.
      • Document all assessments, actions, and responses.

5. See *Fundal Height* section; consider woman's position, type of measuring tape used, measurement method (Fig. 8-7), and conditions of the examination such as an empty bladder and relaxed or contracted uterus.

6. a. See *Body Mechanics* section, Fig. 8-12, and Home Care box—*Posture and Body Mechanics.*

b. See Patient Teaching box, *Safety During Pregnancy,* Fig. 8-17, and prevention measures identified in subsections of *Education for Self-Management* section such as physical activity, rest and relaxation, employment, clothing, and travel.

7. See *Preparation for Breastfeeding* in the *Newborn* section.

8. See *Paternal Adaptation—Accepting the Pregnancy* section for a discussion of each phase.

9. a, b, and f; choices c and e are probable signs and choice d is a positive sign, diagnostic of pregnancy.

10. a; use Nägele's rule by subtracting 3 months and adding 7 days and 1 year to the first day of the last menstrual period (September 10, 2013).

11. d; supine hypotension related to compression of aorta and vena cava is being experienced; the first action is to remove the cause of the problem by turning the woman on her side; this should alleviate the symptoms being experienced, including nausea; assessment of vital signs can occur after the woman's position is changed.

12. a and d; ambivalence is a common response when preparing for a new role and mood swings or emotional lability is commonly related to hormonal changes; a woman's partner or the father of the baby is usually the greatest source of support; attachment begins with the pregnancy and intensifies during the second trimester.

13. a, e, and f; intake of at least 2 to 3 liters per day is recommended; she does not have to abstain from intercourse, but she should empty her bladder before and after intercourse and drink a large glass of water; cranberry juice may be helpful, but there is conflicting evidence.

14. d; continuous support is critical and involves praise, encouragement, reassurance, comfort measures, physical contact, and explanations; the doula does not get involved in clinical tasks; she is not a substitute for the father but rather encourages his participation as a partner with her in supporting the laboring woman.

15. a, b, e, and f; she should assume a lateral position and continue to count for one more hour.

III. Thinking Critically

1. See *Initial Visit* and *Follow-up Visits* sections of *Assessment* section.
   a. • Establish therapeutic relationship with the pregnant woman and her family.
      • Plan time for purposeful communication to gather baseline data related to the woman's subjective appraisal of her health status and to gather objective information based on observation of the woman's affect, posture, body language, skin color, and other physical and emotional signs.
      • Update information and compare to baseline information during follow-up interviews.
   b. Be sure questions reflect principles of effective questioning; consider the need to ask follow-up questions to clarify and gather further information when a problem is identified.
   c. Focus on updating baseline information and asking questions related to anticipated events and changes for the woman's gestational age at the time of the visit.

2. See *Care Management* section and the Nursing Care Plan—Adolescent Pregnancy; answer should emphasize the following:
   • Establishing a therapeutic, trusting relationship so the woman will feel comfortable continuing with prenatal care
   • Teaching the woman about the importance of prenatal care for her health and that of her baby
   • Involving her boyfriend in the care process so he will encourage her participation in prenatal care
   • Following guidelines for health history interview, physical examination, and laboratory testing; ensure privacy and comfort during the examination and teach her about how her body is changing and will continue to change with pregnancy
   • Evaluating the couple's reaction (e.g., same or different) to pregnancy and the need for community agency support

3. a. Reliability depends on the accuracy of date used and the regularity of her menstrual cycles; birth can normally occur 2 weeks before or after the date or from week 38 to 42.
   b. See *Kegel Exercises* section and Patient Teaching box *Kegel Exercises* in Chapter 3.
   c. See *Sexual Counseling* section and Home Care box *Sexuality in Pregnancy*; emphasize that intercourse is safe as long as pregnancy is progressing normally and it is comfortable for the woman; sexual expression should be in tune with the woman's changing needs and emotions; inform that spotting can normally occur related to the fragility of the vaginal mucosa and cervix and that changes in positions and activities may be helpful as pregnancy progresses.
   d. See Nursing Care Plan—Discomforts of Pregnancy and Table 8-3; fully assess what she is experiencing; then discuss why it happens, how long it will likely last, and relief measures that are safe and effective (also see *Coping with Nutritional-Related Discomforts of Pregnancy* section of Chapter 9).

4. See *Physical Activity* section and Home Care box *Exercise Tips for Pregnant Women*; assess her usual pattern of exercise and activity and consider their safety during pregnancy; discuss precautions and guidelines for safe, effective exercise; emphasize that moderate physical activity benefits her and her baby and will prepare her for the work of labor and birth; caution her to take note of the effects of exercise in terms of temperature, heart rate, and feeling of well-being.

5. a. Risk for urinary tract infection related to lack of knowledge regarding changes of the renal system during pregnancy (see *Education for Self-Care—Preventing UTI* section and Table 8-3—Frequency and Urgency):
   • Woman will drink at least 2 to 3 liters of fluids per day; woman will empty bladder at first urge.

- Explain changes that occur in the renal system during pregnancy; increase fluid intake, use acid-ash forming fluids, void frequently to keep bladder empty, perform good perineal hygiene, use lateral position to enhance renal perfusion and urine formation.

b. Acute pain in lower back related to neuromuscular changes associated with pregnancy at 23 weeks of gestation (see Table 8-3—Joint Pain, Backache, and Pelvic Pressure):
- Woman will experience lessening of lower back pain following implementation of suggested relief measures.
- Explain basis for lower back pain and relief measures, including back massage, pelvic rock, and posture changes; encourage woman to change her footwear for better stability and safety.

c. Anxiety related to lack of knowledge concerning the process of labor and birth and appropriate measures to cope with the pain and discomfort (See *Maternal and Paternal Adaptation—Preparing for Childbirth, Childbirth and Perinatal Education* sections):
- Couple will enroll in a childbirth education program in the seventh month of pregnancy.
- Explain the childbirth process and describe the many nonpharmacologic and pharmacologic measures to relieve pain; discuss role of coach and possibility of hiring a doula; make a referral to a childbirth education program and assist with the preparation of a birth plan; discuss childbirth options and prebirth preparations.

6. a. See *Fundal Height* section; purpose of fundal height: indirect assessment of how her fetus is growing.

b. See *Education for Self-Management* section and Patient Teaching Box—Safety during Pregnancy; clothing choices during pregnancy: consider safety and comfort in terms of low-heeled shoe and nonrestrictive clothing.

c. Gas and constipation: see Table 8-3 (Constipation and Flatulence section) and Nursing Care Plan—Discomforts; assess problem and lifestyle factors that may be contributing to the problem; discuss why it occurs and appropriate relief measures (fluids, roughage, and activity).

d. Itchiness: if the woman is experiencing noninflammatory pruritus, use Table 8-3 (Pruritus—noninflammatory section) for basis of discomfort and relief measures; be sure to rule out rashes related to infection or allergic reactions.

e. Travel during pregnancy: see *Travel* section; tell her that she may travel if her pregnancy is progressing normally; emphasize importance of staying hydrated, wearing seat belt, doing breathing and lower extremities exercises, ambulating every hour for 15 minutes, and voiding every 2 hours.

7. See Emergency box *Supine Hypotension* for content required to answer each part of this question.

8. a. Assess nipples for eversion; if they are not, the woman can be taught to use a nipple shell to help her nipples protrude; no special exercises are recommended because they could stimulate preterm labor in a susceptible woman as a result of secretion of oxytocin; keep nipples and areola clean and dry; see *Preparation for Breastfeeding the Newborn* section.

b. Ankle edema: see Table 8-3 (ankle edema to lower extremities); discuss basis of the edema and encourage use of lower extremities exercises and elevation of legs periodically during the day (Fig. 8-15); emphasize importance of fluid intake.

c. Leg cramps: see Table 8-3 (leg cramps) and Fig. 11-16; discuss basis of leg cramps, and then demonstrate relief measures such as pressing weight onto foot when standing or dorsiflexing the foot while lying in bed; avoid pointing the toes; ensure adequate intake of calcium.

9. a. Anxiety related to perceived risk for preterm labor and birth; woman will identify signs suggestive of preterm labor and the action to take if they occur.

b. See *Recognizing Preterm Labor* section, Home Care box *How to Recognize Preterm Labor,* and Fig. 11-18; emphasize that signs are vague, so she must be alert for even subtle changes; teach her how to palpate her abdomen to detect uterine contractions.

c. Empty bladder, drink 3 to 4 glasses of water, assume a side-lying position, and count contractions for another hour; if contractions continue, call health care provider.

10. See *Sibling Adaptation* section and Box 8-1, which provides tips for sibling preparation; emphasize importance of considering each child's developmental level; prepare children for prenatal events, time during hospitalization, and the homecoming of the new baby; refer to sibling classes and encourage sibling visitation after birth; suggest books and videos that parents could use to prepare their children for birth; provide opportunities to spend time with newborns/infants if possible.

11. a. Deficient knowledge related to pregnant spouse's mood changes; Tom will explain basis for wife's mood swings and strategies that he can use to cope with these changes and support his spouse.

b. See *Maternal Adaptation* section and Table 8-3 (psychosocial dynamics, mood swings, and mixed feelings); discuss the basis for the mood swings and experiences during the first trimester including ambivalence; identify measures he can use to support her.

12. See Family Centered Care Box—Creating a Birth Plan and *Birth Setting Choices* and *Birth Plans* sections; answer should include:
- Descriptions of each option along with the criteria for use and the advantages and disadvantages.
- Onsite visits and interaction with health care providers responsible for care at each site should be encouraged.
- Speak to couples who gave birth in these settings to get their impressions.

- Emphasize that the decision is theirs and that they should choose what is comfortable for them; a decision should be made on the basis of a full understanding of each option.
- Assist couple with creation of a birth plan to facilitate their control over the childbirth process and a more positive birthing experience.

13. See *Doula* section and Box 8-6 for content required to answer each part of this question.
14. See *Home Birth* section for content required to answer each part of this question.

CHAPTER 9: MATERNAL AND FETAL NUTRITION

I. Learning Key Terms

1. Low birth weight (LBW)
2. Folate (folic acid); neural tube defects, 0.6 mg (600 mcg)
3. Dietary reference intake (DRI)
4. BMI; underweight, normal weight, overweight, obese
5. Ketonuria
6. Physiologic anemia
7. Lactose intolerance
8. Pica
9. Food cravings
10. My Plate
11. Morning sickness (Nausea and Vomiting of Pregnancy)
12. Hyperemesis gravidarum
13. Constipation
14. Pyrosis

II. Reviewing Key Concepts

1. See separate sections for each nutrient in *Nutrient Needs During Pregnancy* section and Table 9-1 to complete this activity.
2. See Box 9-5 to identify the five risk indicators.
3. See *Weight Gain, Pattern of Weight Gain, Hazards of Restricting Adequate Weight Gain,* and *Excessive Weight Gain* sections.
4. See *Vegetarian Diets* section.
   These diets tend to be low in vitamins B_{12} and B_6, iron, calcium, zinc, and perhaps calories; supplements may be needed.
   Food needs to be combined to ensure that all essential amino acids are provided.
5. See Table 9-5 for several signs of good and inadequate nutrition.
6. See *Weight Gain* and *Pattern of Weight Gain* sections and Box 9-2 to determine weight gain patterns based on each woman's BMI; keep in mind that each woman should gain 1 to 2.5 kg in the first trimester; weight gain per week is recommended for the second and third trimester.
   a. June: BMI 21.3 (normal); total 11.5 to 16 kg; 0.4 kg/week
   b. Alice: BMI 29 (overweight); total 7 to 11.5 kg; 0.3 kg/week
   c. Ann: BMI 15.8 (underweight); total 12.5 to 18 kg; 0.5 kg/week

7. b, d, e, and f; bran, tea, coffee, milk, oxalate-containing vegetables (spinach, Swiss chard), and egg yolks all decrease iron absorption; tomatoes and strawberries contain vitamin C, which enhances iron absorption; meats contain heme iron, which also enhances absorption.
8. c; BMI indicates that this woman is obese; she should not consider a weight loss regimen until healing is complete in the postpartum period; she should gain at least 7 kg; increase in calories should reflect energy expenditure of the pregnancy during the third trimester, which would be approximately 462 kcal.
9. b; BMI indicates woman is at a normal weight; total gain should be 11.5 to 16 kg, representing a gain of 0.4 kg/week and 1.6 kg/month during the second and third trimesters.
10. c; small, frequent meals are better tolerated than large meals that distend the stomach; hunger can worsen nausea; therefore, meals should not be skipped; dry, starchy foods should be eaten in the morning and at other times during the day when nausea occurs; fried, fatty, and spicy foods should be avoided; a bedtime snack is recommended.
11. b, d, and e; legumes are a good source for folic acid along with whole grains and fortified cereals, oranges, asparagus, liver, and green leafy vegetables; choices a, c, and f are not good sources of folic acid though they do supply other important nutrients for pregnancy (see Box 9-1).

III. Thinking Critically

1. a. Concern regarding amount of recommended weight gain during pregnancy:
   - Identify components of maternal weight gain (see Table 9-2); use Fig. 9-2 to illustrate how the weight gain is distributed over weeks of gestation.
   - Discuss impact of maternal weight gain on fetal growth and development; association between inadequate maternal weight gain and low birth weight and infant mortality.
   - Discuss weight gain total and pattern recommended for a woman with a BMI of 18 (underweight).
   b. Eating for two during pregnancy:
   - Place emphasis on quality of food that meets nutritional requirements, not on the quantity of food.
   - Discuss expected weight gain total and pattern for a woman with a normal BMI of 21.4.
   - Excessive weight gain during pregnancy may be difficult to lose after pregnancy and could lead to chronic obesity; excessive fetal size and childbirth problems could also result.
   c. Vitamin supplementation during pregnancy: determine what and how much she takes; compare to recommendations for pregnancy; discuss potential problems with toxicity, especially with overuse of fat-soluble vitamins; see *Water-Soluble and Fat-Soluble Vitamins* sections.

d. Factors that increase nutritional needs during pregnancy: growth and development of uterine-placental-fetal unit, expansion of maternal blood volume and RBCs, mammary changes, increased basal metabolic rate (BMR); see *Nutrients* sections and Table 9-1.

e. Weight reduction diets during pregnancy:
   - BMI indicates overweight status; a gain of 7 to 11.5 kg during pregnancy is recommended.
   - Discuss hazards of inadequate caloric intake during pregnancy in terms of growth and development of fetus and pregnancy-related structures; impact of ketoacidosis.
   - Discuss quality of foods and development of good nutritional habits to be used during the postpartum period as part of a sensible weight loss program.
   - Discuss importance of exercise and activity during pregnancy.

f. Reduction of water intake: discuss importance of and types of fluid to meet demands of pregnancy-related changes, regulate temperature, and prevent constipation and urinary tract infections (UTIs); consider possible association between dehydration and preterm labor and oligohydramnios; see *Fluids* section.

g. Lactose intolerance: discuss basis for problem; reduce lactose intake by using lactose-free products, nondairy sources of calcium, and calcium supplements; take lactase supplements; see *Calcium* section and Box 9-6, *Calcium Sources for Women Who Do Not Drink Milk*.

h. Weight loss lactation: discuss weight loss patterns with lactation; emphasize that pregnancy fat stores are used during lactation with a resultant weight loss; inform her of increased need for nutrients, calories, and fluids, which are used up with lactogenesis.

i. Nutrition guidelines for lactation: adequate calcium intake, a balanced intake of nutrients (about 500 kcal above nonpregnant intake) or at least 1800 kcal/day, adequate fluid intake (should not experience thirst), and avoid tobacco, alcohol, and excessive caffeine.

   See *Nutrient Needs During Lactation* section and Table 9-1 (use for h and i).

2. See *Iron* section of *Nutrient Needs* section, Patient Teaching box *Iron Supplementation*, and Table 9-1 for iron sources.
   - Discuss importance of iron.
   - Emphasize importance of vitamin C for iron absorption; discuss food sources high in iron and vitamin C; discuss foods to avoid when taking iron.
   - Discuss ways to take iron supplements to enhance absorption and minimize side effects including GI upset and constipation.

3. See appropriate section for each nutrition-related discomfort in *Coping with Nutritional-Related Discomforts of Pregnancy* section.

a. See *Nausea and Vomiting* section and Box 9-8 for several relief measures.

b. See *Constipation* section; include adequate fluid and roughage/fiber intake, exercise and activity, regular time for elimination.

c. See *Pyrosis* section; small frequent meals, drink fluids between not with meals, avoid spicy foods, remain upright after eating.

4. See *Care Management and Cultural Influences* sections, Table 9-5, and Box 9-7.

a. Counseling approach:
   - Assess her current nutritional status and habits; obtain a diet history.
   - Analyze current patterns as a basis for menu planning.
   - Discuss weight gain pattern for an underweight woman.
   - Use a variety of teaching methods; keep woman actively involved.
   - Emphasize importance of good nutrition for herself and her newborn.

b. Menu plan: use Tables 9-3 and 9-6 for Native-American foods and for servings of required nutrients for a 1-day menu; distribute throughout day—meals/snacks.

CHAPTER 10: ASSESSMENT OF HIGH RISK PREGNANCY

I. Learning Key Terms

1. High risk pregnancy
2. Daily fetal movement count (DFMC) or Kick Count; movement alarm signal (MAS)
3. Ultrasound (sonography); transvaginal, transabdominal
4. Doppler blood flow analysis
5. Biophysical profile (BPP); ultrasound, electronic fetal monitoring; fetal breathing movements, fetal body movements, fetal tone, nonstress test, amniotic fluid volume
6. Magnetic resonance imaging (MRI)
7. Amniocentesis
8. Percutaneous umbilical blood sampling (PUBS)
9. Chorionic villus sampling (CVS)
10. Maternal serum alpha-fetoprotein (MSAFP)
11. Triple-marker; MSAFP, unconjugated estriol, hCG, age; Quadruple-marker, inhibin A
12. Coombs (indirect)
13. Nonstress test
14. Vibroacoustic stimulation test (Fetal Acoustic Stimulation test)
15. Contraction stress test; nipple-stimulated contraction stress, oxytocin-stimulated contraction stress

II. Reviewing Key Concepts

1. See Box 9-1 and *Assessment for Risk Factors* section, which describe several risk factors in each category listed.
2. See *Nurse's Role in Assessment of High Risk Pregnancy* section; answer should emphasize education,

support measures, and assisting with or performing the test and follow-up care for each test discussed in the chapter.

3. See Box 10-2, which lists risk factors for each pregnancy-related problem identified.

4. d; an amniocentesis with analysis of amniotic fluid for the L/S ratio and presence of phosphatidylglycerol (Pg) is used to determine pulmonary maturity; choice b refers to a contraction stress test; choice c refers to serial measurements of fetal growth using ultrasound.

5. c; food/fluid is not restricted before the test; the test will evaluate the response of the fetal heart rate (FHR) to fetal movement—acceleration is expected; external not internal monitoring is used.

6. b; the triple marker test is used to screen the older pregnant woman for the possibility that her fetus has Down syndrome; serum levels of alpha fetoprotein (AFP), unconjugated estriol, and hCG are measured; maternal serum alpha-fetoprotein alone is the screening test for open neural tube defects such as spina bifida; a 1-hour, 50-g glucose test is used to screen for gestational diabetes; amniocentesis and Coombs testing would be used to check for Rh antibodies and sensitization.

7. c; a suspicious result is recorded when late decelerations occur with less than 50% of the contractions; a negative test result is recorded when no late decelerations occur during at least three uterine contractions lasting 40 to 60 seconds each, within a 10-minute period; a positive test is recorded when there are persistent late decelerations with more than 50% of the contractions; unsatisfactory is the result recorded when there is a failure to achieve adequate uterine contractions.

8. a; a supine position with hips elevated enhances the view of the uterus; a lithotomy position may also be used; a full bladder is not required for the vaginal ultrasound but would be needed for most abdominal ultrasounds; during the test the woman may experience some pressure but medication for pain relief before the test is not required; contact gel is used with the abdominal ultrasound; water-soluble lubricant may be used to ease insertion of the vaginal probe.

III. Thinking Critically

1. See *Ultrasonography* section:
   a. This woman was tested to determine location of gestational sac because PID could have resulted in narrowing of fallopian tube, thereby increasing risk for ectopic pregnancy; in addition, a determination of gestational age and estimation of date of birth would be done related to irregular cycles and unknown date of last menstrual period (LMP).
   b. Explain purpose of test, how it will be performed, and how it will feel; assist her into a lithotomy position or supine position with hips elevated on a pillow; point out structures on monitor as test is performed.

2. See *Ultrasonography* section; instruct woman to come for test with full bladder if appropriate; explain purpose of test and method of examination; assist her into a supine position with head and shoulders elevated on pillow and hip slightly tipped to right or left side; observe for supine hypotension during test and orthostatic hypotension when rising to upright position after test; indicate how the fetus is being measured and point out fetus and its movements.

3. See *Biophysical Profile* section and Tables 10-2 and 10-3 for identification of variables tested; scoring:
   a. Anxiety related to unexpected need to undergo a biophysical profile.
   b. Describe how the test will be performed using ultrasound and external electronic fetal monitoring; explain that the purpose of the test is to view the fetus within its environment, to determine the amount of amniotic fluid, and assess the FHR response to fetal activity.
   c. A score of 8 to 10 is a normal result.

4. See *Amniocentesis* including *Safety Alert* section and *Nurse's Role in Assessment of High Risk Pregnancy* section.
   a. Explain procedure, witness informed consent, assess maternal vital signs and health status and FHR before the test; ensure that ultrasound is performed to locate placenta and fetus before the test.
   b. Explain what is happening and what she will be feeling; help her relax; encourage her to ask questions and voice concerns and feelings; assess her reactions.
   c. Monitor maternal vital signs and status and FHR; tell her when test results should be available and whom to call; administer RhoGAM because she is Rh negative; teach her to assess herself for signs of infection, bleeding, rupture of membranes, and uterine contractions; make a follow-up phone call to check her status.

5. See *Nonstress Test* section.
   a. Test measures response of FHR to fetal activity to determine adequacy of placental perfusion and fetal oxygenation.
   b. Tell her that she can eat before and during the test; schedule test at a time of day that fetus is usually active; assist woman into a semirecumbent or seated position.
   c. Attach tocotransducer to fundus and Doppler transducer at site of point of maximum intensity (PMI); instruct woman to indicate when fetus moves; assess change, if any, in FHR following the movement.
   d. See Table 10-7 and Box 10-8 for the criteria to determine the test result.

6. See *Contraction Stress Test* section.
   a. The test is a way of determining how her fetus will react to the stress of uterine contractions as they would occur during labor; uterine contractions decrease perfusion through the placenta leading to fetal hypoxia; late decelerations during this test could be interpreted as an early warning of fetal compromise.

b. Assess woman's vital signs, general health status, and contraindications for the test; attach external electronic fetal monitor and assess FHR and uterine activity; assist woman into a lateral, semirecumbent, or seated position; determine whether an informed consent is required because contractions will be stimulated.

c. See *Nipple-Stimulation Contraction Stress Test* section.

d. See *Oxytocin-Stimulated Contraction Stress Test* section.

e. See Table 10-5 for criteria used to interpret the test results and to document as **negative**-no late decelerations are noted; as **positive**-late decelerations with more than half of the contractions, limited variability; **suspicious or equivocal**-late decelerations with less than half of the contractions; **Equivocal-hyperstimulatory**-late decelerations with excessive uterine contractions or tone; or **unsatisfactory**—recording is inadequate.

CHAPTER 11: HIGH RISK PERINATAL CARE: PREEXISTING CONDITIONS

I. Learning Key Terms

1. Diabetes mellitus
2. Hyperglycemia
3. Euglycemia
4. Hypoglycemia
5. Polyuria
6. Polydipsia
7. Polyphagia
8. Glycosuria
9. Ketoacidosis, acetonuria
10. Type 1 diabetes mellitus
11. Type 2 diabetes mellitus
12. Pregestational
13. Gestational
14. Glycosylated hemoglobin A_{1c}
15. Macrosomia
16. Hydramnios (polyhydramnios)
17. Glucose reflectance meter (glucometer)
18. Cardiac decompensation; 28, 30, childbirth, 24, 48
19. Functional classifications of heart disease; asymptomatic without limitation of physical activity, symptomatic with slight limitation of activity, symptomatic with marked limitation of activity, symptomatic with inability to carry on any physical activity without discomfort
20. Peripartum cardiomyopathy
21. Rheumatic heart disease
22. Mitral valve stenosis; Aortic stenosis
23. Myocardial infarction
24. Infective endocarditis
25. Mitral valve prolapse
26. Anemia; iron
27. Sickle cell hemoglobinopathy (anemia)
28. Thalassemia (Mediterranean or Cooley's anemia)
29. Bronchial asthma
30. Cystic fibrosis
31. Pruritus gravidarum
32. Polymorphic eruption of pregnancy
33. Intrahepatic cholestasis of pregnancy
34. Epilepsy
35. Multiple sclerosis
36. Bell's palsy
37. Systemic lupus erythematosus (SLE)
38. Restless leg syndrome

II. Reviewing Key Concepts

1. See *Maternal Risks/Complications* and *Fetal Risks/Complications* sections for a list of all major complications.

2. See *Gestational Diabetes Mellitus Screening* section.

3. See *Thyroid Disorders* section for a description of hyperthyroidism and hypothyroidism; consider effects of these disorders on reproductive development, sexuality, fertility in terms of ability to conceive and to sustain a pregnancy to viability, and potential fetal/newborn complications related to maternal treatment of her thyroid disorder.

4. See *Cardiovascular Disorders* section; increased risk for miscarriage, preterm labor and birth, IUGR, maternal mortality, and stillbirth.

5. See *Substance Abuse—Screening* section and Box 11-4 for a full description of the tool and why it is used.

6. d; the woman is exhibiting signs of DKA; insulin is the required treatment, with the dosage dependent on blood glucose level; intravenous fluids may also be required; choice a is the treatment for hypoglycemia; choices b and c, although they may increase the woman's comfort, are not priorities.

7. c; a 2-hour postprandial blood glucose should be less than 120 mg/dL; choices a, b, and d all fall within the expected normal ranges.

8. a, b, and c; a minimum of intake of 55% carbohydrates, 20% protein, and 25% fat is recommended daily.

9. d; washing hands is important but gloves are not necessary for self-injection; vial should be gently rotated, not shaken; regular insulin should be drawn into the syringe first; because she is obese, a 90-degree angle with skin taut is recommended.

10. b, e, and f; other signs of cardiac compensation include moist, productive, frequent cough, and crackles at bases of lungs; pulse becomes rapid, weak, irregular.

11. a; this woman is exhibiting signs of cardiac decompensation; further information regarding her cardiac status is required to determine what further action would be needed.

12. c; furosemide is a diuretic; propranolol is a beta blocker that is used to manage hypertension and tachycardia; although warfarin is an anticoagulant, it can cross the placenta and affect the fetus, whereas heparin, which is a large molecule, does not.

13. b; bed rest is not required for a woman with a class II designation; she will need to avoid heavy exertion and stop activities that cause fatigue and dyspnea; actions in a, c, and d are all appropriate and recommended for class II.

III. Thinking Critically

1. See *Preconception Counseling* section.
   - Discuss purpose in terms of planning pregnancy for the optimum time when glucose control is established within normal ranges, because this will decrease incidence of congenital anomalies; diagnose any vascular problems; emphasize the importance of her health before the pregnancy, helping to ensure a positive outcome.
   - Discuss how her diabetic management will need to be altered during pregnancy; include her husband, because his help and support during the pregnancy are important.
2. See Table 11-2, Patient Teaching box *Treatment for Hypoglycemia*, and *Monitoring Blood Glucose Levels* section.
3. See *Pregestational Diabetes* subsections for the content required to answer each part of this question.
4. See *Gestational Diabetes* section, Fig. 11-4, and the Nursing Care Plan for Woman with Gestational Diabetes for the content required to answer each part of this question.
5. See *Cardiovascular Disorders* section, Patient Teaching box—The Pregnant Woman at Risk for Cardiac Decompensation, and Box 11-3 for the content required to answer each part of this question.
6. See *Care Management—Antepartal* section.
   a. Discuss importance of taking an anticoagulant to prevent thrombus formation; inform that Coumadin will cross placenta and could cause congenital anomalies and fetal hemorrhage; heparin does not cross the placenta.
   b. Information to ensure safe use of heparin:
      - Safe administration; teach subcutaneous injection technique to Allison and family.
      - Stress importance of routine blood tests to assess clotting ability; discuss alternative sources for folic acid.
      - Review side effects, including unusual bleeding and bruising and measures to prevent injury (soft toothbrush, no razors to shave legs).
7. See *Epilepsy* section including the Safety Alert; inform her that effects of pregnancy on epilepsy are unpredictable; convulsions may injure her or her fetus and lead to miscarriage, preterm labor, or separation of the placenta; medications that will be given in the lowest therapeutic dose must be taken to prevent convulsions; folic acid supplementation is important because anticonvulsants can deplete folic acid stores.
8. See *Substance Abuse* section and Boxes 11-4 and 11-5 for description of principles to follow; emphasize:
   - Family focus including child care and education and support for parenting
   - Empowerment building
   - A community-based interdisciplinary approach with multiplicity of services, including those related to sexual and physical abuse and lack of social support
   - Continuum of care
   - Pregnancy as a window of opportunity related to motivation for change

CHAPTER 12: HIGH RISK PERINATAL CARE: GESTATIONAL CONDITIONS

I. Learning Key Terms

1. Hypertension
2. Gestational hypertension
3. Preeclampsia
4. Severe preeclampsia
5. Eclampsia
6. Chronic hypertension
7. Arteriolar vasospasm
8. HELLP syndrome; hemolysis, elevated liver enzymes, low platelets
9. Proteinuria
10. Diuresis
11. Hyperemesis gravidarum
12. Miscarriage (spontaneous abortion); early pregnancy loss, late pregnancy loss (second trimester loss)
13. Missed miscarriage
14. Habitual miscarriage (recurrent spontaneous abortion)
15. Reduced cervical competence (recurrent premature dilation of cervix)
16. Cerclage
17. Ectopic pregnancy
18. Gestational trophoblastic disease; hydatidiform mole, invasive mole, choriocarcinoma
19. Complete hydatidiform mole
20. Partial hydatidiform mole
21. Complete placenta previa
22. Marginal placenta previa
23. Placental abruption (premature separation of the placenta, abruptio placentae)
24. Vasa previa; velamentous insertion of the cord; succenturiate placenta
25. Battledore placenta
26. Disseminated intravascular coagulation (DIC)
27. Asymptomatic bacteriuria
28. Cystitis
29. Pyelonephritis
30. Appendicitis
31. Cholelithiasis
32. Cholecystitis

II. Reviewing Key Concepts

1. See Box 12-1 for blood pressure guidelines.
2. See *Nursing Care Management—physical examination* section.
   a. Hyperreflexia and ankle clonus: see Table 12-4, which grades deep tendon reflex (DTR) responses and Fig. 12-5 for illustrations depicting performance of DTRs and ankle clonus.
   b. Proteinuria: describe dipstick and 24-hour urine collection methods to determine level of protein in urine.

   c. Pitting edema: see Figs. 12-3 and 12-4, which illustrate assessment of pitting edema and classifications.

3. e   4. c   5. b   6. a   7. d
8. c   9. g   10. d   11. a   12. h
13. b   14. f   15. e

16. c; the woman should be seated or in a lateral position, she should rest for 5 to 10 minutes, and the cuff should cover 80% of the upper arm.

17. a; with severe preeclampsia, the DTRs would be more than 3+ with possible ankle clonus; the BP would be more than 160/110; thrombocytopenia with a platelet level less than150,000 mm^3.

18. b, d, and f; the loading dose should be an IV of 4 to 6 g diluted in 100 mL of intravenous fluid; maternal assessment should occur every 15 to 30 minutes and FHR and UC continuously; respirations should be less than 12.

19. b; magnesium sulfate is a CNS depressant given to prevent seizures.

20. b, d, and e; magnesium sulfate is administered intravenously in the hospital with severe preeclampsia; a clean catch, midstream urine specimen should be used to assess urine for protein using a dipstick; fluid intake should be 6 to 8 (8 oz.) glasses a day along with roughage to prevent constipation; gentle exercise improves circulation and helps preserve muscle tone and a sense of well-being; modified bed rest with diversional activities is recommended for mild preeclampsia.

21. b; labetalol is a beta blocker used for hypertension; oral hygiene is important when NPO and after vomiting episodes to maintain the integrity of oral mucosa; taking fluids between, not with, meals reduces nausea, thereby increasing tolerance for oral nutrition.

22. a; the woman is experiencing a threatened abortion; therefore, a conservative approach is attempted first; b reflects management of an inevitable and complete or incomplete abortion; blood tests for HCG and progesterone levels would be done; cerclage or suturing of the cervix is done for recurrent, spontaneous abortion associated with premature dilation of the cervix.

23. c; a, b, and d are appropriate nursing diagnoses, but deficient fluid is the most immediate concern, placing the woman's well-being at greatest risk.

24. b; methotrexate destroys rapidly growing tissue, in this case the fetus and placenta, to avoid rupture of the tube and need for surgery; follow-up with blood tests is needed for 2 to 8 weeks; alcohol and vitamins containing folic acid increase the risk for side effects with this medication or exacerbating the ectopic rupture.

25. c; the clinical manifestations of placenta previa are described; dark red bleeding with pain is characteristic of abruptio placentae; massive bleeding from many sites is associated with DIC; bleeding is not a sign of preterm labor.

26. a; hemorrhage is a major potential postpartum complication because the implantation site of the placenta is in the lower uterine segment, which has a limited capacity to contract after birth; infection is another major complication, but it is not the immediate focus of care; b and d are also important but not to the same degree as hemorrhage, which is life threatening.

III. Thinking Critically

1. See *Preeclampsia* section, Box 12-2, Tables 12-1 12-2, 12-3, and 12-5, and Patient Teaching Boxes for the content required to answer each part of this question.

2. See *Preeclampsia and Eclampsia* sections, Emergency Box—Eclampsia, Boxes 12-3 and 12-4, Tables 12-1, 12-2, 12-3, and 12-5, and Nursing Care Plan—Severe Preeclampsia for the content required to answer each part of this question.

3. See *Hyperemesis Gravidarum* section and Patient Teaching Box—Diet for Hyperemesis for content required to answer each part of this question.

4. See *Ectopic Pregnancy* section and Box 12-5 for content required to answer each part of this question.

5. See *Miscarriage—Threatened* section and Table 12-6 for content required to answer both parts of this question.

6. See *Miscarriage—Inevitable* section, Patient Teaching Box—Discharge Teaching for the Woman after Early Miscarriage, and Table 12-6 for content required to answer each part of this question; be sure to determine what she means by a lot of bleeding, and whether she is experiencing any other signs and symptoms related to miscarriage such as pain and cramping; determine the gestational age of her pregnancy and whether there is anyone to bring her to the hospital if inevitable abortion is suspected; priority nursing diagnosis at this time: deficient fluid volume related to blood loss secondary to incomplete abortion; acknowledge her loss and provide time for her to express her feelings; inform her about how she may feel (mood swings, depression); refer her for grief counseling, support groups, clergy; make follow-up phone calls.

7. See *Hydatidiform Mole* section for content required to answer this question.

8. See *Placenta Previa* and *Abruptio Placentae* sections and Table 12-7 to compare findings for each disorder in terms of characteristics of bleeding, uterine tone, pain and tenderness, and ultrasound findings regarding location of placenta and fetal presentation/position; priority nursing diagnoses: consider diagnoses related to major physical problems such as deficient fluid volume related to blood loss, ineffective tissue perfusion (placenta), and risk for fetal injury; major psychosocial nursing diagnoses could include fear/anxiety, interrupted family processes, and anticipatory grieving; comparison of care management approaches: consider home care versus hospital care for woman with placenta previa; hospital care is the safest approach for woman experiencing abruptio placentae; discuss active versus expectant management for each disorder;

postpartum complications include increased risk for hemorrhage and infection as well as the emotional impact of a major pregnancy-related complication.

9. See *Trauma During Pregnancy* section, Table 12-8, Emergency Boxes—CPR for Pregnant Women and Relief of Foreign Body Airway Obstruction, and Fig. 12-20 for the content required to answer each part of this question.

CHAPTER 13: LABOR AND BIRTH PROCESSES

I. Learning Key Terms

1. Passenger (fetus, placenta), passageway, powers, position of the mother, psychologic responses
2. Fontanels
3. Molding
4. Presentation; cephalic, breech, shoulder
5. Presenting part; occiput, sacrum, scapula
6. Lie; longitudinal (vertical), transverse (horizontal, oblique)
7. Attitude (posture); flexion
8. Biparietal; suboccipitobregmatic
9. Position
10. Engagement
11. Station
12. Bony pelvis, soft tissue
13. Effacement
14. Dilation
15. Lightening
16. Involuntary uterine contractions
17. Bearing down (pushing; contraction of abdominal muscles and diaphragm)
18. Bloody show
19. Mechanism of labor (cardinal movements); engagement, descent, flexion, internal rotation, extension, external rotation (restitution), expulsion
20. Valsalva maneuver
21. Labor and birth
22. Ferguson reflex
23. Regular uterine contractions, dilation and effacement; latent, active, transition
24. Dilated and effaced, birth of the baby
25. Birth of the baby, placenta
26. Recovery, hemostasis
27. Position, blood pressure, uterine contractions, umbilical cord blood flow
28. Endogenous endorphins

II. Reviewing Key Concepts

1. See separate sections for each of the five factors in *Factors of Labor* section; consider the factors of passenger, passage, powers, position of mother, psychologic response.
2. a, c, d, and e; station is 1 cm above the ischial spines (−1); 7 cm more to reach full dilation of 10 cm.
3. c, d, e, and f; systolic blood pressure increases with uterine contractions in the first stage, whereas both systolic and diastolic blood pressure increase during contractions in the second stage; WBC increases.

4. a, d, and e; quickening refers to the woman's first perception of fetal movement at 16 to 18 weeks of gestation; urinary frequency, lightening, weight loss of 0.5 to 1 kg occur to signal that the onset of labor is near; backache, stronger Braxton Hicks and bloody show are also noted; shortness of breath is relieved once lightening occurs reducing pressure on the diaphragm.

III. Thinking Critically

1. • Examination I: ROP (right occiput posterior, cephalic [vertex] presentation, longitudinal lie, flexed attitude), −1 (station at 1 cm above the ischial spines), 50% effaced, 3-cm dilated.
   • Examination II: RMA (right mentum anterior, cephalic [face] presentation, longitudinal lie, extended attitude), 0 (station at the ischial spines, engaged), 25% effaced, 2-cm dilated.
   • Examination III: LST (left sacrum transverse, breech presentation, longitudinal lie, flexed attitude), +1 (station at 1 cm below the ischial spines), 75% effaced, 6-cm dilated.
   • Examination IV: OA (occiput anterior, cephalic [vertex] presentation, longitudinal lie, flexed attitude), + 3 (station at 3 cm below the ischial spines near or on the perineum), 100% effaced, 10 cm (fully dilated).

2. a. See *Onset of Labor* section of the *Process of Labor*; explain in simple terms the interaction of maternal and fetal hormones, uterine distention, placental aging, and prostaglandins.
   b. See *Signs Preceding Labor* section and Box 13-1 for the signs that occur before the onset of labor.
   c. See *Postioning of the Laboring Woman* section; include the following points in answer:
      • Emphasize that the position of the woman is one of the 5 Ps of labor.
      • Discuss each position and describe its effect.
      • Demonstrate each position and have her practice them with her partner.
      • Emphasize the beneficial effects of ambulation and changing positions on fetus, circulation, comfort, and progress.
   d. Breathing initiation after birth: see *Fetal Adaptation*, fetal respiration section, for a description regarding the onset of newborn breathing.

CHAPTER 14: PAIN MANAGEMENT

I. Learning Key Terms

1. Uterine ischemia
2. Visceral
3. Somatic
4. Referred
5. Pain threshold
6. Gate control theory of pain
7. Beta endorphins
8. Dick-Read method
9. Lamaze
10. Bradley

11. HypnoBirthing
12. Birthing from within
13. Cleansing breath
14. Slow-paced breathing
15. Modified-paced breathing
16. Patterned-paced breathing (Pant-Blow breathing)
17. Hyperventilation
18. Effleurage
19. Counterpressure
20. Water therapy (hydrotherapy)
21. Transcutaneous electrical nerve stimulation (TENS)
22. Acupressure
23. Acupuncture
24. Biofeedback
25. Aromatherapy
26. Intradermal water block
27. Therapeutic touch

II. Reviewing Key Concepts

1. See *Perception of Pain* and *Factors Influencing the Pain Response* sections for content required to answer each part of this question.
2. See *Gate Control Theory of Pain* section.
3. b   4. f   5. h   6. a   7. g   8. j
9. m   10. d   11. i   12. l   13. c   14. e
15. k   16. n
17. See individual sections for each regional anesthetic listed and *Care Management* section.
18. See *Systemic Analgesics* section including Safety Alert and Medication Guide for Analgesics for content required to answer each part of this question.
19. See *Care Management—Administration of Medications* section; onset of action is faster and more reliable and predictable when administered intravenously.
20. d; woman can and should change her position while in the bath, using lateral and hand-and-knees when indicated; as long as amniotic fluid is clear or only slightly meconium tinged, a whirlpool can continue; there is no limit to the time she can spend in the water—she can stay as long as she wishes.
21. a; promethazine is a phenothiazine, butorphanol is an opioid agonist-antagonist analgesic; fentanyl is an opioid agonist analgesic.
22. c; metoclopramide is used to prevent or treat nausea and vomiting, it does not provide analgesia nor cause respiratory depression; it can increase the effectiveness of opioid analgesics.
23. d; as a pure opioid agonist, meperidine will not cause abstinence syndrome; a 25-mg dose is appropriate for IV administration; this medication is a potent opioid agonist analgesic; while it can cause respiratory depression, that is more likely to occur with morphine.
24. c; administration of Narcan is given to reverse effects of sedation as the client is experiencing potential symptoms and/or in this case delivery is imminent and the provider wants to counteract possible fetal effects as a result of maternal narcotic administration. The nurse should continue to monitor maternal condition for possible side effects of the medication.
25. a, b, d, and f; spinal headache is rare because the dura is not punctured; using a combined anesthetic-analgesic and reducing dosage can allow a woman to push when the time is right.
26. a, b, and c; d, e, and f are not associated with opioid abstinence syndrome.
27. b; changing the woman to a lateral position will enhance cardiac output and raise the blood pressure because compression of the abdominal aorta and vena cava is removed; administering oxygen and notifying the health care provider would follow along with increasing intravenous fluid administration; administration of a vasopressor, if ordered by the physician, would follow if the other measures are not sufficient to restore the blood pressure.

III. Thinking Critically

1. See *Neurologic Origins of Pain* section; describe why pain occurs and its very real basis including the types of pain and their origin; discuss how women experience the pain and factors that influence the experience; identify measures they can use to help their partners reduce and cope with the pain.
2. See *Nonpharmacologic and Pharmacologic Pain Management* and *Nursing Care Management* sections, Box 14-1, and Nursing Care Plan for content required to answer each part of this question; include the following points in your answer:
   - Basis of pain and its potentially adverse effects on the maternal-fetal unit and the progress of labor
   - Discuss a variety of nonpharmacologic and pharmacologic measures that are safe and effective to use during labor and can have beneficial effects on the maternal-fetal unit and can enhance the progress of labor.
   - Emphasize that the mother and fetus will be thoroughly assessed before, during, and after use of any measure to ensure safety.
3. See *Water Therapy (Hydrotherapy)* section for content required to answer each part of this question.
   - Describe the beneficial effects of water therapy and how it can facilitate the labor process thereby decreasing the possibility of cesarean birth; use research findings to substantiate these claims.
   - Describe the successful experiences of other agencies that have implemented water therapy; state how it has affected the number of births.
   - Use favorable reports of women who have used water therapy; consider how this could affect other women preparing for childbirth.
4. See Emergency box *Maternal Hypotension with Decreased Placental Perfusion* for content required to answer each part of this question.
5. See *Epidural Block* and *Care Management* sections including Safety Alerts, Figs. 14-10 and 14-11, and Box 14-7 for content required to answer each part of this question.

CHAPTER 15: FETAL ASSESSMENT DURING LABOR

I. Learning Key Terms

1. Uterine tachysystole
2. Intermittent auscultation (IA)
3. Ultrasound stethoscope (Doppler ultrasound)
4. Electronic fetal monitoring; external, internal
5. Ultrasound transducer
6. Tocotransducer
7. Spiral electrode
8. Intrauterine pressure catheter (IUPC)
9. Intrauterine resuscitation
10. Fetal stimulation
11. Oligohydramnios
12. Anhydramnios
13. Amnioinfusion
14. Tocolytic therapy

II. Reviewing Key Concepts

1. i   2. j   3. h   4. g   5. k   6. f
7. c   8. b   9. d   10. e   11. a   12. l
13. See *Fetal Response* section for a description of each factor that reduces fetal oxygen supply.
14. See *Uterine Activity* and *Fetal Compromise* section, Box 15-1, and Table 15-1 for content required to answer each part of this question.
15. See *Nursing Management of Abnormal Patterns* section and Fig. 15-7; include a description of baseline rate, baseline variability, presence of periodic or episodic changes in FHR, uterine activity pattern, efficiency of equipment.
16. See *Monitoring Techniques* section and Boxes 15-7 and 15-9 for content required to answer each part of this question; be sure to include advantages and disadvantages for each method in answer.
17. See *Legal Tip, Fetal Monitoring Standards* section; evaluate FHR pattern at frequency that reflects professional standards, agency policy, and condition of maternal-fetal unit; correctly interpret FHR pattern as reassuring or nonreassuring; take appropriate action; evaluate response to actions taken; notify primary health care provider in a timely fashion; know the chain of command if a dispute about interpretation occurs; document assessment findings, actions, and responses.
18. d; the average resting pressure should be 10 mm Hg; a, b, and c are all findings within the expected ranges.
19. a, c, d, and e; the tocotransducer is always placed over the fundus but the ultrasound transducer, which requires the use of gel, should be repositioned when the fetus moves or as needed; woman's position should be changed even though it may mean repositioning the transducers.
20. b; see *Nursing Management of Nonreassuring Patterns—Intrauterine Resuscitation* section.
21. b and d; the baseline rate should be 110 to 160 beats/min; late deceleration pattern of any magnitude is nonreassuring (abnormal), especially if it is repetitive.

22. c; the FHR increases as the maternal core body temperature rises; therefore, tachycardia would be the pattern exhibited; it is often a clue of intrauterine infection because maternal fever is often the first sign; diminished variability reflects hypoxia and variable decelerations are characteristic of cord compression; early decelerations are characteristic of head compression and are not considered an abnormal pattern.
23. b; the pattern described is an early deceleration pattern, which is considered to be benign, reassuring, and requiring no action other than documentation of the finding; it is associated with fetal head compression; changing a woman's position and notifying the physician would be appropriate if nonreassuring signs such as late or variable decelerations were occurring; prolapse of cord is associated with variable decelerations as a result of cord compression.

III. Thinking Critically

1. See *Monitoring Techniques—External Monitoring* section and Box 15-9 for content required to answer each part of this question; include the following points in your answer:
   • Discuss how fetus responds to labor and how the monitor will assess these responses.
   • Explain the advantages of monitoring.
   • Show her a monitor strip and explain what it reveals; tell her how to use the strip to help her with breathing techniques.
2. See *Fetal Heart Rate Patterns* section, Boxes 15-5 and 15-8, and Figs. 15-8, 15-15, and 15-16 for content required to answer each part of this question; the pattern described is a late deceleration pattern with baseline variability change.
3. See *Fetal Heart Rate Patterns* section, Boxes 15-6 and 15-8, and Figs. 15-17 and 15-18 for content required to answer each part of this question; discuss variable deceleration patterns associated with cord compression.
4. See *Intermittent Auscultation* section and Box 15-2 for the content required to answer this question.

CHAPTER 16: NURSING CARE OF THE FAMILY DURING LABOR AND BIRTH

I. Learning Key Terms

1. Regular uterine contractions, effacement, dilation; mucous plug
2. 3, 6, 8, 4, 7, 3, 6, 20, 40, 8, 10
3. Infant is born, dilation, effacement, baby's birth
4. Birth of the baby, placenta is expelled, fundus, discoid, globular ovoid, gush of dark blood, lengthening of umbilical cord, vaginal fullness, fetal membranes
5. 1 to 2 hours
6. p   7. f   8. g   9. j   10. h   11. b
12. m   13. a   14. q   15. e   16. k   17. n
18. d   19. o   20. c   21. i   22. r   23. l

24. Uterine contractions
25. Increment
26. Acme
27. Decrement
28. Frequency
29. Intensity
30. Duration
31. Resting tone
32. Interval
33. Bearing-down effort

II. Reviewing Key Concepts

1. See *First Stage of Labor—Assessment* section and Boxes 16-2 and 16-3 for content required to answer each part of this question.
2. See Box 16-9 for content required to answer each part of this question.
3. See Box 16-11 and *Ambulation and Positioning* section for content required to answer each part of this question.
4. See appropriate sections that discuss general systems assessment, vital signs, Leopold's maneuvers, assessment of FHR and pattern, assessment of uterine contractions, and vaginal examination; see Boxes 16-4, 16-7, and 16-15 and Tables 16-1 and 16-3 for content required to answer this question.
5. See *Laboratory and Diagnostic Tests* section for content required to answer this question.
6. See *Second Stage of Labor* section for content required to answer this question.
7. See *Preparing for Birth and Maternal Position* sections for content required to answer this question; include squatting, side-lying, semirecumbent, standing, and hands-and-knees positions in your answer.
8. See *Fourth Stage of Labor* section for content required to answer this question; discuss how breastfeeding will have positive physiologic effects for the mother and enhance attachment and success of breastfeeding.
9. b, c, d, and e; goal is to remove pressure from the cord and keep it intact and functioning; raising a woman's legs will not do this but a knee-chest position will; cord should be wrapped in a sterile compress moistened with warm sterile normal saline (see Chapter 17 for further information on this labor emergency).
10. a; although b, c, and d are all important questions, the first question should gather information regarding whether or not the woman is in labor.
11. c; pH of amniotic fluid is alkaline at 6.5 or higher, ferning is noted when examining fluid with a microscope, and the fluid is relatively odorless; a strong odor is strongly suggestive of infection.
12. b and d; the only indicators of true labor are cervical change. Other statements are subjective based on maternal perception.
13. c; O or occiput indicates a vertex presentation with the neck fully flexed and the occiput in the transverse section (T) of the woman's pelvis; the station is 2 cm below the ischial spines (+2); the woman is entering the active phase of labor as indicated by 4 cm of dilation; the lie is longitudinal (vertical) because the head (cephalic/vertex) is presenting.
14. b; research has indicated that enemas are not needed during labor; according to research findings a, c, and d have all been found to be beneficial and safe during pregnancy.

III. Thinking Critically

1. See *First Stage of Labor—Assessment* section and Patient Teaching box *How to Distinguish True Labor from False Labor* for content required to answer each part of this question.
   a. Determine the status of her labor; if there is any doubt about the information being given or her status, the patient should be advised to come in for evaluation.
   b. Questions should be clear, concise, open-ended, and directed toward distinguishing her labor status and determining the basis for action.
   c. Discuss assessment measures, comfort, distraction, emotional support and who and when to call; it is important that the nurse make follow-up calls to determine how the woman is progressing.
2. a. and b: See Table 16-3 to determine phase; Denise (active); Teresa (transition); Danielle (latent).
   c. See Box 16-4, Tables 16-2 and 16-4, *Nursing Care* section and *Nursing Care Plan for Labor and Birth* for care measures required by each woman according to her phase of labor.
   d. See Box 16-12 and *Support of the Father or Partner* section in *Second Stage of Labor* section for several suggested measures the nurse can use to support the support person of the laboring woman.
3. See Box 16-6, Fig. 16-6, and *Leopold Maneuvers and Assessment of Fetal Heart Rate and Pattern* sections for content required to answer this question; realize that presentation and position affect location of PMI and the PMI will change as the fetus progresses through the birth canal.
4. See *Vaginal Examination* section and Box 16-8 for content required to answer each part of this question; explain to the woman the data obtained from monitoring and the vaginal examination and tell her what she can do to decrease her discomfort; privacy and discussion of the results is critical.
5. See *Assessment of Amniotic Membranes and Fluid* section including the Nursing Alert; immediate assessment of the FHR and pattern (prolapse of the cord could have occurred, compressing the cord and leading to hypoxia and variable deceleration patterns); vaginal examination (status of cervix, check for cord prolapse); assess fluid, document findings and notify primary health care provider; cleanse perineum as soon as possible once status of fetus, mother, and labor are determined; strict infection control measures after rupture because risk for infection increases.

6. See *First Stage of Labor—Care Management* section emphasizing supportive care during labor and birth for content required to answer this question.
   - Nursing diagnosis: anxiety related to lack of knowledge and experience regarding the process of childbirth.
   - Expected outcome: couple will cooperate with measures to enhance progress of labor as their anxiety level decreases.
   - Nursing measures: provide explanations, demonstrate and assist with simple breathing and relaxation techniques; make use of phases of labor to tailor health teaching.
7. See *Cultural Factors, Culture and Father Participation, and the Non–English Speaking Woman in Labor* sections and Cultural Competence Box 16-1 for content required to answer each part of this question.
8. See *Ambulation and Positioning and Preparing for Birth* sections and Box 16-11 for content required to answer each part of this question.
9. See *Mechanism of Birth Vertex Presentation, Immediate Assessment and Care of Newborn*, and *Fourth Stage* sections and Box 16-13, *Guidelines for Assistance at the Emergency Birth of a Fetus in the Vertex Presentation*, for content required to answer each part of this question.
10. See *Maternal Position* and *Bearing-Down Efforts* sections for the criteria to use to determine correctness of the bearing down technique.
11. See *Perineal Trauma related to Childbirth* section; compare episiotomies with spontaneous lacerations in terms of tissue affected, long-term sequelae, healing process, discomfort; compare reasons given for performing an episiotomy with what research findings demonstrate to be true.
12. See *Siblings During Childbirth* section: Include research findings regarding effect of sibling participation on family and on the sibling; consider the developmental readiness of the child and use developmental principles to prepare him or her for the experience; offer family and sibling classes to prepare them for participation in the birth process; evaluate parental comfort with this option; arrange for a support person to remain with the child during the entire childbirth process.
13. See *Fourth Stage of Labor and Family-Newborn Relationships* sections and Box 16-16 for content required to answer each section of this question.

CHAPTER 17: LABOR AND BIRTH COMPLICATIONS

I. Learning Key Terms
1. Preterm labor
2. Preterm birth
3. Low birth weight (LBW)
4. Fetal fibronectins
5. Cervical length
6. Premature rupture of membranes (PROM)
7. Preterm premature rupture of membranes (PPROM)
8. Chorioamnionitis
9. Dystocia (dysfunctional labor)
10. Hypertonic uterine dysfunction *or* primary dysfunctional labor
11. Hypotonic uterine dysfunction *or* secondary uterine inertia
12. Pelvic dystocia
13. Soft tissue dystocia
14. Fetal dystocia
15. Cephalopelvic disproportion (CPD) *or* fetopelvic disproportion (FPD)
16. Occipitoposterior
17. Breech
18. Multifetal pregnancy
19. Prolonged latent phase
20. Protracted active phase—dilation
21. Secondary arrest—no change
22. Protracted descent
23. Arrest of descent
24. Failure of descent
25. Precipitous labor
26. External cephalic version (ECV)
27. Trial of labor
28. Induction of labor
29. Bishop score
30. Amniotomy
31. Augmentation of labor
32. Cervical ripening
33. Tachysystole
34. Forceps-assisted birth
35. Vacuum-assisted birth *or* vacuum extraction
36. Cesarean birth
37. Postterm, postdate (prolonged), postmaturity syndrome
38. Shoulder dystocia; fetopelvic disproportion, excessive fetal size (macrosomia)
39. Prolapse of umbilical cord
40. Amniotic fluid embolism (AFE) *or* anaphylactoid syndrome of pregnancy

II. Reviewing Key Concepts
1. See *Spontaneous versus Indicated Preterm Birth* sections and Boxes 17-1 and 17-2 for content required to answer this question.
2. See *Activity Restriction* section and Box 17-4 for content required to answer this question.
3. b   4. c   5. e   6. a   7. d   8. f
9. e   10. f   11. c   12. d   13. a   14. g
15. h   16. b
17. See *Dystocia/dysfunctional Labor* section and specific sections for each factor for content required to answer this question.
18. See *Hypertonic Uterine Dysfunction* section.
    - Purpose: help woman experiencing hypertonic uterine dysfunction to rest/sleep so active labor can begin usually after a 4- to 6-hour rest period.
    - What: use of shower or warm bath for relaxation, comfort measures, administration of analgesics to inhibit contractions, reduce pain, and encourage rest/sleep and relaxation.

19. See *Abnormal Uterine Activity* section for content required to answer this question.

20. See *Oxytocin* section and Box 17-8 where several indicators and contraindications are listed.

21. b, c, and e are correct; Black women are at higher risk for preterm labor, leukorrhea is a normal finding during pregnancy, and a BMI represents a normal weight for height.

22. a, c, d, and f; weight loss, not gain, occurs and there is a decrease in cardiac output.

23. a; magnesium sulfate is a central nervous system (CNS) depressant; woman should alternate lateral positions to decrease pressure on cervix, which could stimulate uterine contractions; calcium gluconate would be used if toxicity occurs; infusion should be discontinued if respiratory rate is less than 12.

24. c; it is inserted into the posterior vaginal fornix; the woman should remain in bed for 2 hours; induction can begin within 30 to 60 minutes of the insert's removal.

25. d; a Bishop score of 9 indicates that the cervix is already sufficiently ripe for successful induction; 10 units of Pitocin is usually mixed in 1000 mL of an electrolyte solution such as Ringer's lactate; the Pitocin solution is piggybacked at the proximal port (port nearest the insertion site).

26. a; frequency of uterine contractions should not be less than every 2 minutes to allow for an adequate rest period between contractions; b, c, and d are all expected findings within the normal range.

27. c; the presentation of this fetus is breech; the soft buttocks are a less efficient dilating wedge than the fetal head; therefore, labor may be slower; the ultrasound transducer should be placed to the left of the umbilicus at a level at or above it; passage of meconium is an expected finding as a result of pressure on the abdomen during descent; knee-chest position is most often used for occipitoposterior positions.

28. d; the dosage is correct at 12 mg × 2 doses; it should be given intramuscularly; dosages should be spaced 24 hours apart; therefore the next dose should be given at 11 AM the next day.

29. a; the definitive sign of preterm labor is significant change in the cervix.

III. Thinking Critically

1. See *Predicting Preterm Labor and Birth* section and Boxes 17-1, 17-2, and 17-3 for content required to answer this question; keep in mind that as many as 50% of women go into preterm labor without identifiable risk factors.

2. See *Early Recognition and Diagnosis, Prevention, and Suppression of Uterine Activity* sections, Boxes 17-2 and 17-3, Patient Teaching Box—What to Do If Symptoms of Preterm Labor Occur, and Medication Guides for Tocolytic Therapy and Antenatal Glucocorticoid Therapy for content required to answer each part of this question.

3. See *Suppression of Uterine Activity* and *Lifestyle* sections, Nursing Care Plan for Preterm Labor, Medication Guide for Tocolytic Therapy, Box 17-3, and Patient Teaching Boxes for content required to answer each part of this question.

4. See *Malposition* section and Box 17-11 for the content required to answer this question; LOP indicates that the fetus is in a posterior position—the most common type of malpresentation.

5. See *Cesarean Birth and Trial of Labor and VBAC* sections, Box 17-3, OB Emergencies Box—Meconium Stained Amniotic Fluid, and Patient Teaching Boxes for the content required to answer each part of this question.

   a. Implement typical preoperative care measures as for any major surgery in a calm and professional manner, explaining the purpose of each measure that must be performed; use a family-centered approach.

   b. Assess for signs of hemorrhage, pain level, respiratory effort, renal function, circulatory status to extremities, signs of postanesthesia recovery, emotional status, and attachment/reaction to newborn.

   c. Measures include assessment of recovery, pain relief, coughing and deep breathing, leg exercises and assistance with ambulation, nutrition and fluid intake (oral, IV); provide opportunities for interaction and care of newborn, assisting her as needed; provide emotional support to help her deal with her disappointment and feelings of failure; help her and her family prepare for discharge, making referrals as needed.

   d. Situational low self-esteem related to inability to reach goal of a vaginal birth secondary to occurrence of fetal distress.

   • Discuss and review why Anne needed a cesarean birth, how she performed during labor, and that she had no control over the fetal distress.

   • Discuss vaginal birth after cesarean (VBAC) and likelihood of it being an option because the reason for her primary cesarean (fetal distress) may not occur again; discuss trial of labor next time to determine her ability to proceed to vaginal birth.

   • Use follow-up phone calls to assess progress in accepting cesarean birth.

6. See *Malpresentation* section; right sacrum anterior (RSA) indicates a breech presentation; consider that descent may be slower, meconium is often expelled, increasing danger of meconium aspiration, and risk for cord prolapse is increased; depending on progress of labor and maternal characteristics, cesarean or vaginal birth may occur or external cephalic version (ECV) may be attempted.

7. See *Induction of Labor* section.

   a. See Table 17-3 for factors assessed to determine degree of cervical ripening in preparation for labor process.

   b. Her score should be greater than 9 to ensure a successful induction; cervical ripening will be needed before induction.

c. See *Cervical Ripening Methods* section and *Medication Guide* for guidelines for use and adverse reactions; consider how and where it is inserted, protocol to follow after the insertion, and adverse reactions and what to do if they occur.

d. See Box 17-9, *Procedure: Assisting with Amniotomy*; explain what will happen, how it will feel, and why it is being done; assess maternal-fetal unit before and after the procedure; document findings; support woman during procedure telling her what is happening; document procedure and outcomes/reactions appropriately.

e. Induction protocol:
   1. A   2. NA   3. A   4. A   5. A
   6. NA   7. NA   8. A   9. NA   10. NA

f. See Box 17-9—focus on factors related to mother, fetus, and labor process.

g. See Emergency box, *Uterine Tachysystole with Oxytocin.*

8. See *Postterm Pregnancy, Labor, and Birth* section and Patient Teaching Box—Postterm Pregnancy for content required to answer each part of this question.

9. See *Obesity* section for content required to answer this question.

CHAPTER 18: MATERNAL PHYSIOLOGIC CHANGES

I. Learning Key Terms

1. Postpartal diaphoresis
2. Afterpains/afterbirth pains
3. Prolactin; oxytocin
4. Episiotomy
5. Uterine atony
6. Hemorrhoid
7. Involution
8. Autolysis
9. Puerperium; fourth trimester
10. Diastasis recti abdominis
11. Lochia
12. Lochia rubra
13. Lochia serosa
14. Lochia alba
15. Engorgement
16. Subinvolution; retained placental fragments, infection
17. Exogenous oxytocin (Pitocin)
18. Dyspareunia
19. Kegel exercises
20. Colostrum
21. Postpartal diuresis
22. Striae gravidarum

II. Reviewing Key Concepts

1. See *Urethra and Bladder* section of *Urinary System* for content required to answer each part of this question.
2. See *Bowel Evacuation* section for content required to answer this question.
3. See *Blood Volume* section for content required to answer this question.

4. See *Coagulation Factors* section for content required to answer this question.

5. See Box 18-1 for the information to complete your answer.

6. d; fundus should be at midline; deviation from midline could indicate a full bladder; bright to dark red uterine discharge refers to lochia rubra; edema and erythema are common shortly after repair of a wound; decreased abdominal muscle tone and enlarged uterus result in abdominal protrusion; separation of the abdominal muscle walls, diastasis rectus abdominis, is common during pregnancy and the postpartum period.

7. b; the woman is describing the normal finding of postpartum diaphoresis, which is the body's attempt to excrete fluid retained during pregnancy; documentation is important but not the first nursing action; infection assessment and physician notification are not needed at this time.

8. d; afterpains are most likely to occur in the following circumstances: multiparity, overdistention of the uterus (macrosomia, multifetal pregnancy, hydramnios), breastfeeding (endogenous oxytocin secretion), and administration of an oxytocic.

III. Thinking Critically

1. a. Afterpains: breastfeeding with newborn sucking causes the posterior pituitary to secrete oxytocin, stimulating the let-down reflex; uterine contractions are also stimulated, leading to afterpains, which will occur for the first few days postpartum.

   b. See *Involution Process* section; progress of uterine descent in the abdomen is described.

   c. See *Lochia* section; discuss characteristics of rubra, serosa, and alba lochia in terms of color, consistency, amount, odor, and duration.

   d. See *Abdomen* section for content required to answer question—focus on reason for the occurrence and what can be done to restore abdominal muscle tone safely.

   e. See *Postpartal Fluid Loss* section; discuss normalcy of these processes designed to rid the body of fluid retained during pregnancy. Be sure to ask questions regarding characteristics of urine, including amount and any pain with urination, to rule out a bladder infection or urinary retention evidenced by frequent voiding of small amounts of urine (overload).

   f. See *Pituitary Hormones and Ovarian Function* section; emphasize that breastfeeding is not a reliable method because return of ovulation is unpredictable and may precede menstruation; discuss appropriate contraceptive methods for a breastfeeding woman, taking care to avoid hormonal based methods until lactation is well established.

   g. See *Nonbreastfeeding Mothers* section for content required to answer this question; discuss the process of natural lactation suppression, why it is used now, and what she can do to enhance her comfort and facilitate the process.

   h. See *Vagina and Perineum* section for content required to answer this question.

CHAPTER 19: NURSING CARE OF THE FAMILY DURING THE POSTPARTUM PERIOD

I. Learning Key Terms

1. Couplet care; mother-baby care, rooming-in
2. Early postpartum discharge; shortened hospital stay, one-day maternity stay
3. Oxytocic
4. Uterine atony
5. Sitz bath
6. Afterpains (after-birth pains)
7. Splanchnic engorgement, orthostatic hypotension
8. Kegel
9. Engorgement
10. Rubella
11. RhoGAM (Rh immune globulin)
12. Warm line

II. Reviewing Key Concepts

1. See *Promotion of Breastfeeding* section for the content required to answer this question.
2. See *Prevention of Bladder Distention* section for content required to answer this question.
3. See *Promotion of Ambulation* section including safety alert for content required to answer this question; in addition to activity include the use of support hose (if varicosities are present) and importance of remaining well hydrated.
4. See *Lactation Suppression* section for content required to answer this question.
5. See *Prevention of Excessive Bleeding* section; include each measure in your answer:
   • Maintain uterine tone
   • Prevent bladder distention
6. See Box 19-2 and *Psychosocial Needs* section for the content required to answer the question.
7. c; the woman should be assisted into a supine position with head and shoulders on a pillow, arms at sides, and knees flexed; this will facilitate relaxation of abdominal muscles and allow deep palpation.
8. a; Methergine as an oxytocic that contracts the uterus, thereby preventing excessive blood loss; lochia will therefore reflect expected characteristics.
9. b; a direct and indirect Coombs' must be negative, indicating that antibodies have not been formed, before RhoGAM can be given; it must be given within 72 hours of birth; the newborn needs to be Rh+; it is often given in the third trimester and then again after birth.
10. d; this is a medical aseptic procedure; therefore, clean, not sterile, equipment is used; the water should be warm at 38° to 40.6° C; it is often used 2 to 3 times a day for 20 minutes each time.
11. d and e; the sitz bath should be used 2 to 3 times per day for 20 minutes each time; topical medications should be used sparingly only 3 to 4 times per day.
12. b and d; temperature of 38° C during the first 24 hours may be related to deficient fluid and is therefore not a concern; fundus should be firm not boggy; saturation of the pad in 15 minutes or less would be a concern; usually women have a good appetite after birth; each voiding should be at least 100 mL.

III. Thinking Critically

1. See *Promotion of Comfort—Nonpharmacologic and Pharmacologic Interventions* sections, Nursing Care Plan "Acute Pain"; assess characteristics of pain and relief measures already tried and effectiveness; use a combination of pharmacologic and nonpharmacologic measures as indicated by the nature of the pain being experienced; if breastfeeding, administer a systemic analgesic just after a feeding session; make sure medication is not contraindicated for breastfeeding women.
2. See *Prevention of Excessive Bleeding* section, Emergency box *Hypovolemic Shock*, and Nursing Care Plan "Risk for Deficient Fluid Volume" for content required to answer each part of this question.
3. See *Rubella* section including Legal Tip for the content required to answer this question.
4. See *Prevention of Rh Isoimmunization* section including Nursing Alert and *Medication Guide* for content required to answer this question.
5. See *Sexual Activity and Contraception* section and the Home Care Box: Resumption of Sexual Intercourse for content required to answer this question.
6. a. Nursing diagnosis: risk for infection of episiotomy related to ineffective perineal hygiene measures.
      Expected outcome: episiotomy will heal without infection.
      Nursing management: see *Prevention of Infection* section and Box 19-1 for full identification of measures to enhance healing and prevent infection.
   b. Nursing diagnosis: constipation related to inactivity and lack of knowledge.
      Expected outcome: woman will have soft formed bowel movement.
      Nursing management: see *Promotion of Bowel Function* section.
   c. Nursing diagnosis: acute pain related to episiotomy and hemorrhoids.
      Expected outcome: woman will experience a reduction in pain following implementation of suggested relief measures.
      Nursing management: see *Promotion of Comfort* section and Box 19-1.
7. See *Prevention of Bladder Distention* section and Nursing Care Plan "Risk for Impaired Urinary Elimination"; most likely basis for finding is bladder distention—discuss implications of bladder distention and measures to facilitate emptying of the bladder.
8. See *Promotion of Ambulation* section including safety alert for content required to answer this question.
9. See *Planning for Discharge, Discharge Teaching,* and *Follow-up after Discharge Services* sections for the content required to answer each part of this question.
10. See *Impact of Cultural Diversity* section and Box 19-3 for the content required to answer each part of this question.

11. See Chapter 18 and Table 19-1 for the content required to answer each part of this question.
    a. Position for fundal palpation: supine, head and shoulder on pillow, arms at sides, knees slightly flexed.
    b. Fundal characteristics to assess: consistency (firm or boggy), height (above, at, below umbilicus), location (midline or deviated to the right or left).
    c. Position for assessment of perineum: lateral or modified Sims position with upper leg flexed on hip.
    d. Episiotomy characteristics to assess: REEDA (redness, edema, ecchymosis, drainage, approximation); presence of hematoma; adequacy of hygiene, including cleanliness, presence of odor, method used to cleanse perineum and to apply topical preparations.
    e. Characteristics of lochia to assess: stage, amount, odor, clots.
12. See *Transfer from Recovery Area* section for a discussion of essential information that should be reported regarding the woman, the baby, and the significant events and findings from her prenatal and childbirth periods.
13. See *Prevention of Infection* section and Box 19-1 for content required to answer each part of this question.

CHAPTER 20: TRANSITION TO PARENTHOOD

I. Learning Key Terms
1. Attachment; bonding
2. Acquaintance
3. Mutuality
4. Signaling behaviors
5. Executive behaviors
6. Claiming
7. En face (face to face)
8. Entrainment
9. Biorhythmicity
10. Reciprocity
11. Synchrony
12. Transition to parenthood
13. Dependent (taking-in)
14. Dependent-independent (taking-hold)
15. Interdependent (letting-go)
16. Becoming a mother
17. "Pink" period; "blue" period (postpartum blues; baby blues)
18. Engrossment
19. Responsivity

II. Reviewing Key Concepts
1. See *Parental Attachment, Bonding, and Acquaintance* and *Assessment of Attachment* sections, Tables 20-1, 20-2, and 20-3, and Box 20-1 for content required to answer each part of the question.
2. See *Parental Tasks and Responsibilities* section for content required to answer this question.

3. See *Parent-Infant Contact—Early Contact and Extended Contact* section for the content required to answer each part of this question.
4. See *Touch* section for a description of touch as it progresses from an exploration with fingertips to gentle stroking, patting, and rubbing.
5. Factors influencing parental responses to the birth of their child: see section for each factor in the *Diversity in Transition to Parenthood* and *Parental Sensory Impairment* sections.
6. d; choice a reflects the first phase of identifying likenesses; choice b reflects the second phase of identifying differences; choice c reflects a negative reaction of claiming the infant in terms of pain and discomfort; choice d reflects the third or final stage of identifying uniqueness.
7. b; early close contact is recommended to initiate and enhance the attachment process.
8. a; engrossment refers to a father's absorption, preoccupation, and interest in his infant; b represents the claiming process phase I, identifying likeness; c represents reciprocity; d represents en face or face-to-face position with mutual gazing.
9. b; taking-in is the first 1 to 2 days of recovery following birth; other behaviors exhibited include reliance on others to help her meet needs, being excited, and being talkative.
10. c; approximately 50% to 80% of women experience postpartum blues; new parents should be reassured that their skills as parents develop gradually and they should seek help to develop these skills; postpartum blues that are self-limiting and short lived do not require psychotropic medications; support and care of the postpartum woman and her newborn by her partner and family is the most effective prevention and coping strategy; feelings of fatigue from childbirth and meeting demands of newborn can accentuate feelings of depression.

III. Thinking Critically
1. See *Communication Between Parent and Infant* section and Tables 20-1 and 20-2 for the content required to answer each part of this question.
2. See *Parental Attachment, Bonding, and Acquaintance* and *Parent-Infant Contact* sections for the content to answer this question; be sure to emphasize that the process of attachment is ongoing and the delay in interacting with her newborn will not affect this process.
    • Help her meet her own physical and emotional needs so that she develops readiness to meet her newborn's needs.
    • Help her get to know her baby and interact with and care for him; point out newborn characteristics, including how the baby is responding to her efforts.
    • Show her how to communicate with her newborn and how her newborn communicates with her.
    • Arrange for follow-up after discharge to assess how attachment is progressing.

3. See *Sibling Adaptation* section and Family-Centered Care box, which identifies strategies parents can use to help their other children accept a new baby; caution her that adjustment takes time and is strongly related to the developmental level and experiences of the sibling(s); give mother suggestions regarding what she can do now and what she did previously.

4. See *Parental Attachment, Bonding, and Acquaintance* and *Communication Between Parent and Infant* sections and Tables 20-1, 20-2, and 20-3 for content required to answer each part of this question; Nursing diagnosis: Risk for impaired parent-infant attachment related to lack of knowledge and feeling of incompetence regarding infant care.

5. See *Parental Tasks and Responsibilities* section; foster attachment, acquaintance, and claiming; help parents get acquainted with the infant and to reconcile the real child with the fantasy child; discuss the basis of molding, caput succedaneum, and forceps marks and how they will be resolved; be alert for problems with attachment and care so follow-up can be arranged.

6. See *Grandparent Adaptation* section; observe interaction between grandparents and parents taking note of signs of effective interaction and conflict; involve grandparents in teaching sessions as appropriate for this family; spend time with grandparents to help them be supportive without "taking over" or being critical; help the new parents recognize the unique role grandparents can play as parenting role models, nurturers, and providers of respite care.

7. See *Becoming a Mother* and *Postpartum Blues* sections and Patient Teaching Box—Coping with Postpartum Blues for content required to answer this question; Nursing diagnosis: ineffective maternal coping related to hormonal changes and increased responsibilities following birth; Expected outcome: woman will report feeling more contented with her role as mother following use of recommended coping strategies.

8. See *Becoming a Father* section and Table 20-5 to discuss the transition process to fatherhood and nursing measures that provide the father with support, teaching, demonstrations, and practice and interaction time with the newborn.

CHAPTER 21: POSTPARTUM COMPLICATIONS

I. Learning Key Terms

1. Postpartum hemorrhage (PPH); Early (acute, primary) PPH; Late (secondary) PPH
2. Uterine atony
3. Pelvic hematoma; vulvar hematomas, vaginal hematomas
4. Placental accreta
5. Placenta increta
6. Placenta percreta
7. Inversion

8. Subinvolution
9. Hemorrhagic (hypovolemic) shock
10. Idiopathic thrombocytopenic purpura
11. von Willebrand disease
12. Disseminated intravascular coagulation
13. Thrombosis
14. Thrombophlebitis
15. Superficial venous thrombosis; Deep vein thrombosis (DVT)
16. Pulmonary embolism
17. Postpartum, puerperal infection
18. Endometritis
19. Mastitis
20. Uterine prolapse
21. Cystocele
22. Rectocele
23. Stress incontinence
24. Fistula
25. Vesicovaginal fistula
26. Urethrovaginal fistula
27. Rectovaginal fistula
28. Pessary
29. Anterior colporrhaphy
30. Posterior colporrhaphy
31. Mood disorders
32. Postpartum depression without psychotic features
33. Postpartum psychosis (postpartum depression with psychotic features)
34. Bipolar (manic-depressive) disorder
35. Grief (bereavement)
36. Bittersweet grief

II. Reviewing Key Concepts

1. See *Hemorrhagic (Hypovolemic) Shock—Medical Management* section: restore circulating blood volume to enhance perfusion of vital organs and treat the cause of the hemorrhage.

2. See *Postpartum Hemorrhage—Nursing Interventions* and *Hemorrhagic Shock* sections for content required to answer this question; cite interventions related to improving and monitoring tissue perfusion, treating the cause of the hemorrhage, enhancing healing, supporting the woman and her family, fostering maternal-infant attachment as appropriate, and planning for discharge.

3. See *Legal Tip—Standard of Care for Bleeding Emergencies* for content required to answer this question.

4. See *Nursing Care Management* section of *Postpartum Infections* and Box 21-4 for a list of prevention measures including good prenatal nutrition to control anemia and intrapartal hemorrhage, perineal hygiene, and adherence to aseptic techniques.

5. See *Loss and Grief Responses* section.
   a. Acute distress - denial and disbelief
   b. Intense grief - guilt
   c. Intense grief - disorganization
   d. Reorganization - "why"; searching for meaning
   e. Reorganization - recovery

6. See *Communicating and Caring Techniques* and *Help Mother, Father, and other Family Members*

Actualize the Loss sections including the Nursing Alert for the content required to answer this question.

7. See *Postpartum Psychologic Complications—Nursing Care in the Home and in the Community* and *Providing Safety* sections including the Nursing Alert for the content required to answer each part of this question; identify possibility of woman harming herself, her baby, or both of them.

8. b; although a, c, and d are correct actions, the woman's hypertensive status would be a contraindicating factor for its use; therefore, the order should be questioned as the nurse's first action.

9. d; Hemabate is a powerful prostaglandin that is the third-line medication given to treat excessive uterine blood loss or hemorrhage related to uterine atony; it has no action related to pain, infection, or clotting.

10. a; puerperal infections are infections of the genital tract after birth; pulse will increase, not decrease, in response to fever; lochia characteristics will change, but this will not be the first sign exhibited; WBC count would already be elevated related to pregnancy and birth.

11. b, c, d, and f; heparin and warfarin (Coumadin) are safe for use by breastfeeding women; heparin, which is administered intravenously or subcutaneously, is the anticoagulant of choice during the acute stage of DVT; warfarin is administered orally, not parenterally.

12. a; although the other questions are appropriate, the potential for harming herself or her baby is the most serious and very real concern.

13. a; telling her to be happy that one twin survived may be interpreted that she should not grieve the loss of the daughter who died—the loss must be acknowledged and the tasks for mourners accomplished; b, c, and d are all appropriate responses by the nurse, with choices b and c helpful in actualizing the loss.

14. b, d and e; f represent the intense grief phase, and a and c represent the reorganization phase.

15. b; see Box 21-6; note that a, c, and d are in the category of what not to say, whereas b represents a response that acknowledges the difficulty of the loss and offers an opportunity for expression of feelings.

16. a, b, e, and f; c and d are helpful for postpartum depression.

17. d; doxepin should not be administered to women who are breastfeeding; a, b, and c are safe; see Table 21-1.

III. Thinking Critically

1. See *Postpartum Hemorrhage* section, Nursing Care Plan—Postpartum Hemorrhage, Medication Guide for Drugs Used to Manage Postpartum Hemorrhage, Box 21-1, and Emergency Box—Hemorrhagic Shock for the content required to answer each part of this question.
   a. Risk factors for early postpartum hemorrhage: parity (5-1-0-7), vaginal full-term twin birth 1 hour ago; hypotonic uterine dysfunction treated with oxytocin (Pitocin); use of forceps for birth; increased manipulation with birth of twins.

   b. Nurse's response to excessive blood loss: most common cause of the excessive blood loss 1 hour after birth would be uterine atony, especially because woman exhibits several risk factors.
   - Assess fundus for consistency, height, and location; massage if boggy.
   - Express clots, if present, once uterus is firm.
   - Check bladder for distention (distended bladder will reduce uterine contraction); check perineum for swelling and ask woman about experiencing perineal pressure (hematoma formation is possible related to use of forceps for birth).

   c. Guidelines for administering Pitocin IV: use Medication Guide.

   d. Signs of developing hemorrhagic shock: see Emergency box.

   e. Nursing measures to support the woman and family:
   - Explain progress, including meaning of findings and need for treatment measures being used, including their purpose and effectiveness.
   - Use a calm, professional, organized approach that incorporates periods of uninterrupted rest.
   - Initiate comfort measures.
   - Provide opportunities for interaction with newborn and updates on newborn's status.

2. See *Postpartum Infections* section and Box 21-4 for the content required to answer each part of this question.

3. See *Mastitis* section and Fig. 21-3 for the content required to answer each part of this question; Nursing diagnoses: acute pain related to inflammation of right breast; ineffective breastfeeding OR anxiety related to interruption of breastfeeding while taking antibiotics or related to concerns regarding transmission of infection to newborn; emphasize correction of breastfeeding techniques and breast care measures to prevent recurrence.

4. See *Thromboembolic Disease* section and Medication Guide for warfarin sodium (Coumadin) for content required to answer each part of this question.
   a. Risk factors: in addition to hypercoagulability of pregnancy continuing into the postpartum period, other risk factors for this woman would be cesarean birth, obesity, age over 35 years, multiparity, smoking habit, and varicosities in both legs.
   b. Signs and symptoms indicative of DVT: see *Clinical Manifestations* section.
   c. Nursing diagnosis: anxiety related to unexpected development of a postpartum complication.
   d. Expected care management: see *Medical Management and Nursing Interventions* sections including Nursing Alert.
   e. Discharge instructions:
   - How to assess leg and to assess for signs of unusual bleeding
   - Proper use of elastic/support stockings
   - How to take anticoagulant safely and importance of follow-up to assess progress
   - Practices to prevent bleeding while taking an anticoagulant and importance of avoiding pregnancy because warfarin is teratogenic

- Importance of avoiding aspirin and NSAIDs for pain and food/vitamin supplements that are sources of vitamin K because they can interact with warfarin (Coumadin)

5. See *Sequelae of Childbirth Trauma—Cystocele and Rectocele and Care Management* sections for content required to answer each part of this question.
   a. Signs and symptoms most likely exhibited: see *Clinical Manifestations* section.
   b. Two priority nursing diagnoses with expected outcomes:
      - Constipation or diarrhea related to displacement of rectum into posterior rectal wall; woman will experience regular, soft, formed bowel elimination.
      - Impaired urinary elimination related to displacement of bladder into anterior vaginal wall; woman will fully empty bladder every 2 to 3 hours.
      - Ineffective sexuality patterns related to vaginal changes associated with cystocele and rectocele; woman will openly discuss measures to enhance sexual function.
   c. Management of cystocele and rectocele: see *Care Management* section; answer should include Kegel exercises, diet (fiber and fluids), stool softener, mild laxative, genital hygiene measures, emotional support.
   d. Using a pessary (see Fig. 21-9); Nursing diagnosis: risk for infection related to insertion of foreign object into vagina.

6. See *Postpartum Psychological Complications—Mood Disorders* section, Patient Teaching Boxes—Signs of Postpartum Blues, Depression, and Psychosis and Preventing Postpartum Depression, and Box 21-5 for content required to answer each part of this question.

7. See *Loss and Grief* section and Box 21-6 for content required to answer each part of this section.
   a. Approach to individualize support measures: see *Assessment* section.
      - Begin with assessment to determine best approach to take for this couple.
      - Determine nature of the parental attachment with the pregnancy and the meaning of the pregnancy and birth to the parents—their perception of the loss—recognizing that responses of father and mother may differ.
      - Understand circumstances surrounding the loss—listen to their story.
      - Observe the immediate response of each parent to the loss—do they match?
      - Identify persons comprising their social network and how can they support them; do the parents want their support?
   b. Cite questions and observations to gather information required to create an individualized plan of care: use each of the areas identified in section "a" of this critical thinking situation to formulate questions and organize observations.

   c. See *Communicating and Caring Techniques* section and Box 21-6 for examples of therapeutic communication techniques that include encourage expression of feelings by leaning forward, nodding, reflection, saying "tell me more"; observe nonverbal cues; use touch as appropriate; listen patiently and use silence while couple tell their story.
   d. See Box 21-6; 1 – N, 2 – T, 3 – N, 4 – N, 5 – T, 6 – T, 7 – N, 8 – N, 9 – T, 10 – T

8. See *Meet the Physical Needs of the Postpartum Bereaved Mother* section for the content required to answer this question.

9. See *Help Parents with Decision Making and Help Mother, Father, and Other Family Members Actualize the Loss* and *Create Memories for the Parents to Take Home* sections for content required to answer each part of this question.

CHAPTER 22: PHYSIOLOGIC AND BEHAVIORAL ADAPTATIONS OF THE NEWBORN

I. Learning Key Terms

1. Neutral thermal environment
2. Thermogenesis
3. Nonshivering thermogenesis
4. Convection
5. Radiation
6. Evaporation
7. Conduction
8. Hyperthermia
9. Nevus simplex (telangiectatic nevi)
10. Molding
11. Caput succedaneum
12. Cephalhematoma
13. Mongolian spots
14. Acrocyanosis
15. Vernix caseosa
16. Milia
17. Jaundice
18. Meconium
19. Erythema toxicum (neonatorum)
20. Uric acid crystals (brick dust)
21. Wink reflex
22. Hydrocele
23. Ecchymosis
24. Murmur
25. Lanugo
26. Subgaleal hemorrhage
27. Desquamation
28. Nevus flammeus (port wine stain)
29. Nevus vascularis (strawberry hemangioma)
30. Pseudomenstruation
31. Prepuce
32. Surfactant
33. Epstein (epithelial) pearls
34. Polydactyly; oligodactyly
35. Syndactyly
36. Sleep-wake states

37. Deep; light; increasing
38. Drowsy, quiet alert, active alert, crying
39. Quiet alert
40. State regulation
41. Habituation
42. Orientation
43. Consolability
44. Temperament
45. Easy child
46. Slow to warm up child
47. Difficult child

II. Reviewing Key Concepts

1. See *Respiratory System* section for a description of how a newborn begins to breathe; include chemical, mechanical, thermal, and sensory factors in your answer.
2. j   3. f   4. b   5. i   6. d   7. h
8. a   9. e   10. g   11. c   12. k
13. See *Transition to Extrauterine Life* section at beginning of chapter for identification of each phase and description of timing/duration and typical newborn behaviors for each phase.
14. a, b, and c; the newborn at 5 hours old is in the second period of reactivity, during which tachycardia, tachypnea, increased muscle tone, skin color changes, increased mucus production, and passage of meconium are normal findings; temperature should range between 36.5° and 37.2° C, and respiratory rate should range between 30 and 60 BPM; expiratory grunting and nasal flaring and retractions of the sternum are signs of respiratory distress.
15. a; the rash described is erythema toxicum; it is an inflammatory response that has no clinical significance and requires no treatment because it will disappear spontaneously.
16. b; physiologic jaundice does not appear until 24 hours after birth; further investigation would be needed if it appears during the first 24 hours, because that would be consistent with pathologic jaundice; a, c, and d are all expected findings.
17. d; b and c are common newborn reflexes used to assess integrity of neuromuscular system; syndactyly refers to webbing of the fingers.
18. c; telangiectatic nevi (nevus simplex) are also known as stork bite marks and can also appear on the eyelids; milia are plugged sebaceous glands and appear like white pimples; nevus vasculosus or a strawberry mark is a raised, sharply demarcated, bright or dark red swelling; nevus flammeus is a port-wine, flat red to purple lesion that does not blanch with pressure.

III. Thinking Critically

1. See *Thermogenesis—Cold Stress and Heat Loss* section and Fig. 22-2 for the content required to answer each part of this question. Nursing Diagnosis: Risk for imbalanced body temperature—hypothermia related to immature thermoregulation associated with newborn status; Expected outcome: newborn's temperature will stabilize between 36.5° and 37.2° C within 8 to 10 hours of birth.
2. See *Integumentary System* and *Skeletal System* sections; discuss each finding in terms of cause, significance for the newborn's health status and adjustment, and how/when it will be resolved; refer to Fig. 22-10 to facilitate parental understanding.
3. See *Respiratory System* section for the content required to answer this question; you should also consult Table 23-3 for further information to answer this question.
4. See *Sensory Behaviors* section including vision, hearing, smell, taste, and touch:
   a. Discuss and demonstrate newborn's capability regarding vision, hearing, touch, taste, and smell.
   b. Face-to-face/eye-to-eye contact, objects (bright or black-and-white changing, complex patterns), sound (talking to infant, music, heartbeat simulator), touch (infant massage, cuddling).
5. Discuss the characteristics and cause of Mongolian spots (see *Mongolian Spots* section and Fig. 22-5).
6. See *Conjugation of Bilirubin and Newborn Jaundice* sections for the content to compare and contrast each type of jaundice listed.

CHAPTER 23: NURSING CARE OF THE NEWBORN AND FAMILY

I. Learning Key Terms

1. Apgar score; heart rate, respiratory effort, muscle tone, reflex irritability, color
2. Bulb syringe
3. Thermistor probe
4. Ophthalmia neonatorum; Erythromycin, tetracycline
5. Vitamin K
6. New Ballard score
7. Appropriate for gestational age (AGA)
8. Large for gestational age (LGA)
9. Small for gestational age (SGA)
10. Late preterm
11. Preterm
12. Term
13. Postterm
14. Post mature
15. Early term
16. Petechiae
17. Bilirubin
18. Physiologic jaundice
19. Blanch test
20. Pathologic hyperbilirubinemia
21. Kernicterus
22. Transcutaneous bilirubinometer (TcB)
23. Phototherapy
24. Hypoglycemia
25. Hypocalcemia
26. Bradypnea
27. Tachypnea
28. Handwashing (hand hygiene)

29. Bilirubin (fiberoptic) blanket
30. Circumcision

II. Reviewing Key Concepts

1. See *Protective Environment* section; discuss each of the following in your answer:
   a. Environmental modifications
   b. Infection control measures
   c. Safety in terms of security precautions and identification measures
2. See *Baseline Measurement of Physical Growth* section, Table 23-3 Measurements section, and Figs. 23-1, 23-2, 23-3, and 23-4 for content required to answer this question.
3. See *Discharge Planning* and *Discharge Teaching* sections and Home Care boxes—Safety and Bathing, Cord Care, Skin Care, and Nail Care for content required to answer each part of this question.
4. See *Collection of Specimens* section and Figs. 23-12 and 23-13 for content required to answer this question.
5. See *Intervention—Airway Maintenance* and *Maintaining an Adequate Oxygen Supply* sections and Box 23-4 for the content required to answer each part of this question.
6. d, e, and f; thinning of lanugo with bald spots, descent of testes, and absence of scarf sign are consistent with full-term status; pulse and weight are not part of the Ballard scale; the popliteal angle for a full-term newborn would be 90 degrees or less.
7. c and f; glucose should be 40 to 60 mg/dL and calcium should be at least 7.8 mg/c; a, b, d, and e all fall within the expected range (see Table 23-4).
8. b; signs of hypoglycemia include cyanosis along with apnea, hypothermia, jitteriness/twitching, irregular respirations, high-pitched cry, difficulty feeding, hunger, lethargy, eye rolling, and seizures.
9. a; the control panel should be set between 36° to 37° C; the probe should be placed in one of the upper quadrants of the abdomen below the intercostal margin, never over a rib; axillary, not rectal, temperatures should be taken.
10. b; acetaminophen should be given every 4 hours for a maximum of 5 doses in 24 hours; the site should be checked every 15 to 30 minutes for the first hour and then every hour for the next 4 to 6 hours; diaper wipes should not be used on the site because they contain alcohol, which would delay healing and cause discomfort; the yellow exudate is a protective film that forms in 24 hours, and it should not be removed.
11. b, c, and d; mother does not have to be hepatitis B positive for the vaccine to be given to her newborn; use a 5/8-inch 25-gauge needle and insert it at a 90-degree angle.
12. b, c, e, and f; administer within 1 to 2 hours and squeeze a 1- to 2-cm ribbon of ointment into the lower conjunctival sac.

III. Thinking Critically

1. See Table 23-1 and *Apgar Scoring* section for the content to answer this question.
   a. Baby boy Smith: heart rate: 160 (2); respiratory effort: good, crying (2); muscle tone: flexion, active movement (2); reflex irritability: cry with stimulus (2); color: acrocyanosis (1); score is 9 and is within normal limits; interpretation: score of 7 to 10 indicates that the infant is not having difficulty adjusting to extrauterine life.
   b. Baby girl Doe: heart rate: 102 (2); respiratory effort: slow, irregular, weak cry (1); muscle tone: some flexion (1); reflex irritability: grimace with stimulus (1); color: pale (0); score is 5; interpretation: score of 4 to 6 indicates moderate difficulty adjusting to extrauterine life.
2. See Tables 23-1 and 23-2 and *Initial Physical Assessment, Apgar Scoring, Immediate Care after Birth, Protective Environment,* and *Promoting Parent-Infant Intervention* sections for the content to answer each part of this question; be sure to include the following in your answer:
   • Assessment of physical status and stabilization of respiration and airway patency
   • Maintenance of body temperature
   • Immediate interventions in terms of identification, prophylactic medications, infection control measures, security, promotion of bonding/attachment
3. See *Discharge Planning, Discharge Teaching, Protective Environment,* and *Promoting Parent-Infant Interactions* sections, Table 23-3, and Patient Teaching Box—Signs of Illness for the content required to answer each part of this question; by including the parents you have a chance to observe parent-infant interactions and to identify and meet learning needs; foster active involvement in assessment and care of their newborn; encourage discussion of concerns and asking of questions; chance to explain and demonstrate newborn characteristics and capabilities.
4. See *Airway Maintenance* and *Maintaining an Adequate Oxygen Supply* sections and Guidelines Box—Suctioning with a Bulb Syringe for the content required to answer each part of this question; Nursing Diagnosis: Impaired gas exchange related to upper airway obstruction with mucus.
5. See *Discharge Planning* and *Discharge Teaching* sections, Patient Teaching Box—Care for the Circumcised Newborn at Home, and Home Care Box—Bathing, Cord Care, Skin Care, and Nail Care for the content required to answer each part of this question; Nursing Diagnosis: Risk for infection related to removal of foreskin and healing umbilical cord site; Expected Outcome: Cord and circumcision site will heal without infection.
6. See *Phototherapy* and *Physiologic Problems—Jaundice* and *Parent-Infant Interaction* sections and Chapter 22 for a full discussion of the basis for physiologic (nonpathologic) jaundice for the content required to answer each part of this question. Be sure that your answer includes the importance of telling parents in simple terms that their newborn is exhibiting physiologic jaundice, explaining

why it occurs, what impact it will have on their newborn's health, and how it will be resolved; in addition ensure that they are given time to interact with their newborn during feeding times when the infant is out of the lights and even when under the lights.

7. See *Circumcision and Neonatal Responses to Pain* sections, Box 23-5, and Table 23-6 for the content required to answer this question.

CHAPTER 24: NEWBORN NUTRITION AND FEEDING

I. Learning Key Terms

1. Lobes
2. Alveoli
3. Milk ducts
4. Montgomery glands
5. Nipple erection reflex
6. Myoepithelial cells
7. Areola
8. Lactation (lactogenesis)
9. Prolactin
10. Oxytocin
11. Everted; inverted (flat)
12. Breast (nipple) shell
13. Galactogogue
14. Colostrum
15. Nipple confusion
16. Feeding readiness cues
17. Let down; milk ejection
18. Rooting reflex
19. Latch (latch-on)
20. Engorgement
21. Football hold
22. Cradle (traditional) hold
23. Lactation consultant
24. Mastitis
25. Thrush
26. Tongue-tie
27. Weaning
28. Foremilk
29. Hindmilk
30. Early onset jaundice (breastfeeding-associated jaundice)
31. Late onset jaundice (breast milk jaundice)

II. Reviewing Key Concepts

1. See *Benefits of Breastfeeding* section and Table 24-1; emphasize the importance and benefits of breastfeeding for infants, mothers, and family/society.
2. See *Positioning* section and Fig. 24-5; describe the positions of football hold, cradle (traditional), modified cradle (across the lap), and side-lying.
3. See *Supporting Breastfeeding Mothers* section for the content required to answer each part of this question.
4. See *Latch* section and Figs. 24-6 and 24-7 for the content required to answer each part of this question.
5. b; birth weight is regained in 10 to 14 days; 6 to 8 wet diapers are expected at this time; should be fed every 2 to 3 hours for a total of 8 to 10 times per day.

6. d; mother should be encouraged to let her newborn begin to suck on her clean finger until the baby begins to calm down then switch to the breast; a, b, and c are all appropriate actions to calm a fussy baby.
7. d; no soap should be used because it could dry the areola and increase the risk for irritation; vitamin E should not be used because it is a fat-soluble vitamin that the infant could ingest when breastfeeding; lanolin or colostrum/milk are the preferred substances to be applied to the area; plastic liners can trap moisture and lead to sore nipples.
8. b; a combination hormonal contraceptive could decrease the milk supply if given before lactation is well established during the first 6 weeks after birth; after 6 weeks, a progestin-only contraceptive could be used because it is the least likely hormonal contraceptive to affect lactation; even complete breastfeeding is not considered to be a reliable method because ovulation can occur unexpectedly even before the first menstrual period; diaphragm used before pregnancy would have to be checked to see whether it fits properly before the woman uses it again.
9. b; supplements are not required when using prepared formulas; a 2-week-old infant should consume approximately 90 to 150 mL of formula at each feeding; formula should never be heated in the microwave because it could be overheated or unevenly heated.
10. a, c, and d; nipples should not be washed using soap; plastic liners can keep nipples and areola moist and increase the risk for tissue breakdown; bring baby to breast, not breast to baby.
11. c; limiting length of feeding does not protect the nipples and areola; b and d are correct actions but not the most important.

III. Thinking Critically

1. See *Choosing an Infant Feeding Method* section.
   a. Decisional conflict regarding feeding method for their newborn related to lack of knowledge and experience with newborn feeding methods.
      Couple will choose the feeding method for their newborn that is most comfortable for them.
   b. Both should learn about the pros and cons of feeding methods with an emphasis on the benefits of breastfeeding and how the partner can help with the method.
   c. The prenatal period is a less stressful time, allowing for full consideration of options, how feeding methods would be incorporated into life activities (such as work outside the home), and learning about breastfeeding by attending a prenatal breastfeeding class and reading.
   d. Provide information about feeding methods in a nonjudgmental manner while still emphasizing the importance of breastfeeding as the preferred method, dispel myths, address personal concerns of the couple, and make needed referrals to WIC, lactation consultant, breastfeeding classes, and the La Leche League.

2. See *Anatomy of the Lactating Breast, Uniqueness of Human Milk,* and *Insufficient Milk Supply sections* for the content to answer parts a and b.
   a. Breast size: discuss development of lactation structures during pregnancy; emphasize the importance of this development and not the breast size for successful lactation.
   b. Let-down reflex: explain what it is and why it happens (including physical and emotional triggers); emphasize its importance in providing the infant with hindmilk.
   c. See *Indicators of Effective Breastfeeding* section and Box 24-2, which identify maternal and newborn indicators of effective breastfeeding; put the indicators in writing and go over each one; provide contact person if mother is concerned.
   d. See *Sore Nipples* section and Fig. 24-15; discuss and demonstrate measures to prevent and treat sore nipples, including, most importantly, good breastfeeding techniques such as latch-on, removal, and alternating starting breast and positions; discuss effective and recommended breast care measures.
   e. See *Engorgement* section; begin by describing engorgement, what it is, why it occurs, and when, and then discuss prevention and relief measures.
   f. See *Lactogenesis* section for the content required to answer this question—focus on the impact of oxytocin secretion.
   g. See *Breastfeeding and Contraception* section; emphasize that breastfeeding is not an effective contraceptive method; although ovulation may be delayed, its return cannot be predicted with accuracy and may occur before the first menstrual period; discuss contraceptive methods that are safe to use with breastfeeding and resuming sexual intercourse during the postpartum period.
   h. See *Expressing and Storing Breast Milk, Working and Breastfeeding,* and *Weaning* sections; discuss how she can continue breastfeeding if she wishes to do so and how to wean when she is ready emphasizing that weaning needs to be a gradual process.
3. See *Frequency and Duration of Feeding* and *Sleepy Baby* sections for the content required to answer each part of this question.
   a. Nursing diagnosis: imbalanced nutrition less than body requirements related to infrequent feeding of newborn.
      Expected outcome: mother will awaken infant every 2 to 3 hours during the day and every 4 hours at night to feed the infant, achieving at least 8 feedings per day.
   b. Nursing approach: discuss feeding readiness cues to facilitate proper timing of feedings; discuss techniques to wake sleeping baby and signs indicating adequate intake.
4. See *Formula Feeding* section and Home Care box *Formula Preparation and Feeding* for the content required to answer each part of this question.

   a. Discuss how the mother can facilitate close contact and socialization with the infant during feeding; reassure that properly prepared formulas will fully meet her newborn's need for nutrients and fluid.
   b. Discuss how to choose a formula type; amount and frequency of feedings; how to prepare formula, safety measures, cues of feeding readiness and satiety, and burping.
5. See *Nursing Care Management—Assessment* section and Box 24-2 to determine what to assess; formulate questions that address the assessment factors; in addition ask questions about such areas as frequency and duration of feedings, breastfeeding techniques used, how she feels about breastfeeding and how well she feels she is doing, family support for breastfeeding; her ability to rest; and nutrient and fluid intake.

CHAPTER 25: THE HIGH RISK NEWBORN

I. Learning Key Terms

1. m 2. n 3. o 4. p 5. q 6. i
7. a 8. l 9. r 10. j 11. k 12. h
13. g 14. c 15. e 16. f 17. b 18. s
19. d 20. t 21. u 22. v
23. TORCH
24. Herpes simplex virus
25. Cytomegalovirus
26. Hand washing
27. Fetal alcohol spectrum disorder (FASD)
28. Hemolytic disease of the newborn
29. Erythroblastosis fetalis; hydrops fetalis
30. Indirect Coombs'
31. Direct Coombs'
32. Neonatal Abstinence Syndrome
33. Meconium
34. Toxoplasmosis
35. Inborn errors of metabolism
36. Phenylketonuria (PKU)
37. Galactosemia
38. Congenital hypothyroidism
39. Clavicle
40. Phrenic nerve paralysis
41. Therapeutic hypothermia
42. Retinopathy of Prematurity
43. Necrotizing enterocolitis
44. Patent ductus arteriosus
45. Bronchopulmonary dysplasia
46. Respiratory distress syndrome
47. Persistent Pulmonary Hypertension of the Newborn

II. Reviewing Key Concepts

1. See also Box 25-2
   CNS—irritability, hyperactivity, tremors, high-pitched cry, seizures, exaggerated Moro reflex
   Gastrointestinal—poor feeding, diarrhea, vomiting
   Respiratory—tachypnea, nasal congestion
   Autonomic—diaphoresis, disrupted sleep patterns, temperature instability

2. With maternal diabetes there is an increase in maternal insulin production as a result of hyperglycemia; insulin does not cross the placental circulation to the fetus, thus the fetus increases insulin production to manage the added glucose which easily passes from the maternal circulation to the fetus. At birth the newborn pancreas continues to produce large amounts of insulin and glucose stores are rapidly depleted thus resulting in hypoglycemia.

3. Metabolic—hypoglycemia, hypocalcemia

   Cardiac—ventriculoseptal defect, cardiomyopathy,

   Central Nervous system—anencephaly, spina bifida, holoprosencephaly, sacral agenesis and caudal regression

   Hematologic—polycythemia, hyperbilirubinemia

4. Encourage woman to seek pregestational care because euglycemia before and during pregnancy is a major factor in preventing complications including congenital anomalies associated with diabetes during pregnancy.

5. See also section on Rh incompatibility and ABO incompatibility. Basically human blood cells contain a variety of antigens, also known as agglutinogens, substances capable of producing an immune response if recognized by the body as foreign. The reciprocal relationship between antigens on RBCs and antibodies in the plasma causes agglutination (clumping). In other words, antibodies in the plasma of one blood group (except the AB group, which contains no antibodies) produce agglutination when mixed with antigens of a different blood group. In the ABO blood group system, the antibodies occur naturally. In the Rh system, the person must be exposed to the Rh antigen before significant antibody formation takes place and causes a sensitivity response known as isoimmunization. If the Rh (D)-negative mother conceives an Rh (D)-positive fetus and the fetus' blood cells enter into the maternal circulation, the antibody formation sequence (anti-Rh) is initiated. Fetal blood cells are destroyed by the maternal antibodies if maternal cells (anti-Rh) come in contact with the fetal circulation thus causing fetal anemia and an increased production of fetal erythrocytes, which are immature red cells. See the discussion on isoimmunization for further discussion of erythroblastosis fetalis. The placenta processes the bilirubin produced by destroyed fetal red cells, but at birth the newborn liver is immature and cannot handle the circulating volume of bilirubin, thus jaundice ensues. In ABO incompatibility the immune response and production of antibodies to fetal cells is less dramatic than the Rh response, thus the fetal red cell destruction is less severe in the majority of cases. See Table 25-6 for ABO group incompatibilities.

6. d; RhoGAM should be administered to the mother within 72 hours of birth; pathologic jaundice is unlikely because Coombs' test results indicate that antibodies have not been formed to destroy the newborn's RBCs; RhoGAM is given to prevent formation of antibodies; it would not be given if antibodies have already been formed, as indicated by positive Coombs' test results.

7. b and c; risk of transmission of HIV is greater than the benefits of breastfeeding; isolation is not required, nor are gloves, for routine care measures; the nurse should be using standard precautions as would be used with all patients; antiviral treatment begins after birth before HIV status is known; opportunistic pulmonary infections are a concern when the infant is diagnosed with HIV infection.

8. Physiologic functions and potential problems are discussed in specific sections of *Preterm Infant* and *Late Preterm Infant—Nursing Care Management* sections.

   Respiratory function—immature alveolar development and function leading to respiratory distress; decreased chest wall musculature; decreased diaphragmatic excursion.

   Cardiovascular function—delayed closure of functional fetal shunts such as the ductus arteriosus which increases blood flow to the lungs by mixed oxygenated and deoxygenated blood, thus placing an increased workload on the heart and lungs; hypoxemia and high circulating levels of prostaglandins keep the ductus arteriosus from closing in neonatal period.

   Thermoregulation—decreased subcutaneous fat tissue and immature CNS thermoregulatory function contribute to poor thermoregulation with ensuing increased glucose metabolism and often poor glucose stores; nonshivering thermogenesis increases glucose metabolism and oxygen consumption; eventual outcome in a cold preterm infant is a metabolic acidosis, respiratory compromise, and possibly death if no interventions occur.

   CNS function—immature CNS regulation; stimulation capable of taxing neonate and causing stress as neonate is unable to self-regulate and respond to environmental stimuli; pain sensation is enhanced.

   Nutritional status—functional immaturity of GI system in relation to ability to physically consume the amount of caloric intake required to maintain positive nitrogen balance and promote growth; increased susceptibility to feeding intolerance due to poor absorption of formula or breast milk; low stomach capacity; increased transit time through GI system and decreased absorption and metabolism of milk.

   Renal status—delayed glomerular filtration with inability to concentrate urine in first month of life; unable to compensate for increased water losses through the immature skin; immature renal function further compromises electrolyte balance since this is primarily determined by circulating fluid volume.

   Hematologic status—increased turnover of red blood cells, in comparison to adult or older child, and decreased oxygen carrying capacity in hemoglobin place infant at risk for hyperbilirubinemia, anemia, and hypoxemia; decreased rate of erythropoiesis further compromises infant red cell volume.

   Immune status and infection prevention—immaturity of cellular and humoral immune system prevents rapid recognition of foreign virus and bacteria and localization and phagocytosis of same; thus immature infants are susceptible to common pathogens; decreased skin maturity also contributes to infection susceptibility as does the immature gut mucosal barrier, making the neonate more susceptible to certain viruses and bacteria that enter the GI system; increased invasive procedures place the infant at higher risk for infection.

9. b, d, and e; retractions, nasal flaring reflect increased effort and work to breathe; a, c, and f are all expected findings consistent with efficient respiratory effort in the preterm newborn.

10. b; although a, c, and d are appropriate and important, respiration with adequate gas exchange takes precedence, especially because adequate surfactant is not produced before 32 weeks of gestation.

11. c; fracture from trauma is more common in the upper body (e.g., humerus, clavicle); hypocalcemia is common; the newborn of a gestational diabetic mother is more likely to experience congenital anomalies such as heart defects.

III. Thinking Critically

1. See *Nutrition* and *Gavage Feeding* sections.
   a. Observe for ability to suck and swallow and the coordination of each; signs of respiratory distress during the feeding; length of time for the feeding and the amount ingested; presence of regurgitation, vomiting, or abdominal distention after feeding; daily weight gains and losses and elimination patterns.
   b. Emphasize tubing choice and measurement of tubing length, insertion without trauma and securing to maintain placement, checking placement.
   c. Imbalanced nutrition: less than body requirements related to weak suck associated with premature status.
   d. Initiate measures to prevent aspiration with proper tube insertion, removal, and position check techniques.
      • Instill breast milk or formula by gravity rather than pushing syringe barrel to expedite feeding.
      • Cuddle, swaddle infant during feedings; involve parents; use nonnutritive sucking.
      • Document assessment findings and specifics of the procedure.
   e. Proceed cautiously, checking for gastrointestinal, respiratory (signs of distress, decreased pulse oximetry), nutritional, and signs of tolerance or intolerance for advancement; decrease gavage feedings as ability to suck improves; alternate oral feedings and gavage feedings according to infant tolerance.

2. Current practice dictates a radiograph as the only certain way to determine nasogastric (NG) tube placement in the stomach. Methods such as auscultation of an air bubble, neck-ear-xiphoid (NEX) measurements for insertion depth, and pH measurements are considered imprecise when used as the *only* method for determination of placement. See also section on Gavage Feeding.

3. See *Developmental Outcome* section and Nursing Care Plan *High Risk Infant*.
   a. • Infant stressors: continuous exposure to light and noise; administration of sedatives and pain medications; invasive procedures and medications required for treatment
      • Family stressors: infant size and compromised and often fluctuating health status of their newborn; difficulty interacting with newborn and making eye contact; increased learning needs regarding status of newborn and care needs; concern regarding potential disabilities
   b. See *Developmental Outcome* section for a description of these behaviors.
   c. See *Developmental Outcome* section for many ideas, including waterbeds, kangaroo care, swaddling, coordinated plan of care to provide for period of interrupted rest and sleep, use pain medications and sedatives as needed, provide diurnal light patterns, decrease noise level, and use stroking, talking, mobiles, decals, music, and windup toys for stimulation.
   d. Change position frequently, observing effect of position change on breathing and oxygenation and preventing aspiration; consider boundaries, body alignment, sense of security and comfort when positioning; teach parents; use facilitated tucking and blanket swaddling.

4. See *Postterm Infant* section.
   a. Rationale for increased mortality: increased oxygen demands are not met and likelihood for impaired gas exchange occurs, leading to hypoxia and passage of meconium into amniotic fluid; risk for aspiration of meconium into lungs.
   b. Typical assessment findings: thin, emaciated appearance (dysmature) caused by loss of subcutaneous fat and muscle mass; peeling of skin; meconium staining on fingernails; long hair and nails; absence of vernix.
   c. Two major complications: meconium aspiration syndrome and persistent pulmonary hypertension of the newborn (PPHN); see separate section that describes each complication.

5. Minimal enteral (trophic gastrointestinal priming) feedings have been shown to stimulate the infant's gastrointestinal tract, preventing mucosal atrophy and subsequent enteral feeding difficulties. Enteral feedings with as little as 0.1 to 4 mL/kg of breast milk or preterm formula may be given by gavage as soon as the infant is medically stable. These enteral feedings have been shown to simulate the infant's gastrointestinal tract, preventing mucosal atrophy and subsequent enteral feeding difficulties.

6. See *Facilitating Parent-Infant Relationships*.
   a. Measures should include ideas regarding helping parents get to know their newborn, informing of status, educating regarding care needs, providing emotional support and help with the grieving process, making referrals to parents groups and

home care agencies, mobilizing family support system.

b. See *Parental Responses* and *Parental Maladaptation* sections and attachment content in Chapter 20 to formulate your answer; include progress of touch, eagerness to help with care, asking questions and demonstrating interest in status, visiting practices, and bringing items from home to identify the newborn as their own and part of a family.

CHAPTER 26: 21st CENTURY PEDIATRIC NURSING

I. Learning Key Terms

1. c	2. f	3. k	4. a	5. u	6. b
7. h	8. d	9. j	10. t	11. g	12. m
13. i	14. e	15. l	16. o	17. p	18. n
19. q	20. s	21. r			

II. Reviewing Key Concepts

1. b   2. d   3. d   4. d

5. Possible answers: homelessness; poverty; low birth weight; chronic illnesses; foreign-born adopted; day care centers.

6. a   7. a

8. e	9. a	10. b	11. g	12. f
13. d	14. c	15. h	16. j	17. k	18. i

19. Quality of care refers to the degree to which health services for individuals and populations increase the likelihood of desired health outcomes and are consistent with current professional knowledge (Institute of Medicine, 2000).

20. Examples given by the National Quality Forum are:
   1. Death among surgical inpatients with treatable serious complications (failure to rescue)—The percentage of major surgical inpatients who experience a hospital-acquired complication and die
   2. Pressure ulcer prevalence—Percentage of inpatients who have a hospital-acquired pressure ulcer
   3. Falls prevalence—Number of inpatient falls per inpatient days
   4. Falls with injury—Number of inpatient falls with injuries per inpatient days
   5. Restraint prevalence—Percentage of inpatients who have a vest or limb restraint
   6. Urinary catheter–associated urinary tract infection for intensive care unit (ICU) patients—Rate of urinary tract infections associated with use of urinary catheters for ICU patients
   7. Central line catheter–associated bloodstream infection rate for ICU and high risk nursery patients—Rate of bloodstream infections associated with use of central line catheters for ICU and high risk nursery patients
   8. Ventilator-associated pneumonia for ICU and high risk nursery patients—Rate of pneumonia associated with use of ventilators for ICU and high risk nursery patients

III. Thinking Critically

1. Responses could include ideas such as the following:
   - Education about prevention of heart disease, cancer, or obesity related to nutrition in order to educate the public about foods offered in public schools
   - Dental health care clinics in the public school system
   - Program to immunize children at the time of admission to the public schools, rather than just requiring proof of immunization
2. Responses could include ideas such as the following:
   a. Family advocacy/caring: In home health, a nurse helps the family of a child recently diagnosed with type 1 diabetes prepare for the long-term care of their child with insulin by identifying community resources, teaching the technical skills that will be needed for the care, and expressing compassion for the family.
   b. Disease prevention/health promotion: During a clinic visit, the nurse takes time to teach a young mother about early childhood caries for her expected child when discussing methods of infant feeding.
   c. Health teaching: A school nurse discusses hypoglycemia—its symptoms, causes, and treatment—of a child with type 1 diabetes mellitus who is beginning to make independent decisions about his or her disease and who has just experienced a hypoglycemic episode.
   d. Support/counseling: A pediatric nurse practitioner meets with children and their parents to help foster expression of feelings and thoughts after the death of a classmate from leukemia.
   e. Coordination/collaboration: A pediatric clinical specialist who practices in a small community hospital helps a family plan care for a child with cerebral palsy who needs surgery at a large medical center. Transportation, housing for the family, financial needs, and community services for cerebral palsy are all planned for.
   f. Ethical decision making: A staff nurse on the infant-toddler surgical division at a large metropolitan children's hospital is a member of an interdisciplinary team for a liver transplant patient and a primary nurse for two patients who were both born with biliary atresia; both children are dying. The nurse is instrumental in providing information to help decide which of the two patients will receive the transplant.
   g. Research: A pediatric clinical nurse specialist (CNS) sees differences in the recovery rates of children who are admitted with acute appendicitis. The CNS works with the staff nurse to identify differences in the care methods used and begins a clinical research project.
   h. Health care planning: A community health nurse is a member of the local nurses' association governmental affairs committee and speaks regularly with the congressman for the area where the community clinic is located.

CHAPTER 27: FAMILY, SOCIAL, CULTURAL, AND RELIGIOUS INFLUENCES ON CHILD HEALTH PROMOTION

I. Learning Key Terms

1. g	2. d	3. h	4. f	5. e	6. b
7. i	8. j	9. a	10. c	11. n	12. o
13. l	14. m	15. k	16. q	17. r	18. p
19. e	20. b	21. c	22. d	23. a	24. h
25. f	26. g	27. k	28. j	29. l	30. i

II. Reviewing Key Concepts

1. c	2. c	3. c	4. a	5. a	6. e
7. c	8. b	9. a	10. d	11. b	12. T
13. F	14. T	15. F	16. T	17. T	18. T
19. a	20. c	21. b			

III. Thinking Critically

1. a. Promote physical survival and health of the children (e.g., reassure the parents as you examine each of the infants that they are healthy and that the parents are doing a good job). Foster the skills and abilities necessary to be a self-sustaining adult (e.g., complete a family assessment. Using the assessment, identify the family's capabilities and look at basic attributes of the family, resources within the family, and family's perceptions of the situation.). Foster behavioral capabilities for maximizing cultural values and beliefs (e.g., assess the participation of the extended family for advice and assistance).
   b. Immediate needs include providing emotional support for the family during the stressful newborn period, ensuring infant safety and protection, positive reinforcement for correct parenting behaviors, education, and skill training for infant's needs.
   c. Establish a functional healthy family unit.
   d. Seek support from extended family, provide parenting instruction, attend support group for parents with twins, and identify community resources available for the family.
2. a. First determine Noemi's knowledge of English and determine if a translator is needed. Questions which may be asked include but are not limited to the following:
   "How do you feel about immunizations for your children?" "How did you travel to the clinic?" "Do you prefer written instructions in English or Spanish?" "Who usually cares for the child during the day?" "Are your children in a day care or are they cared for in your home?"
   b. Shake hands and provide a clear introduction. Sit down close to Noemi. Use pictures and models for more clear communication. Identify any concerns or questions Noemi might have about her children's welfare and health, in addition to immunization status.
   c. Children are seen as gifts from God. Illness may be seen as a sign from God. The male is the dominant figure and influences many practices.

Folk healing and remedies used by older family members may be tried. Perception of time may interfere with keeping appointments. Family is highly valued, and there is often a multigenerational family structure. Personal interests are often subordinate to family needs.

3. The 5 components of cultural competence are:
   a. Cultural awareness—A cognitive process through which the nurse appreciates and is sensitive to the cultural values of the patient and family
   b. Cultural knowledge—The foundation the nurse builds through formal and informal education that includes world views of different cultures, values, beliefs, and perceptions about health and illness
   c. Cultural skill—The ability to include cultural data in the nursing assessment through the collection of cultural data in the health interview and observations
   d. Cultural encounter—The process through which the nurse seeks opportunities to engage in cross-cultural interactions directly or indirectly
   e. Cultural desire—The genuine and sincere motivation to work effectively with minority clients; can only be achieved if the individual wants to engage in the process of acquiring cultural competence

CHAPTER 28: DEVELOPMENTAL AND GENETIC INFLUENCES ON CHILD HEALTH PROMOTION

I. Learning Key Terms

1. c	2. a	3. s	4. l	5. b	6. r
7. k	8. j	9. q	10. i	11. h	12. p
13. g	14. o	15. f	16. n	17. e	18. t
19. m	20. d				

II. Reviewing Key Concepts

1. c	2. a	3. c	4. b	5. a	6. b
7. b	8. c	9. c	10. d	11. c	12. d
13. a	14. e	15. c	16. b	17. f	18. a
19. d	20. i	21. h	22. g	23. a	24. d
25. b	26. c	27. d	28. a	29. c	30. d
31. d	32. g	33. d	34. c	35. e	36. f
37. j	38. b	39. a	40. i	41. h	42. b
43. a	44. d	45. c	46. b	47. a	

III. Thinking Critically

1. Factors should include watching television for 4 to 5 hours a day, family history of heart disease, aggressiveness, overweight, and elevated cholesterol.
2. Strategies should be described that restrict the child's viewing of violent programs, increase the parents' awareness of the content of the shows that are viewed, help the child correlate consequences with the actions, point out subtle messages, and help the child explore alternatives to aggressive conflict resolution.
3. Outcomes described should include the child selecting more healthful snacks, watching television for about 1 hour per day, increasing physical activity, and exploring the possibility of adding out-of-the-home activities, such as scouting, sports, and music.

CHAPTER 29: COMMUNICATION, HISTORY, AND PHYSICAL ASSESSMENT

I. Learning Key Terms

1. f	2. a	3. d	4. b	5. c	6. e
7. n	8. p	9. w	10. l	11. v	12. o
13. u	14. i	15. m	16. t	17. k	18. s
19. h	20. r	21. g	22. q	23. j	

II. Reviewing Key Concepts

1. b	2. d	3. d	4. T	5. T	6. T
7. b	8. a	9. c	10. d	11. d	

12. Components of a pediatric health history: identifying information, chief complaint, present illness, past history, review of systems, family medical history, psychosocial history, sexual history; it also may include a family history and a nutritional history.

13. b	14. c	15. a	16. d	17. b	18. c
19. d	20. a	21. c	22. b	23. b	24. a
25. d					

26. body mass index, race, ethnicity, very low birth weight

27. a	28. F	29. T	30. T	31. b

32. apical, 1 full minute

33. d	34. c	35. a

36. Pupils Equal, Round, React to Light and Accommodation

37. b	38. b	39. b	40. b	41. c	42. c
43. d					

III. Thinking Critically

1. Responses should include the following:
   a. Parents, as well as children, are involved, and the nurse must decide whether to address the adult or the child.
   b. Relationships with the child are often mediated via the parent, whereas with adults, the communication is usually with one person only. Refocusing may be needed more often with family communication, because family issues may surface during the communication process if the parent is involved in the interview. Developmental stage and age must be considered. Play and nonverbal or abstract communication techniques may need to be used with families, whereas communication is usually solely verbal with adults.
   c. The informant for the child may be the parent, whereas the adult usually is his or her own informant. If the child is the informant, little may be known of the birth history, milestones, and immunization status. Birth history, immunizations, growth and development, family assessment, and nutritional assessment are all included in every child's assessment. In the adult these are usually not included or not included with the same depth.
2. In the infant the ear canal curves upward. In older children the ear canal curves downward and forward.
3. Cyanosis will appear bluish in light skin and ashen gray in dark skin. Pallor will show as a loss of rosy glow in light skin and ashen gray or yellowish in dark skin. Pallor is difficult to assess in dark skin. Erythema is easily seen in light skin but difficult to see except in the mouth or conjunctiva in dark-skinned individuals. Do not rely on this sign in dark skin. Ecchymosis is purplish yellow-green in light skin. In dark skin it is difficult to see except in the mouth or conjunctiva. Jaundice is seen easily in light skin. In dark skin assess the sclera, palms, soles, and hard palate.

CHAPTER 30: PAIN ASSESSMENT AND MANAGEMENT

I. Learning Key Terms

1. c	2. e	3. a	4. l	5. m	6. f
7. h	8. i	9. g	10. j	11. k	12. d
13. b					

II. Reviewing Key Concepts

1. b	2. d	3. a	4. b	5. d	6. T
7. T	8. F	9. T	10. F	11. T	12. F
13. T	14. b	15. T			

16. 7 to 10
17. mother, primary caregiver
18. cognitive impairment
19. Hispanic
20. a. Biologically based (foods, special diets, herbal or plant preparations, vitamins, other supplements)
   b. Manipulative treatments (chiropractic, osteopathy, massage)
   c. Energy based (Reiki, bioelectric or magnetic treatments, pulsed fields, alternating and direct currents)
   d. Mind-body techniques (mental healing, expressive treatments, spiritual healing, hypnosis, relaxation)
   e. Alternative medical systems (homeopathy; naturopathy; ayurvedic; and traditional Chinese medicine, which includes acupuncture and moxibustion)

III. Thinking Critically

1. Behavioral assessment. Behavioral assessment may provide a more complete picture of the total pain experience when administered in conjunction with a subjective self-report measure.
2. Suitable pain assessment scales include: Wong-Baker FACES Pain Rating Scale, Oucher, poker chip tool, word graphic rating scale, visual analogue scale, and color tool.
3. They have an increased frequency in quiet sleep, longer duration of quiet sleep, and decreased crying in the neonatal intensive care unit. Pain scores are also significantly lower in kangaroo-held infants.
4. A ceiling effect means that dosages higher than the recommended doses will not produce greater pain relief. A major difference between opioids and non-opioids is that non-opioids have a ceiling effect.

CHAPTER 31: THE INFANT AND FAMILY

I. Learning Key Terms

1. h	2. f	3. j	4. g	5. m	6. b
7. e	8. a	9. i	10. c	11. l	12. d
13. k	14. n				

II. Reviewing Key Concepts

1. b	2. b	3. c	4. c	5. b	6. c
7. d	8. a	9. b	10. c	11. a	12. c
13. c	14. b				
15. F	16. T	17. F	18. F	19. F	20. F
21. e	22. b	23. c	24. d	25. f	26. a

III. Thinking Critically

1. Descriptions should include the following: lifts head off table when supine, sits erect momentarily, bears full weight on feet, transfers objects from hand to hand, rakes at a small object, bangs a cube on the table, produces vowel sounds and chained syllables, vocalizes four distinct vowel sounds, plays peek-a-boo, fears strangers when mother disappears, and imitates simple acts.
2. Vitamin D—All infants (including those exclusively breast-fed) should receive a daily supplement of 400 international units of vitamin D beginning in the first few days of life to prevent rickets and vitamin D deficiency.

    Iron—If the infant is being exclusively breast-fed after 4 months (when fetal iron stores are depleted), iron supplementation (1 mg/kg/day) is recommended until appropriate iron-containing complementary foods such as iron-fortified cereal are introduced.
3. Low birth weight, Low Apgar scores, Recent viral illness, Siblings of two or more SIDS victims, Male sex, Infants of Native American or African-American ethnicity
4. Breastfeeding, current immunizations, and supine sleep position
5. Genetic factors, maternal smoking, prone sleeping, sleeping on a soft surface, sleeping with an adult or child, sleeping on a non-infant bed surface such as a couch

CHAPTER 32: THE TODDLER AND FAMILY

I. Learning Key Terms

1. c	2. i	3. d	4. h	5. b
6. e	7. g	8. f	9. a	10. j

II. Reviewing Key Concepts

1. d	2. b	3. c	4. a	5. a	6. c
7. d	8. d	9. d	10. a	11. c	12. d
13. b	14. b	15. d			

16. convertible car restraints, rear-facing
17. c
18. a. Foods: hot dogs, nuts, dried beans, pits from fruits
    b. Play objects: anything with small parts
    c. Common household objects: thumbtacks, nails, screws, coins, jewelry, old refrigerators, storage chest
    d. Electrical items: outlets, garage doors, car windows

III. Thinking Critically

1. A few questions and clinical data from the following areas should be described: nutrition, sleep and activity, dental health, injury prevention, temperament, and psychologic development.
2. Gross motor development milestones include the ability to go up and down stairs alone, using both feet on each step; run fairly well with a wide stance; pick up objects without falling; kick a ball forward without overbalancing.
3. Fine motor development milestones include the ability to build a tower of six to seven cubes; align two or more cubes in a row like a train; turn the pages of a book one at a time; imitate vertical and circular strokes when drawing; turn doorknobs; and unscrew lids.
4. Language development milestones include having a vocabulary of 300 words; using two- or three-word phrases; using the pronouns I, me, and you; understanding directional commands; giving first name; verbalizing the need for toileting; and talking incessantly.
5. Negativism contributes to the toddler's acquisition of a sense of autonomy by the assertion of self-control and serving as an attempt to control the environment and a way to increase independence.

CHAPTER 33: THE PRESCHOOLER AND FAMILY

I. Learning Key Terms

1. h	2. p	3. g	4. o	5. u	6. w
7. f	8. n	9. e	10. t	11. m	12. d
13. l	14. x	15. v	16. c	17. s	18. k
19. b	20. r	21. j	22. a	23. q	24. i

II. Reviewing Key Concepts

1. 3, 5
2. 2 to 3; 4.5 to 6.5
3. b   4. c   5. d

6. T	7. T	8. F	9. F	10. T
11. d	12. a	13. c	14. c	15. b	16. d

III. Thinking Critically

1. The child will need some preparation for this new preschool experience. One cannot guarantee that the child will have less trouble adjusting than a child who has never attended day care. A change such as this, although not drastic, could cause disruption because of differences in the programs, as well as differences between the day care "caregiver" and the preschool "teacher" and styles used by each. The amount and quality of the attention may differ from the day care to the preschool. The

preschool may have more expectations for the child to be independent and autonomous than the day care center does.

2. An example: The mother will verbalize at least five strategies that can be used to help prepare her child for the preschool experience.

3. Possible responses might include visit the school ahead of time, introduce the child and the teacher, begin to talk about the new school, refer to the new school in a positive way, and maintain confidence on the first day.

4. Characteristics that indicate that the child is ready for preschool include social maturity, good attention span, and academic readiness.

CHAPTER 34: THE SCHOOL-AGE CHILD AND FAMILY

I. Learning Key Terms

1. i   2. j   3. h   4. e   5. d   6. k
7. a   8. b   9. m   10. c   11. f   12. g
13. l   14. n

II. Reviewing Key Concepts

1. c
2. shedding the first deciduous tooth; puberty, with the acquisition of permanent teeth
3. T   4. F   5. T   6. F   7. T   8. F
9. 10; 12; 8
10. T
11. a   12. c   13. d   14. d   15. c   16. b
17. personal hygiene, nutrition, exercise, recreation, sleep, safety
18. d
19. T

III. Thinking Critically

1. Response should include nutritional assessment and his knowledge and use of safety precautions when riding his bike.

2. Response should include support for the mother by reassuring her that her child is healthy and that playing soccer will allow him to increase strength and develop motor skill performance.

3. Response should outline the information about nutrition related to good lifelong dietary habits.

4. Response should include ideas about how to give the child recognition and positive feedback for his accomplishments.

CHAPTER 35: THE ADOLESCENT AND FAMILY

I. Learning Key Terms

1. e   2. o   3. f   4. q   5. p   6. g
7. d   8. h   9. n   10. c   11. b   12. m
13. i   14. a   15. j   16. l   17. k

II. Reviewing Key Concepts

1. 10½, 15; 12, 4
2. a
3. c
4. pubertal delay, 4
5. b   6. b
7. 2, 8; 15½, 55; 4, 12; 15½, 66
8. c   9. d   10. a   11. d   12. d   13. a
14. d   15. c   16. d   17. T   18. T

III. Thinking Critically

1. Nonlean body mass, primarily fat, increases in adolescence. Fatty tissue deposition is more pronounced in girls, particularly in the regions over the thigh, hips, buttocks, and breast tissue. Using the 95th percentile as the top of the normal range, nutritional counseling to prevent additional weight gain and/or eating disorders should be instituted whenever there is concern.

2. A sense of group identity is essential to the later development of personal identity. Younger adolescents must resolve questions concerning relationships with peer groups before they are able to resolve questions about who they are in relation to the family and society. Peer groups serve as a strong support to the adolescent, individually and collectively, providing a sense of belonging and a feeling of strength and power. They form a transitional world between dependence and autonomy.

3. Show respect for the adolescent's privacy; show honest and sincere interest in the adolescent's beliefs and feelings; and listen without interrupting the adolescent.

4. Benefits include exercise for growing muscles and interactions with peers; a "socially acceptable" means to enjoy stimulation and conflict.

5. Reasons include the emphasis on slimness as a standard for beauty and femininity and increased family stress.

6. Behavior modification programs that include consistency in approach, involvement of all team members, continuity of caregivers, clear communication among team, clear communications with the patient, and support of patient are most effective.

7. Factors that might be noted include a disturbed family situation, economic stresses, family disintegration, medical problems, psychiatric illness, abandonment, or alcoholism. Adolescent girls make more unsuccessful suicide attempts than boys and are likely to ingest pills as the method.

CHAPTER 36: CHRONIC ILLNESS, DISABILITY, AND END-OF-LIFE CARE

I. Learning Key Terms

1. b   2. h   3. e   4. g   5. i   6. c
7. d   8. f   9. k   10. a   11. j

II. Reviewing Key Concepts

1. b   2. d
3. Support the family's coping and/or promote the family's optimum functioning throughout the child's life
4. Possible strategies include providing education regarding what can reasonably be expected of the child, assistance in identifying the child's strength, praise for a parental job well done, and finding respite care so that parents can renew their energies.
5. a
6. Possible tasks include accept the child's condition; manage the child's condition on a day-to-day basis; meet the child's normal developmental needs; meet the developmental needs of other family members; cope with ongoing stress and periodic crises; assist family members to manage their feelings; educate others about the child's conditions; and establish a support system.
7. d   8. d
9. Shock/denial, adjustment, and reintegration/acknowledgment
10. b   11. c
12. Possible answers include loss of senses, confusion, muscle weakness, loss of bowel and bladder control, difficulty swallowing, change in respiratory pattern, and weak/slow pulse.
13. d   14. c   15. c   16. d   17. c

III. Thinking Critically

1. Responses should include the following:
   - Using the development approach emphasizes the child's abilities and strengths rather than his or her disability. Under the developmental model, attention is directed to the child's functional development, changes, and adaptation to the environment.
   - Families are supported in their natural caregiving and decision-making roles by building on their unique strengths as individuals.
   - By applying the principles of normalization, the environment for the child is normalized and humanized.
   - The school has now become an essential component of the child's overall physical, intellectual, and social development.
2. Assessment aids in evaluating the individual's ability to cope with various aspects of the crisis and identifies possible areas for intervention.
3. Children between the ages of 3 years and 5 years see death as a departure. They may recognize the fact of physical death but do not separate it from living abilities. They view death as temporary and gradual.
4. A preschooler is likely to perceive illness as punishment for past thoughts or actions.
5. Developmentally the adolescent's task is to establish an identity by finding out who he is, what his purpose is, and where he belongs. Any suggestion of being different, or of not being at all, is a tremendous

threat to accomplishing this task. The adolescent's concern is for the present much more than the past or the future.

CHAPTER 37: COGNITIVE AND SENSORY IMPAIRMENT

I. Learning Key Terms

1. u   2. i.   3. t   4. j   5. h   6. k
7. g   8. l   9. f   10. m   11. s   12. e
13. n   14. d   15. r   16. c   17. o   18. b
19. p   20. v   21. a   22. q

II. Reviewing Key Concepts

1. b   2. d   3. c   4. a   5. b   6. d
7. Task analysis is the process of breaking a skill into its components; it is used when teaching cognitively impaired children to help them master one part of the skill at a time, beginning with the parts the child has mastered already. Each task is separated into its necessary components and each step is taught completely before proceeding to the next activity.
8. c   9. b   10. a
11. genetic counselling
12. b   13. d   14. b   15. a   16. d   17. h
18. f   19. d   20. c   21. g   22. b   23. e
24. a   25. d   26. d   27. d
28. Possible strategies include the following: talk to child about everything that is occurring; emphasize aspects of procedures that are felt/heard; approach the child with identifying information; explain sounds; encourage parents to room in; encourage parents' participation; bring familiar objects from home; orient child to surroundings. (If the child has sight on admission but will lose sight during hospitalization [e.g., as a result of eye surgery], point out significant aspects of the room's layout and practice ambulation with eyes closed before the procedure.)
29. b   30. b

III. Thinking Critically

1. Responses should include the following nursing interventions: ensure that the child has appropriate toys for entertainment; place the child in a room with other children of the same approximate developmental age; treat the child with dignity and respect; explain procedures using methods of communication appropriate for the child's cognitive level; focus on growth-promoting experiences for the child.
2. The hearing-impaired child is often unable to proceed past parallel play within a group, because of an inability to follow the direction of cooperative play. Also, a hearing deficit may not allow the child to interpret enough of the conversation to join in. As a result, the hearing-impaired child may stay on the periphery or avoid social interaction altogether.

3. Speech is learned through a multisensory approach, and the usual mechanisms are not available to the deaf child.

4. Responses should include the following: avoid excessive eye strain when doing close work; periodically look into the distance to relax the muscles of accommodation; use proper lighting; light should not be glaring or cast shadows on reading material; get sufficient amounts of rest and nutrition; have eyes checked at least yearly by a licensed optometrist or ophthalmologist; teach safety regarding common eye injuries.

CHAPTER 38: FAMILY-CENTERED CARE OF THE CHILD DURING ILLNESS AND HOSPITALIZATION

I. Learning Key Terms
1. f   2. b   3. e   4. a   5. c   6. d

Ii. Reviewing Key Concepts
1. e
2. b   3. c   4. a
5. T   6. T
7. c   8. a   9. a   10. a
11. Answers could include: initial aloofness toward parents, followed by tendency to cling to parents, demands for parents' attention, vigorous opposition to any separation. Other negative behaviors include new fears, resistance to going to bed, night waking, withdrawal and shyness, hyperactivity, temper tantrums, food finickiness, attachment to blanket or toy, regression in newly learned skills.
12. e   13. b   14. c   15. a   16. b   17. c
18. seriousness of the threat to the child, previous experience with illness or hospitalization, medical procedures involved in diagnosis and treatment, available support systems, personal ego strengths, previous coping abilities, additional stresses on the family system, cultural and religious beliefs, and communication patterns among family members.
19. intense emotional upset and physical resistance.
20. aggression, verbal expression, and dependency.
21. precise verbalization of pain, passive requests for support or help, and procrastination.

III. Thinking Critically
1. Recognize that family members know the child best and are most aware of the child's needs. Welcome unlimited family presence. Encourage family to bring other significant family members to visit. Arrange for family members to have a meal together.
2. Some recommended toys for a 4-year-old child include the following: large puzzles, blocks, dress-up materials, puppets, crayons, blunt scissors and paper.
3. Be positive in your approach to the child. Be honest with the child. Convey to the child the behaviors expected. Be consistent in expectations and relationships

with the child. Treat the child fairly, and help the child feel this. Encourage parents to maintain a truthful relationship with the child. Make certain the child has a call light or other signal device within reach. Help children maintain their usual contacts. Protect the child from unfamiliar sights, sounds, and equipment.

CHAPTER 39: PEDIATRIC VARIATIONS OF NURSING INTERVENTIONS

I. Learning Key Terms
1. m   2. d   3. l   4. c   5. e
6. f   7. b   8. k   9. g   10. j
11. h   12. a   13. i

II. Reviewing Key Concepts
1. d   2. b   3. c
4. Possible supportive strategies include the following: Expect success; have extra supplies handy; involve the child; provide distraction; allow expression of feelings; praise the child; use play in preparation of and after the procedure.
5. a. Give a toddler a push-pull toy.
   b. Touch or kick Mylar balloons.
   c. Make creative objects out of needleless syringes.
   d. Practice band instruments.
   e. Move the patient's bed to the playroom, activity room, or lobby (within reasonable expectations of child's condition).
   f. Put toys at the bottom of bath container.
   g. Make freezer pops using the child's favorite juice.
6. a   7. b   8. c   9. a   10. c   11. a
12. b   13. c   14. d   15. b   16. d   17. d
18. a   19. a   20. c   21. d   22. b   23. c
24. b   25. d   26. c   27. a   28. d   29. d

III. Thinking Critically
1. Medical-surgical restraints are used for children with an artificial airway or airway adjunct for delivery of oxygen, indwelling catheters, tubes, drains, lines, pacemaker wires, or suture sites. Medical-surgical restraints may be instituted for any of the following reasons:
   • Risk for interruption of therapy used to maintain oxygenation or airway patency
   • Risk of harm if indwelling catheter, tube, drain, line, pacemaker wire, or sutures are removed, dislodged, or ruptured
   • Patient confusion, agitation, unconsciousness, or developmental inability to understand direct requests or instructions
   • Medical-surgical restraints can be initiated by an individual order or by protocol; the use of the protocol must be authorized by an individual order. The order for continued use of restraints must be renewed each day. Patients are monitored at least every 2 hours and documentation of such monitoring is required.

2. Traditional methods for verifying NG tube placement in the stomach have been shown to be inadequate in the determination of safe placement. Auscultation alone is not sufficient as tube placement in the stomach is not guaranteed with the auscultation of a swoosh of air. The measure most commonly used by clinicians, nose-ear-xiphoid distance, is often too short to locate the entire tube pore span in the stomach. However, the nose-ear-midxiphoid umbilicus span approaches the accuracy of the age-specific prediction equations and is easier to use in a clinical setting. The best option is to adapt the nose-ear-midxiphoid umbilicus measurement for NG or OG tube length. Testing the aspirate pH is another adjunct to verifying proper tube placement but there are limitations with medication use. The radiograph is the only foolproof method of verifying safe placement but exposure to radiation is a concern. Current evidence and best practice suggests that a combination of verification methods to confirm NG tube placement will reduce the required number of x-rays in children.

3. ETCO$_2$ is noninvasive and more sensitive to the mechanics of ventilation than pulse oximetry and thus hypoxic episodes can be prevented through the early detection of hypoventilation, apnea, or airway obstruction. Normal ETCO$_2$ values are 30 to 43 mm Hg, which is slightly lower than normal arterial PCO$_2$ of 35 to 45 mm Hg. A special sampling nasal cannula can be used in nonintubated patients. Changes in wave form and numeric display follow changes in ventilation by a very few seconds and precede changes in respiratory rate, skin color, and pulse oximetry values.

CHAPTER 40: RESPIRATORY DYSFUNCTION

I. Learning Key Terms

1. g   2. f   3. p   4. e   5. m   6. k
7. d   8. j   9. b   10. i   11. c   12. h
13. a   14. o   15. n   16. l

II. Reviewing Key Concepts

1. b   2. c   3. c   4. b   5. b   6. c
7. d   8. a   9. c   10. a   11. b   12. a
13. a   14. c   15. c   16. d   17. c   18. a
19. b   20. d   21. b   22. c   23. b   24. d
25. c   26. d   27. c   28. b   29. d   30. d
31. d   32. c   33. a   34. d   35. d   36. d
37. c   38. b
39. Restlessness, tachypnea, tachycardia, diaphoresis
40. d
41. h   42. b   43. e   44. c   45. l   46. a
47. d   48. i   49. k   50. j   51. g   52. f

III. Thinking Critically

1. Child sweats profusely, remains sitting upright, and refuses to lie down. A child who suddenly becomes agitated or suddenly becomes quiet may be seriously hypoxic.

2. a. Respiratory symptoms include obstruction of bronchioles and bronchi with abnormally thick mucus.
   b. Delayed growth and development as a result of decreased absorption of nutrients, including vitamins and fat; increased oxygen demands for pulmonary function; and delayed bone growth.
   c. Anorexia is common in children with CF due to poor absorption and passage of intestinal waste; large amount of mucus and sputum which is often swallowed; at times violent coughing episodes; frequent respiratory treatments; and the large amounts of medications in pill form which must be taken (these are filling).

3. The child may return to school. There is no need for isolation because the disease is almost always noninfectious in children. Child should refrain from vigorous activity/sports and be protected from stress during the active stage of primary tuberculosis.

CHAPTER 41: GASTROINTESTINAL DYSFUNCTION

I. Learning Key Terms

1. e   2. d   3. k   4. j   5. i   6. c
7. h   8. b   9. l   10. g   11. a   12. f

II. Reviewing Key Concepts

1. b   2. d   3. c   4. c   5. c
6. c   7. d
8. Isotonic
9. hypotonic, less
10. hypertonic; loss, intake; greater
11. b   12. c
13. Skin turgor, capillary refill, body weight, level of consciousness, activity level, respiratory pattern, status of oral mucosa (dry), thirst (in older child), urine output in last 24 hours
14. c   15. c   16. d   17. b   18. c   19. d
20. a   21. d   22. c
23. Absorbing the toxin with activated charcoal, performing gastric lavage, [or] increasing bowel motility to expel the toxins
24. d   25. c   26. a   27. c
28. handwashing
29. rotavirus
30. a   31. b   32. e   33. d   34. c
35. b   36. d
37. Pruritis
38. c   39. b   40. d   41. d   42. a   43. a
44. c   45. a   46. b   47. d   48. d   49. c
50. d   51. b   52. T   53. T   54. F
55. Assessment, support respiratory system; other supportive measures; gastric decontamination with assessment; monitoring and supportive measures; family support; prevention of recurrence

56. Phase 1— expand ECF volume quickly and improve circulatory and renal function; an isotonic solution is used at a rate of 20 mL/kg, given as an IV bolus over 20 minutes and repeated as necessary after assessment of the child's response to therapy.

    Phase 2— replace deficits, meet maintenance water and electrolyte requirements, and catch up with ongoing losses. Water and sodium requirements for the deficit, maintenance, and ongoing losses are calculated at 8-hour intervals, taking into consideration the amount of fluids given with the initial boluses and the amount administered during the first 24-hour period. With improved circulation during this phase, water and electrolyte deficits can be evaluated, and acid–base status can be corrected either directly through the administration of fluids or indirectly through improved renal function. Potassium is withheld until kidney function is restored and assessed and circulation has improved.

    Phase 3— begin oral fluids slowly and advance as tolerated to full feedings (see below). The BRATT diet is no longer recommended.

57. When the child is alert, awake, and not in danger, correction of dehydration may be attempted with oral fluid administration. Mild cases of dehydration can be managed at home or in the ED or urgent care by this method. Oral rehydration management consists of replacement of fluid loss over 4 to 6 hours, replacement of continuing losses, and provision for maintenance fluid requirements. Clear fluids are preferred initially; breastfeeding may be resumed, and the child tolerating clear fluids can be advanced to solid foods after tolerance is demonstrated. Avoid fatty foods like French fries and pizza during this phase. In general, a mildly dehydrated child may be given 50 mL/kg of oral rehydration solution (ORS), and a child with moderate dehydration may be given 100 mL/kg of ORS.

III. Thinking Critically

1. Assessment should include accurate history of bowel habits; diet and events that may be associated with the onset of constipation; drugs or other substances that the child may be taking; and consistency, color, frequency, and other characteristics of the stool.

2. Ulcerative colitis (UC) is a chronic inflammatory reaction involving the mucosa and submucosa of the large intestine. Mucosa becomes hyperemic and edematous with patchy granulation that bleeds easily and leads to superficial ulceration. Crohn disease (CD) affects the terminal ileum and involves all layers of the bowel wall. Edema and inflammation progress to deep ulceration with fissure and obstruction.
   - Rectal bleeding: common in UC; uncommon in CD
   - Diarrhea: often severe in UC; moderate to absent in CD
   - Pain: less frequent in UC; common in CD
   - Anorexia: mild to moderate in UC; can be severe in CD

- Weight loss: moderate in UC; severe in CD
- Growth restriction: usually mild in UC; often pronounced in CD

CHAPTER 42: CARDIOVASCULAR DYSFUNCTION

I. Learning Key Terms

1. o	2. r	3. n	4. p	5. m
6. l	7. q	8. k	9. t	10. e
11. d	12. u	13. f	14. c	15. j
16. a	17. g	18. s	19. b	20. h
21. i				

II. Reviewing Key Concepts

1. b	2. a	3. a	4. e	5. a
6. c	7. b			

8. The most significant complications include stroke, seizures, tamponade, and death. The patient may also suffer loss of circulation to the affected extremity, dysrhythmias, hemorrhage, cardiac perforation, hematoma, hypovolemia and dehydration, hypoglycemia in infants, and changes in the temperature and color of the affected extremity.

9. d	10. d	11. b	12. d	13. a	14. b
15. c	16. b	17. c	18. d	19. c	20. d
21. a	22. b	23. c			
24. c	25. d	26. c	27. d	28. b	
29. c	30. d				
31. a	32. d	33. a	34. d	35. b	36. c
37. b					
38. c	39. b	40. d	41. c	42. b	43. a
44. a	45. d	46. d	47. d	48. a	49. d
50. b					
51. d	52. d	53. c			

54. 3, yearly
55. e

III. Thinking Critically

1. Responses should include the following clinical manifestations: growth delay; feeding difficulty; dyspnea; weak cry, cyanosis; and dry, hot skin.

2. Components of a child's history that could indicate a high risk for congenital heart disease include the following: maternal rubella; poor nutrition; maternal type 1 diabetes; maternal age over 40 years; maternal alcoholism; a sibling or parent with a congenital heart defect; a chromosomal abnormality, especially Down syndrome or other noncardiac congenital anomalies.

3. Digitalis improves cardiac functioning by increasing cardiac output, decreasing heart size, decreasing venous pressure, and decreasing edema. Diuretics remove accumulated fluid and sodium, thereby decreasing the work of the heart.

4. Responses should include the following: encourage parents to express their fears and concerns regarding the child's cardiac defects and physical symptoms; encourage family to participate in child's care;

encourage family to include others in child's care to prevent exhaustion; and assist family in determining appropriate physical activity.

CHAPTER 43: HEMATOLOGIC AND IMMUNOLOGIC DYSFUNCTION

I. Learning Key Terms

1. e   2. c   3. a   4. f   5. b   6. d

II. Reviewing Key Concepts

1. a
2. iron deficiency
3. a   4. b
5. Administer between meals; administer with a fruit juice; administer through a straw or with a medication syringe
6. a   7. d   8. d   9. d   10. b   11. d
12. immune thrombocytopenia
13. c   14. a   15. c   16. c   17. c   18. d
19. b   20. d   21. a   22. d   23. c
24. *pneumocystis carinii* pneumonia
25. d   26. d   27. a

III. Thinking Critically

1. Analyze the drug and dosage and administer medication on a regular schedule. Suggest changes to prevent rather than treat pain after it occurs.
2. Apply pressure to area of bleeding for 10 to 15 minutes to allow for clot formation. Immobilize and elevate area above the level of the heart to decrease blood flow. Apply cold to promote vasoconstriction.
3. Provide meticulous skin care, especially in the mouth and perianal regions, because they are prone to ulceration. Change position frequently to stimulate circulation and relieve pressure. Encourage adequate calorie/protein intake to prevent negative nitrogen balance.

CHAPTER 44: GENITOURINARY DYSFUNCTION

I. Learning Key Terms

1. q   2. a   3. j   4. i   5. l   6. h
7. b   8. p   9. k   10. c   11. o   12. f
13. d   14. n   15. g   16. m   17. e

II. Reviewing Key Concepts

1. d
2. Uncircumcised
3. d   4. a   5. b   6. b
7. corticosteroid
8. a   9. c   10. c   11. c   12. b   13. a
14. c   15. e   16. c   17. b   18. b
19. hemodialysis, peritoneal dialysis, hemofiltration
20. Hemodialysis
21. Peritoneal
22. a   23. e   24. e

III. Thinking Critically

1. Interventions should include the following: offer a nutritious diet; limit salt during edematous phase; enlist the aid of the child and parents in formulation of a diet; provide a cheerful, relaxed environment during meals; provide special and preferred foods; serve food in an attractive manner; serve small quantities.
2. Response should include the following: encourage the parents to room in with the child, spend time with the child, provide opportunities for the child to socialize with other children who have no infection, and provide age-appropriate play activity in the room or in a playroom.
3. Protein is restricted in children with acute renal failure to prevent the accumulation of nitrogenous wastes.
4. Nursing interventions should include the following: assess home situation, teach the family home care, help the family acquire needed drugs and equipment, assist the family in problem solving and diet planning, prepare the child and family for home peritoneal dialysis and/or kidney transplantation, maintain periodic contact with the family, and refer the family to special agencies and support groups.

CHAPTER 45: CEREBRAL DYSFUNCTION

I. Learning Key Terms

1. j   2. f   3. k   4. g   5. m   6. e
7. i   8. l   9. d   10. a   11. c   12. b
13. h

II. Reviewing Key Concepts

1. d   2. c   3. b   4. c   5. d   6. c
7. b   8. b   9. b   10. d   11. c   12. a
13. Meningococcal meningitis
14. b   15. d   16. b   17. d   18. e   19. d
20. a   21. e   22. f   23. d

III. Thinking Critically

1. Assessment parameters should include vital signs, pupillary reactions, and level of consciousness. Interventions should include the following: elevate head of bed 15 to 30 degrees, avoid positions or activities that increase intracranial pressure (ICP), prevent constipation, minimize emotional stress and crying, prevent or relieve pain, schedule disturbing procedures to take advantage of therapies that reduce ICP, and monitor ICP.
2. Assessment data should include a description of the child's behavior before and during a seizure, the age of onset of the first seizure, the usual time at which seizures occur, any factors that precipitate seizures, any sensory phenomena that the child can describe, duration and progression of the seizure, and postictal feelings and behavior.

3. Consumption of such a diet forces the body to shift from using glucose as the primary energy source to using fat, and the individual develops a state of ketosis. The ketogenic diet has been shown to be an efficacious and tolerable treatment for medically refractory seizures. Studies have shown that as many as 56% of children on the diet had greater than a 50% reduction in seizure episodes.

4. Glasgow Coma Scale (GCS) of 8, GCS evaluation of less than 8 with respiratory assistance, deterioration of condition, subjective judgment regarding clinical appearance, and response.

CHAPTER 46: ENDOCRINE DYSFUNCTION

I. Learning Key Words

1. e   2. j   3. d   4. n   5. i
6. m   7. k   8. c   9. l   10. g
11. b   12. h   13. a   14. f

II. Reviewing Key Concepts

1. b   2. c
3. Constitutional growth
4. Acromegaly results from hypersecretion of growth hormone that occurs after epiphyseal closure. If hypersecretion occurs before epiphyseal closure, the disorder is called *pituitary hyperfunction*, and physical features do not become distorted as in acromegaly.
5. 7, 6; 9
6. c   7. a   8. b   9. b
10. d   11. b   12. c   13. b
14. insulin, oral diabetic agents
15. d   16. b   17. c   18. d
19. polyuria (increased urination); polydipsia (increased thirst); polyphagia (increased hunger)
20. b
21. rapid-acting, intermediate-acting; before breakfast, the evening meal
22. c   23. b

III. Thinking Critically

1. Clinical manifestations of hypopituitarism include short stature but proportional height and weight, well-nourished appearance, a tendency to be relatively inactive and to shun aggressive sports, restricted bone-age proportional to height-age, and eruption of permanent teeth is delayed and teeth are overcrowded and malpositioned. Sexual development is delayed but normal.
2. a. Clinical manifestations: polyuria, possible enuresis; polydipsia, with intense thirst in some children; infants may be irritable; dehydration may occur if unable to drink (older children).
   b. Therapeutic management: The usual treatment is hormone replacement, either with an intramuscular or subcutaneous injection of vasopressin tannate in peanut oil or with a nasal spray of aqueous lysine vasopressin.

3. Expected symptoms include irritability, shaky feeling, sweating, pallor, tremors, tachycardia, and shallow respirations. Weakness, dizziness, headache, drowsiness, irritability, loss of coordination, seizures, and coma are more severe responses and reflect CNS glucose deprivation and the body's attempts to elevate the serum glucose levels.

4. Treat hypoglycemia by giving the child simple sugar or carbohydrate (milk, fruit juice, glucose tablet, table sugar). Ensure child is able to swallow before administering any of these to prevent aspiration or airway compromise.

CHAPTER 47: INTEGUMENTARY DYSFUNCTION

I. Learning Key Terms

1. d   2. m   3. c   4. l   5. b   6. k
7. a   8. j   9. s   10. i   11. h   12. n
13. r   14. g   15. p   16. f   17. o   18. q
19. e   20. w   21. t   22. v   23. bb   24. u
25. aa   26. z   27. ee   28. x   29. y   30. dd
31. cc

II. Reviewing Key Concepts

1. c   2. a   3. c   4. a   5. d
6. pull parallel to the skin
7. b   8. b   9. a   10. a   11. a
12. b   13. b   14. T   15. c   16. b
17. c   18. d   19. d   20. e   21. c
22. thermal, electrical, chemical
23. Hot water scald
24. b   25. d   26. a   27. c   28. c   29. b
30. d   31. a   32. a   33. c   34. c
35. a   36. b

III. Thinking Critically

1. Possible diagnoses include the following: impaired skin integrity related to eczematous lesions, risk for infection related to risk of secondary infection of primary lesions, interrupted family processes related to child's discomfort and lengthy therapy.

2. Suggested interventions include the following: use superabsorbent disposable diapers, change diapers as soon as they become wet or soiled, expose the affected area to light and air, do not use rubber pants or cloth diapers, wipe off the stool after soiling occurs but do not wipe off all of the barrier paste, use a barrier paste, use a corn starch powder instead of baby powder, and avoid overwashing the skin.

3. School-age children are more susceptible because of their social nature and their proximity to other children in school and at play.

4. Infection is a leading cause of death in the patient with thermal injury and is a serious complication. Adhering to sterile technique lessens the chance of infection. The skin normally acts as a barrier to infection, and because it is compromised by thermal

injury it cannot effectively resist many organisms that are common to the skin surface.

5. Have all materials ready before beginning, administer appropriate analgesics and sedatives, remind the child of the impending procedure to allow sufficient time to prepare, allow the child to test and approve the temperature of the water, allow the child to select the area of the body on which to begin, allow the child to request a short rest period during the procedure, allow the child to remove the dressings if desired, provide something constructive for the child to do during the procedure, inform the child when the procedure is near completion, and praise the child for cooperation.

CHAPTER 48: MUSCULOSKELETAL OR ARTICULAR DYSFUNCTION

I. Learning Key Terms

1. g	2. o	3. f	4. h	5. n	6. e
7. d	8. i	9. m	10. c	11. l	12. j
13. a	14. k	15. b			

II. Reviewing Key Concepts

1. d	2. d	3. b	4. h	5. i	6. a
7. c	8. b	9. d	10. e	11. f	12. g
13. b	14. c				

15. lower extremities; track and field; runners

16. d	17. b	18. d	19. a	20. d	21. b
22. d					

23. lordosis, kyphosis

24. d	25. a	26. b	27. a	28. b	29. d
30. a	31. d	32. a	33. c	34. a	35. d

III. Thinking Critically

1. The straps should be checked in the beginning of therapy and every 1 to 2 weeks for adjustments. It is important that parents understand the correct use of the appliance, which may or may not allow for its removal during bathing. Do not remove the harness unless approved by the practitioner. Parents are instructed to not adjust the harness.

   Skin care is an important aspect of the care of an infant in a harness. Stress these instructions:

   Always put an undershirt (or a shirt with extensions that close at the crotch) under the chest straps and put knee socks under the foot and leg pieces to prevent the straps from rubbing the skin.

   Check frequently (at least two or three times a day) for red areas under the straps and the clothing.

   Gently massage healthy skin under the straps once a day to stimulate circulation. In general, avoid lotions and powders because they can cake and irritate the skin.

   Always place the diaper under the straps.

   Encourage parents to hold the infant with a harness and continue care and nurturing activities.

2. The six Ps of ischemia from a vascular, soft tissue, nerve, or bone injury should be included in an assessment of any injury.
   1. Pain
   2. Pallor
   3. Pulselessness
   4. Paresthesia
   5. Paralysis
   6. Pressure
3. a. Compartment syndrome is a serious complication that results from compression of nerves, blood vessels, and muscle inside a closed space. This injury may be devastating, resulting in tissue death and disuse.

   The signs and symptoms are:

   Pain: Severe pain that is not relieved by analgesics or elevation of the limb; movement increases pain

   Pulse: Inability to palpate a pulse distal to the fracture or compartment

   Pallor: Pale-appearing skin, poor perfusion, capillary refill greater than 3 seconds

   Paresthesia: Tingling or burning sensations

   Paralysis: Inability to move extremity or digits

   Pressure: Involved limb or digits may feel tense and warm; skin is tight, shiny; pressure within the compartment is elevated

   Pallor, paralysis, and pulselessness are late signs.

   b. Tight, restrictive, and limb-encircling devices such as flexible bandage (Ace), cast, splint, or immobilization device (e.g., traction boot)

   c. Fasciotomy—the pressure on the compartment is released by surgically cutting open the muscle longitudinally.

CHAPTER 49: NEUROMUSCULAR OR MUSCULAR DYSFUNCTION

I. Learning Key Terms

1. g	2. c	3. f	4. d	5. b
6. a	7. e			

II. Reviewing Key Concepts

1. a	2. e	3. b	4. d	5. d	6. b
7. b	8. a	9. b			

10. latex allergy; latex sensitivity

11. b	12. a	13. c	14. c
15. a	16. e	17. d	18. b

III. Thinking Critically

1. Suggested interventions include the following: helping parents develop a balance between limiting the child's activity because of muscular weakness and allowing the child to accomplish goals independently (refer to Chapter 41).
2. Interventions aimed at preventing the complications of Guillain-Barré syndrome include the following: observe for difficulty swallowing and respiratory

involvement; monitor vital signs frequently; monitor level of consciousness; maintain good postural alignment; change position frequently; perform passive range of motion every 4 hours; ensure adequate nutrition; provide bowel and bladder care to prevent constipation and urine retention.

3. Nursing goals include the following: stabilize the entire spinal column with a rigid cervical collar with supportive blocks on a rigid backboard. Ensure airway patency and continually assess neurologic function to prevent further deterioration. Prevent complications and maintain bodily functions. Assist with diagnostic exams. Provide information for adolescent and parents about the patient's status and allow expression of feelings, most of which will initially be shock and denial.

4. This autonomic phenomenon is caused by visceral distention or irritation, particularly of the bowel or bladder. Sensory impulses are triggered and travel to the cord lesion, where they are blocked, which causes activation of sympathetic reflex action with disturbed central inhibitory control. Clinical manifestations of autonomic dysreflexia include a drastic increase in systemic blood pressure, headache, bradycardia, profuse diaphoresis, cardiac arrhythmias, flushing, piloerection, blurred vision, nasal congestion, anxiety, spots on the visual field, or absent or minimum symptoms.